OMEGA SIX

THE DEVIL'S FAT

Why excess Omega 6, and lack of Omega 3,
promotes CHD, aggression, depression, ADHD,
weight gain, obesity, poor sleep, PCOS, breast
cancer, infertility, arthritis, and 'western' illnesses.

ROBERT ANDREW BROWN

Les Creux Limited

Disclaimer
The information in the book has been compiled from sources believed to be reliable
and true. However, fats are an evolving science in which much is still unknown, and
controversy exists as to the role of Omega Six and Omega Three. If the scientific
community all accepted that excess Omega Six was a health issue, then it would not
be on the shelves without a health warning! The book includes elements of original
thought, conjecture, and trials, that are not yet generally accepted. This book is to
inform and foster debate. This book is not in any way intended to take the place
of medical advice and consultation. Please consult a qualified physician before
undertaking significant changes in diet.

Published by Les Creux Limited
The Cottage,
Le Coin Farm,
Mont Cochon,
St. Lawrence
Jersey JE3 1ND

ISBN No. : 978-0-9557074-0-7

E-mail enquiries@omegasixthedevilsfat.com
Web sites www.omegasixthedevilsfat.com and www.thedevilsfat.com

10 9 8 7 6 5 4 3 2 1

Cover design Quadrant Infotech (India) Pvt. Ltd. and the Author.
Typesetting by Quadrant Infotech (India) Pvt. Ltd and the Author.
Design and production Consultation, Jill Ronsley, Sun Editing & Book Design.
Thanks to Barnes Publishing for assistance.
Bound and printed by Lightning Source.

I dedicate this book to all those who have a passion for, and give their lives to, research into the truly fundamental field of fats.

We ARE truly the fats we digest. This work wobbles tentatively on the shoulders of research giants, who have spent lifetimes fighting to bring simple tidings of dietary hope, to a wider public audience.

The message lives in the shadows, waiting to be heard, because it has no visible corporate bottom line value. This discovery of the researchers, may prove to be a fundamental dietary truth of enormous consequence.

Become passionate about your physical essence, fats.

Please help illuminate the elephant in the global room.

CONTENTS

1. Introduction

2. Disease of prosperity

3.   The elephant in the room – Stark truths

11. Dietary basics of Omegas Three, Six, Nine, and other fats

22. Immune regiments

23. Pregnancy, postnatal depression, chronic fatigue, depression, PMT, fertility issues, osteoporosis, PCOS, uterine and breast cancers

24.   The brain–DHA, EPA, Omega Threes and–ADHD, aggression, Bipolar disorder, depression, dementia, dyslexia, dyspraxia, intelligence, PMT, suicide, schizophrenia, and some psychiatric conditiions.

26. Omega Three – Sources, environmental implications

27. Sleep, Omega 3, and 6

28. Omega Six–ultimate hormone controller, and link to nature

29. Omega Three, Omega Six and 'western' conditions–Overview

30   Terminology

(* Inherited conditions included as EFA have been shown to have some impact.)

THANKS

This book would not have happened or been possible without the Internet. Google, Wikipedia, NCBI, and PubMed were invaluable research tools, and provided very useful search and cross reference facilities.

A number of books and trials provided invaluable background and insights. Particular insights in my journey were found in articles by J. M. Bourre, R. Brueggemeier, L. Cordain, M. A. Crawford, U. N. Das, J. R. Hibbeln, S. M. Innis, Y. Kagawa, W. Lands, M. de Lorgeril, R. Lupu, J. Menendez, L. C. Reis, N Salem, A. Simopoulos, W. L. Smith, and their colleagues who are to numerous to name.

The following books generally share a passion for prevention. Recognition of their contribution is not necessarily to agree with the entire contents. They provided individual gems, issues, seeds of understanding, or great knowledge;

☞ *Breaking the Vicious Cycle* – Elaine Gottschall [Insights into digestion].

☞ *The China Study* – T. Colin Campbell – [Links between disease diet and different populations, with insight to attitudes to prevention].

☞ *The Driving Force* – Michael Crawford, David Marsh – [Insights into evolution and food].

☞ *Essential Reproduction* – Martin H. Johnson – [Insights into reproduction and fats, a very useful reference work].

☞ *Fatty Acids in Foods and their Implications* – Ching Kuang Chow - [Wide ranging very useful reference work].

☞ *Fats that Heal Fats that Kill* – Udo Erasmus – [The importance of vegetable oil and relevance of the processing of oils].

☞ *Fish, Omega-3 and Human Health* by William E. M. Lands – [Man of particular vision - Fundamental insights and a reference book].

☞ *Know Your Fats* – Dr Mary Enig – [The benefit and importance of saturated fats, and an understanding of the huge impact of manufactured fats].

☞ *Nutrition and Physical Degeneration* – Weston A Price – [Reference – brilliant man of vision - A global comparative observation of primitive and western dietary impact on health and jaw formation in the 1920s].

☞ *Omega 3 Fatty Acids in Clinical Nutrition* - Axel R Heller, S N Stehr, T Koch - [Reference and important practical applications in medicine].

☞ *The Omega-3 Connection* – Andrew L Stoll – [Brain and mental health]

☞ *Our Stolen Future* - Theo Colburn, Dianne Dumanoski, John Peterson Myers [Synthetic chemicals health gender and reproduction]

☞ *The Queen of Fats* – Susan Allport [Lots of useful gems – a history].

☞ *Smart Fats* – Michael A. Schmidt [Importance of fats to mental health and wider implications – now replaced by *Brain Building Nutrition*].

☞ *Fish Oil The Natural Anti-Inflammatory* - Joseph C. Maroon MD, Jeffrey Bost PAC [Found after completion of this book - a work of clarity].

Lands, is clearly a man well ahead of his time, his insights are key, and his book fascinating if complex. I thank him for permission to use his graph, featured below. Online National Institutes of Health (NIH USA) lectures on fats in the eicosanoid pathway including a lecture by Smith were a huge help. Hibbeln's thoughts on behaviour have been key. Weston Price's 1920's book on the holistic relevance of diet as reflected in dental arch formation and dental health, is immensely thought provoking.

I have read a significant number of trials and other books, too many to mention here. I sincerely thank all the authors, and institutions they represent.

I would like to thank all those who have given me help advice and encouragement on the way, AndiBB, the Angel of the warming frozen north, Amber, Cliff, Rachel and Viv. My thanks to those that gave views on the cover, including the local library, health shop, local book shops and coffee shop.

The source of the basis of many of the diagrams is Wikipedia, and I thank those who have generously contributed them to Wikipedia on an open source basis.

The writing researching, editing, and organisation of this book prior to the production stage, been has been very largely a one-person effort. The spelling and terminology reflects the trials, and is a mix of English and American. It is my first book and has been a steep learning curve. I apologise for any errors. Please advise me and I will get them corrected.

My enormous thanks to Jill Ronsley Sun Editing & Book Design for valuable advice and her professionalism, the team of Quadrant Infotech (India) for their hard work patience and dedication in setting text and illustrations, copy reading, and cover design, and Barnes Publishing Jersey for early advice and help.

This book only happened, because of the very large number of people around the world, who dedicate their lives, to science and research in this field. The credit for discoveries in, and illumination of the very fundamental and under-recognised field of lipids, properly belongs to the researchers. I again dedicate this book to them.

Finally, thank you for reading and buying this book. I hope you find this book thought provoking, and it helps you better understand the importance of balancing Omega Three and Six in your diet.

Robert Andrew Brown

PREFACE

The credit for this book must go to those who dedicate their lives to lipid research. I by a stroke of fate have had the time and impulse, to try and bring the importance of lipid research, to a wider audience. I tentatively and respectfully advance some original material, in that I have not seen the theories elsewhere, but I would be surprised if they have not crossed the minds of others. I am constantly reminded of how complex the subject is, and how very little I know.

WE ARE ARGUABLY OMEGA THREE/SIX CENTRIC. OMEGA 3 AND 6 MOTHER FATS CAN ONLY BE OBTAINED FROM DIET. WE CANNOT MAKE THEM FROM SCRATCH. WE AND ANIMALS CANNOT CONVERT OMEGA SIX TO OMEGA THREE.

Plants can make them and convert them, we cannot. The body has a limited ability to convert Omega 3 and 6 mother fats, into longer fats of the same family. Western dietary elements, stop people converting the mother fats, to the long chain fats. The body uses its ability to manufacture, elongate, and disassemble fats, their effects, and availability, to control body systems. These systems include sex hormones, steroids, metabolism and sleep.

The message of the book, 'balance the Omega Threes and Sixes', is founded in extensive and solid research of others, but is still a matter of debate. The need to balance Omega Threes and Sixes is arguably fundamental to human health.

I am no medical Luddite. I am immensely grateful to western medicine. However, the very successful commercial market model, does not sit well, with determination of cause and prevention. There is no commercial benefit in pointing out simple preventive strategies. For example economically successful drugs, COX blockers, seek to reverse or moderate, the downstream impact of excess Omega 6 on inflammatory conditions like arthritis, asthma, and pain.

This dichotomy applies from top to bottom. It is not the decision of an individual, but the sum of all the knee-jerk reactions. Researchers cannot insist to their bosses, that a discovery suggests prevention would be a better starting point, or parallel path option to a drug; they would not have a job. The conclusion of commercial trials will always be, "this mechanism could provide a target for a drug". The conclusion will not be "this is an effective prevention mechanism— we had better tell everybody".

That is the consequence of profit as a sole market driver. It is untenable to allow people to become ill, as an inevitable consequence, of there being no corporate profit driver for prevention. The cost of illness to individuals, nations, and humanity, is too high. Prevention has to take a higher priority. With more effective prevention, the need for medical intervention will not disappear, it will just shift focus to areas beyond prevention.

The balance of Omega 3 and 6, is absolutely key to health and behaviour. We are badly distorting intake ratios, primarily through excess Omega Six in vegetable oils. We also change the fat profiles of the animals we eat, by feeding them heavily on grain, which is high in Omega 6. We are breeding crops low in Omega 3, to achieve longer shelf lives. We remove Omega Three from the food chain to extend shelf life. We block the body's internal fats elongation pathways, with excess Omega Six intakes from vegetable oils, excess sugar, trans fats, etc.

Omega 3 intake in the West, is recorded as falling over the last 15 years. DHA in breast milk in Canada and Australia, has fallen by about 50 per cent in the last 15 years. DHA in Canadian breast milk was .17 per cent, compared with .99 per cent in Japan. In Canada in 2005, only 10 per cent of women met the dietary DHA intake recommendation. Twenty per cent had only traces of DHA in their diet. [Average DHA - Canadian breast milk 0.14 per cent - Japan .99 per cent].

Omega Six really does alter behaviour, metabolic rate, sleep, sex hormone and steroid production. Omega 6 levels in the cell membranes of the body, influence behaviour and mood, by controlling chemicals in the brain such as dopamine, serotonin, and melatonin. Omega 3 and 6 fats impact on immune function, T-cells, natural killer cells, and macrophages[i]. Omega 3 and 6 have a role in regulating stress responses, through the hormone steroid pathways, lipid rafts, and gene expression. For example DHA reduces norepinephrine[ii] [iii][AKA noradrenaline, a chemical released during a stress response]. Omega Six makes inflammatory chemicals. It is now accepted inflammation and stress response are linked, and a factor in neurological conditions such as depression and mania.

Omega Six products and pathways have fundamental consequences. Omega Six chemical products, PGE2s, have been shown to influence, and even maybe control, the enzymes by which cholesterol is turned into the sex hormones and steroids [Fig. 23.11b]. Cox blockers shut off legs of the Omega Six pathways.

---

i   The immunostimulating and antimicrobial properties of lithium and antidepressants LIEB Julian ; The Journal of infection (J. infect.) 2004, vol. 49, n°2, pp. 88–93 [6 page(s) (article)] (102 ref.).

ii Auditory Brainstem Evoked Response in Juvenile Rats Fed Rat Milk Formulas with High Docosahexaenoic Acid Auestad N.; Stockard-Sullivan J.; Innis S.M.; Korsak R.; Edmond J. Nutritional Neuroscience, Volume 6, Number 6, December 2003 , pp. 335–341(7).

iii Intravenous fish oil blunts the physiological response to endotoxin in healthy subjects. Intensive Care Med. 2007 May; 33(5):789–97. Epub 2007 Mar 22. Pluess TT, Hayoz D, Berger MM, Tappy L, Revelly JP, Michaeli B, Carpentier YA, Chioléro RL. Department of Intensive Care Medicine, CHUV, 1011, Lausanne, Switzerland.

The most shocking revelation on my journey, was that common COX blocking drugs given at a critical period in the gestation of rats, changed hormone levels, which, changed the mental sexual orientation and 'homosexualised' the offspring. Inappropriate hormones at a critical time near birth, actually altered the physical structure of key parts of the brain from male to female, or female to male.

Rats were turned homosexual by drugs intervention. The same drugs are used in humans, in pregnancy, but no research has been done in humans. Similar alterations of brain configuration linked to sexual orientation have been observed in humans. Could there be wider implications of such drug interventions, at critical pregnancy developmental points, in humans? Opioid analgesics (Codeine is a weak one) and antifungal agents, also affect PGE2, and so potentially the sex hormone pathways[iv]. It is acknowledged more research is required.

I suggest Omega Six consumption and availability, connects humans to the fecundity of nature via the body's sex hormones, brain messengers, and chemical pathways. These fats alter the very structure of the brain. Omega Six confers essentially male behavioural attributes. Omega Three confers essentially female attributes. Omega Six and Three intake levels modify behaviour in fundamental ways, through known chemical pathways such as dopamine and serotonin.

I suggest the fats conversion pathways, and Omega Three-Six balance, are fundamental to sleep and body repair. The Omega Six PGE2, has been shown to be higher in daytime. DHA with melatonin appears to be central to sleep, and may be higher at night. Melatonin and DHA, close down the Omega 6 pathways at night. Many of the body chemicals follow a day night rhythm. Lack of DHA, and excess Omega Six, may impair melatonin activity, and so prevent proper body shutdown, sleep, and repair. Lack of sleep is linked to many 'Western' conditions.

I postulate Omega Three-Six levels and balances, are the prime controlling factors, and external regulators, of the fertility cycle. Omega Six enzymes control steroid and hormone production. DHA closes down Omega 6 production. Oestrogen increases DHA production. The ability of women to make more DHA, helps define behavioural and physical differences, between the sexes. Building cells needs DHA. The baby's need for DHA is a key part of hormone regulation.

The Omega Three-Six balance, and Omega Six availability, DHA, sleep and melatonin, alters the time of puberty, which also links to brain development.

Does excess Omega 6 delicately alter maleness and femaleness of offspring, and the sexual outlook and profile, at a very subtle level, of whole generations.

I suggest Omega 3 and 6 have a key role to play in obesity, by a combination of metabolic changes with Omega 6 forcing the body to store fat, interaction with fructose, and the lack of Omega 3, leading to a blocking of insulin and leptin functions. I tentatively suggest a possible mechanism, based on the desaturase pathways, for insulin and leptin blocking, and so 'metabolic syndrome'.

---

iv   Med Hypotheses. 2007;69(4):829–35. Epub 2007 Mar 23. Sex, drugs and sports: Prostaglandins, epitestosterone and sexual development. Sanders BK.

Omega Six works with fructose, which also forces fat storage. Omega Six and fructose were originally scarce resources found together in fruits and berries.

Like smoking, it will take time to 'prove' that excess Omega Six, and the lack of Omega Three is bad for you. The body is so complex, so multifaceted and multilayered, that you are never going to get absolute 'proof' in the foreseeable future. Mankind cannot live on Omega 3s and 6s alone, so it is not possible to isolate their effect. That is the nature of these complex issues of human biology. As with smoking, there will simply be a growing consensus of opinion over time.

The chemical pathways and mechanisms do exist, to explain the extensive negative effects of **excess** Omega Six. However, demonstrating that many of the necessary pathways exist, it is not the same as proving cause and effect.

This book does not have many solutions for different conditions just three basic rules are applicable to everything;

☞ ***Balance the Omega Three and Six mother fats.***
☞ ***Do not block the conversion pathways.***
☞ ***Ensure an adequate supply of long chain fats.***

Once you accept they reduce one health risk, for instance heart related mortality, all the rest is a bonus.

This diagram represents, graphically in both senses, the impact of excess long chain Omega Six, on the risk of death from heart disease. This graph is from work by William Lands[v]. He is a respected pioneer in the world of lipids, constant advocate,

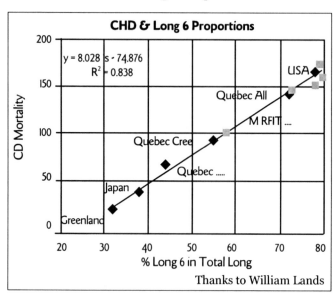

Thanks to William Lands

and originator of the need to balance the Omega Threes and Sixes. William Lands has been working in this field since the mid 1950s. The graph looks at the percentage of long chain Omega Six in tissue, against heart related death rates. The higher the proportion of Omega Sixes, the greater is the risk of death from a coronary related event.

---

v   "Fish, Omega-3 and Human Health" by William Lands and in an article in the journal "Lipids" (Lands, Lipids 2003 (Apr.); 38: 317–321).

Mr. Lands put it; you can pick your risk of a fatal heart condition by selecting your Omega Six intake level.

Bill Lands is the author of a fascinating book *Fish, Omega -3 and Human Health,* which passionately sets out arguments as to the need for education on the importance of Omega 3 and 6 in biological function, and the exciting and meaningful potential for disease prevention.

Long chain and mother Omega Threes in diet, also reduce the risk of cardiac events. This is accepted by the medical profession, and is backed with intake recommendations. *Reduced cardiac risk is a reason to balance your Omega Threes and Sixes. All the rest is a bonus.*

The question is, how long will it take for there to be wider medical recognition of the need to balance the Omega Threes and Sixes? How many children do you want give furred arteries, mental issues, compromised intelligence, asthma, diabetes, acne, and early puberty, before this simple truth is recognised?

It took a very long time for both scurvy and smoking to be fully recognised as issues, 50 or 60 years. Are you prepared to condemn another generation, to increasing early illness, increased global aggression, reduced intelligence, and take 'western' conditions to the less affected parts of the world?

Please do not discard out of hand that balancing the Omega Threes and Sixes can reduce the risks of 'western' conditions, improve our intelligence, and reduce aggression, impulsiveness, because it sounds too easy and simple.

There is nothing simple about Omega Three and Omega Six. The chemistry is immensely mind numbingly incomprehensibly complex. Omega Three and Six are arguably amongst a limited number of master controllers of body processes.

The worst culprits of excess Omega Six supply are vegetable oils. World vegetable oil consumption is rising rapidly. The "Undeveloped" world too is seeing huge growth in 'western' conditions.

Good digestion is a massive health issue. Fat absorption is complex, and multi-stage. If you have adequate Omega 3 in your diet but do not absorb it, you have a problem. Omega 3 DHA intake levels for many are already low, below 100 mg day. It is clearly very important to absorb the already limited Omega 3 in the average diet. There are different absorption routes for different fats [11.20]. I was not aware, at the time I wrote 11.20, that long chain Omega 3s, may in fact not enter the body by the lymphatic system, but by direct absorption that takes place in the small intestine. It appears much is not known.

Digestive disturbances are common, and Omega 3 is scarce. Fat blockers may present much greater risks than is currently appreciated.

If the primary intake of Omega 3 is by direct absorption, a healthy intestinal tract[vi] may be immeasuably important.

---

vi   Effects of Dietary Fatty Acids on Lipid Metabolism Gary J Nelson United States Department of Agriculture, University of California, Davis California. From Fatty Acids in Foods and their Health Implications edited by Ching Kuang Chow.

We chemically adulterate fats to sell foods. The latest fat adulteration is interesterified fats [11.23]. Fats in nature come in particular configurations. Fats exist commonly in a chemical toast rack of three fats, a triglyceride. During processing in the body, the centre fat remains attached to the rack. The fats on each side are released, for processing and re-manufacture into new toast rack combinations. In nature, short chain saturated fats may not generally be found in the middle of the toast rack[vii].

We make artificial fats with saturated short fats in the middle of the toast rack, so you can have flaky crumbly pastries [11.21], and biscuits, that last on the shelf. These are called interesterified fats. They are being used to replace hydrogenated fats. As yet we do not know the full consequence of this reorganisation of fats.

This is effectively another long term human dietary experiment you are about to become part of. Is it good or bad? Some suggest not so good, but as usual more trials are required to determine if there will be unforeseen future negatives. Given the fundamental importance of fats to healthy body function, is adulteration of fats a risk worth taking for flaky pasty. One for you at the moment I am afraid.

Those who live in the centres of civil organisation and administration are equally affected. Factory farmed chicken eggs in a Washington DC supermarket, have 10 times less DHA than eggs of a true free-range bird.

Nations are in competition. The Japanese have far lower rates of 'western' conditions. Japanese health costs per head are half those of the U.S. The Japanese score higher in IQ tests, and have lower crime. Japan has a far better Omega Three-Six profile. Japan has recognised the balance of Omega Three and Six in the diet is a national health issue, and issued intake guidelines.

We are programmed to alter our behaviour to maximise survival dependent on the fertility of the earth. In nature the availability of Omega 6 reflects the fecundity of the earth. Farming and mechanical extraction of seed oils has allowed us unknowingly to break that link.

Excess Omega 6 and lack of Omega 3 is arguably exaggerating the male traits outside design specifications, and downgrading feminine traits, making us more aggressive and impulsive. Lack of DHA links to poorer neurological function.

A widespread trend to lower intelligence and unbalanced exaggeration of masculine traits could be disastrous for humanity.

Future health costs of burgeoning 'western' conditions are almost unaffordable. To that, you can add wider consequential, more subtle, social and economic costs. The wider costs of illness to, the individual, carers, the wider family and society, are incalculable.

---

vii   Absorption and Transport of Dietary Lipid, Vernon Welch. University of Reading, Whitekinghts, Reading England. Jurgen T Borlak Solday Pharma, Hannover, Germany. From Fatty Acids in Foods and their Health Implications edited by Ching Kuang Chow.

1

INTRODUCTION

1.1 **I want to scream**–I want to scream this. It is for me inescapably obvious. But how do I explain it to you? How do I get you to spend precious time, in a hectic world, to understand a simple truth? **We block our fat conversion pathways with excess Omega Six. We consume;**

- ➤ *Far too much Omega 6* mother fat LA
- ➤ *Far too little Omega 3* mother fat ALA,
- ➤ *Too little long chain Omega 3* EPA and DHA.

A few thought provoking quotes;

- ➤ "The increases in world LA consumption over the past century may be considered *a very large uncontrolled experiment* that may have contributed to increased societal burdens of aggression, depression, and cardiovascular mortality. [1]"

- ➤ "A large body of evidence suggests that there is a significant under consumption of omega–3, long-chain, polyunsaturated fatty acids (LC-PUFAs) and that *this is the cause of multiple chronic diseases and developmental aberrations.* [2]"

- ➤ "According to the World Health Organisation, there are more than *one billion overweight adults globally* and at least 300 million of them are obese"

- ➤ "In the UK, recent figures from the Department of Health based on the Health Survey for England 2003 predict that by 2010, *one in three adults will be obese*, whilst 27 per cent of girls (11–15 years old) will be obese approaching child-bearing age (Department of Health, 2006). [3]"

ABBREVIATIONS

To save using the long names of the fats in this book, the **abbreviations** are used. You will need these as you read this book.

LA	Linoleic acid	Omega Six mother	18:2 n6
ALA	Linolenic Acid	Omega Three mother	18:3 n3
AA	Arachidonic acid	Omega Six	20:4 n6
EPA	Eicosapentaenoic	Omega Three	20:5 n3
AD	Adrenic acid	Omega Six	22:4 n6
DPA	Docosapentaenoic	Omega Six	22:5 n6
DPA	Docosapentaenoic	Omega Three	22:5 n3
DHA	Docosahexaenoic Acid	Omega Three	22:6 n3

THE SHAPES

It is important to grasp what saturated, monosaturated, and polyunsaturated means in terms of structure. I know this sounds silly but hold your arm out straight in front of you. Wiggle your hand about 5–10 degrees. Your straight arm with little movement or ability to change shape is a saturated fat.

Now imagine straight-armed hugs, or baby holding. (Please do not try with real babies or strangers on the tube/subway). It is not possible to hold a baby, or have a proper hug if you cannot bend your arm. Saturated fats cannot get close and personal with other chemicals, but are good for making structures rigid.

Bend your elbow and imagine the joint will do a Meryl Streep 360–degree unrestricted head turn. Your arm is now a monosaturate. This gives you more ability to hug.

You can now flex your arm AND wrist. Your arm is now a polyunsaturate. If you were DHA, you would have 12 points of rotation creating 'bends' [30.10]. Unlike your arm, the angles are relatively fixed. These bonds it is suggested have 360-degree rotation. Imagine the shapes you could make with your arm and finger joints if you could rotate them all through 360 degrees.

For fats, meeting the right mate is like life, keep on moving, and sooner or later, you may bump into someone suitable. Fats are always in motion, a cross between molecular disco dancers[i] and Billy Whizz, looking for their place in life.

These shapes allow the fats to get up close and personal, and react in tight spaces only they can fit in—super hugs. The more shapes you can make the more chance there is of fitting in. Straight arms do not hug as well as bent arms. A straight arm can't replace an arm that bends—and vice versa—so it is with fats.

Double bonds are less chemically stable than single bonds. Using different pairs of strings [bonds] makes different shapes. The combination of shape, position, and contact points between double bonds allows chemical reaction.

---

i   Susan Allport The Queen of Fats.

A carbon atom makes four bonds. For a carbon atom, imagine a tennis ball with four evenly distributed elastic strings attached. The strings, known as bonds, are attachment points for other chemicals. An attachment can have one or more strings. A one string attachment is a single bond. A two string attachment is a double bond. One string bonds are much more stable than two string bonds. The stretched "strings" of a double bond are more likely to unknot.

One bond, a single string, can rotate. Double bonds of two strings resist rotation, and so help determine the shape [30.10]. Different chemicals have different number of strings (bonds). Hydrogen has one and oxygen two.

Just like in the intimacies of life, if the right bits are not in contact with the right places, you are not going to get a reaction. A double bond out of contact with its opposite number will produce no reaction. So the chemical interaction of fats is about shape, fit, and close contact of reactive bits.

1.2 **Gunk in the frying pan—*RESPECT!*** These fats Omega Three and Omega Six fats are the very essence of life.

1.3 **Dumber and sicker**—We are becoming dumber, sicker, more aggressive impulsive selfish humans, because of excess of mother Omega 6, and lack of mother Omega 3 and long Omega 3s. Dumber, sicker, more aggressive impulsive selfish humans, are more likely to extinguish themselves as a species.

In this complex resource-pressured world, we need as much intelligence, goodwill, reserve and tolerance as we can access. Omega Six brings out our acquisitive behaviour, linked to sex, aggression, and territorial breeding rights. Omega Six is a mind altering "drug".

How do we judge if the whole of society is changing? We are seeing higher rates of a huge range of 'western' disease particularly in the young, including previously unseen trends like rising ADHD, higher levels of depression, suicide, diabetes 1 and 2, asthma, and the list goes on.

We are all different but there are inescapable facts. FACT: STRAIGHT FORWARD SIMPLE AND INESCAPABLE = Brains and eyes, testes and women's reproductive systems, do not function properly without adequate DHA.

If you want a part of the explanation for a more dysfunctional sicker society, it is excess Omega Six and lack of Omega Three. If you want a part of the explanation for falling intelligence and fertility, it is excess of Omega 6 and lack of 3.

If you want a part of the explanation for educational deficits in the poorest sector with the most vegetable oil dependent nutrition, it is maybe at least in part excess of Omega 6 and lack of Omega 3.

Trials have shown lack of Omega Three connects to crime, violence, aggression, paedophilia, and behavioural disorders. The U.S.A. spends 15 per cent of their economy on health care. The Japanese spend half the amount spent in the USA per capita on health care.

So the Japanese have more money to spend on other things. Based on IQ tests, the Japanese are one of the brightest nations. The Japanese have greater intake of fish and Omega 3. The Chinese are the world's biggest fish farmers.

1.4   The Devil's Fat? The seven deadly sins—Is Omega Six LA linoleic acid 18:2 n6 the Devil's Fat? Certainly it has plenty of 6s, and Omega 6 pushes us unknowingly towards the seven deadly sins, lust, gluttony, greed, wrath, envy, pride, and sloth.

Trials suggest that aggression, impulsiveness, criminal behaviour, depression, suicide, and illness, all are increased by higher levels of Omega 6. So maybe excess Omega 6 is the Devil's work.

Excess Omega Six increases testosterone, and reduces serotonin, which induces aggression, impulsiveness and criminal behaviour. Tendencies toward acquisitiveness aggression and impulsiveness, would be consistent with territorial defence for breeding.

We have responsibility for our excess consumption of Omega Six. It is a choice we make. In its correct proportion, Omega Six allows us to breed. It activates our reproductive pathways. At natural Omega Six dosages, we can balance the relationship survival seesaw.

But in excess, Omega Six tips us to aggression, selfishness, impulsiveness, less cooperative spirit, lower intelligence, smaller brains, and illnesses (all magnified in the absence of adequate Omega Three).

The Devil (Real or construct, I leave to you) has found a really neat subversive mechanism here. Unobtrusive, seemingly beneficial, simple, freely chosen, and yet with scarcely imaginable negative consequences.

Increasing aggression, acquisitiveness, selfishness, and loss of female virtues, are consequences of Omega Six, which could subtly lead to our destruction.

Vegetable oils generally have a very high Omega 6 content. Vegetarian, Kosher, Halal and related diets, all over the world, are prone to excess Omega Six intake, due to the substitution of high levels of vegetable oils for other fats.

Omega Six in body fat in the middle east, where figures are available, is reported as around 25 per cent, compared with national averages of 16 per cent in the U.S.A. and 10 per cent in Europe.

Clearly such things are complex and dependent on very many factors, but it is an unavoidable fact that the general biology of all of us humans is similar. Could diets high in Omega 6, and low in Omega 3, subtly contribute to the potential for a more conflicted world?

1.5   Lord of the Fats—Omega Six is 'Environmental Master' of us all. Arguably, Omega Six is the "Lord of the Fats". Misused Omega Six is a disaster.

Omega Six intake controls breeding patterns, breeding behaviour, and our fertility. Somebody joked, if the title was changed to 'Omega Sex', the book would sell better.

For a moment I seriously considered 'Omega Sex' as title. After all, Omega Six is the ultimate controller of the sex hormones. Omega Six is a gauge in all of us, of food in the environment. When our Omega Six was low, there were insufficient food resources available for us to breed.

Omega Six intake controls sexual drive, reproduction, protection of family, and acquisition of breeding rights. Omega Six is the mechanism by which nature controls our behaviour for our own good. Nature turns off our breeding capability to improve our survival chances when food is short.

The problem is we have managed to break nature's links and rules – but without knowing it.

1.6   **Mistress of the Fats** – Humans start life as 'brain female'. Brains are turned male towards the end of pregnancy [See 24.29]. Omega Three underlies the feminine virtues of nurture, caring, sharing, cooperation, women's neural function, as well as "intelligence" (more neurons in less brain space).

If Omega Six is the Devil's Fat, then Omega Three is arguably God's response. DHA, an Omega Three, increases serotonin, and reduces male behaviour, including aggression and impulsiveness. Omega Three moderates and cools the Omega Six chemical products, and reduces production of them. Omega Three reduces depression and psychiatric disorders.

L.C. Reis and J.R. Hibbeln, well respected and prolific lipid researchers, produced a thesis on the cultural importance and symbolism of fish. Fish is important as a moderator of mental function, and wellbeing. Treatment of illness with food, has a long recorded history, in many cultures including the Chinese, Ancient Greeks, Indians, Egyptians, Sumerians, and Babylonians.

Fish is accorded religious recognition in many cultures. It is logical that the special regard in which fish is held, was due to recognition over many thousands of years of its dietary importance, and impact on wellbeing and society.

Fish is sacred in Christianity, forms part of the iconographic symbolism, was talked about in parables, and traditionally was part of the Christian diet.

Fish is sacred or features prominently in Judaism, Hinduism, Buddhism, Shinto, and ancient Middle Eastern Religions. Reis and Hibbeln said fish is "yin" in Chinese culture, and associated with peace and calm. Aggression is Yang.

"Peace, order, and the reduction of impulsive aggression tend to knit societies together", and "fish as a food calms aggression, reduces distressful emotions and promotes peacefulness in conscious and unconscious associations"[ii].

---

ii   Cultural symbolism of fish and the psychotropic properties of omega–3 fatty acids L.C. Reis and J.R. Hibbeln. Prostaglandins, Leukotrienes and Essential Fatty Acids 75 (2006) 227–236 National Institute on Alcohol Abuse and Alcoholism, NIH, MD USA.

1.7   Way outside our design parameters—Your excess consumption of Omega Six has tremendous consequences for you, your family, and arguably the survival of the species. We are "breaking down".

You are unknowingly participating in a huge dietary experiment. This experiment is making us sicker, more depressed, more stupid, less fertile, fatter, and more aggressive. The impact is magnified in children. There are sufficient trials on the Omega Three to make this conclusion almost unavoidable. Far less work has been done on excess Six, but there have been a number of trials and there are experts who write on the subject.

The actions of fats in the body are very complex. Prevention research is not very sexy or rewarding in financial profit terms. I am hoping to convince you that reducing your Omega Six intake makes strong sense and NOW.

This could be like smoking. It could take 30 years for it to be accepted that excess Omega Six is harmful at best, and deadly at worst. So, get ahead of the game, read on, and make up your own mind.

1.8   Not lords of the environment—By design, creation or evolution, animals have an intimate relationship with their environment. We are no different. We are coming to think that we are above our environment. The reality is that our environment forged our design parameters.

We are programmed to acquire, fight when we needed to, and protect a patch of land that provides good berries. We are not free to do as we wish. We require oxygen. We require water. We require certain nutrients.

We have evolved, or been designed, to nutrients being available within certain tolerance. Omega 3 and 6 are building blocks, fuel, chemicals raw materials, and hormones controllers. They are fundamental to function.

If we do not get Omega 3 and 6 in the right fuel mix, we do not function properly. Put the wrong fuel in a car, and it will breakdown. Put the wrong utensils in a microwave, and it will break.

We humans are breaking down. ADHD, Alzheimer's, osteoporosis, digestive problems, depression, aggression, intelligence, and many more conditions all link to lack of Omega Three and excess Omega Six.

1.9   Omega Six and obesity—OK, you are more interested in the getting rid of the love handles and spare tyre.

Omega Six instructs the body to store fat. It tells the body to make bigger and more fat cells available. Omega Six historically comes with fruit sugar. The body is instructed to store fructose as fat too. Omega Six switches down the metabolism.

Excess Omega Six fat sets the body in an inflammatory mode. Too much Omega Six, and your hormones and steroids may be out of balance. Omega Six is a key raw material, and a consequential controller of hormone and steroids.

Omega Six says get ready to breed! Whoopee time. Save Omega Six and accompanying sugars, put on some weight for reserves, and go and reproduce. The fat switch is set to on.

You can turn the store fat switch off with Omega 3. You can rebalance your hormones with Omega Three. You can switch down inflammatory tendencies. Omega Threes encourage the body to burn fat and make small fat cells.

Increasing your long chain Omega Threes, and heavily cutting down your Omega Six intake, will switch off the "store fat" button. Your body will be pushed towards burn and not store. It will help you lose weight.

Omega Three will improve your hair, eyes, skin, nails, and possibly fertility and sex life. It will help reduce the risk of PCOS and hirsuteness. It will help sort out your kids' ADHD, improve sleep, delay puberty, and reduce their long term risk of osteoporosis, arthritis, asthma, diabetes, dementia, heart disease, and depression, to name but a few (see back cover)–Or just an easy way to assist tip the balance in weight loss–Now are you more interested?

1.10   **Fundamental to function at every level**–There are lots of environmental factors we respond to, like light, minerals, vitamins, etc... But arguably there are none to which we are so sensitive as Omega Six. Excess of Omega Six has far reaching consequences.

WHY? Because these fats are fundamental parts of the structure of the body. These fats are fundamental to function at every level. The structure of your brain is 60 per cent fat. Your cell membranes are made in significant part of fat. Fats are the source of hormones and steroids.

Fats have a part in controlling sex hormones. Fats are cellular messengers. Fats are energy sources. Fats are your fuel depot. Fats are the raw materials for massive families of very influential chemicals.

1.11   **Divorced from nature**–We have divorced our diet from nature. We have broken our link with nature. We now operate outside our design parameters. Omega Six was always a scarce, seasonal, and precious resource. Now Omega Six comes by the bottle and fryer full. Independence from nature is not all bad, as long as we understand our actions, the link to nature, and the consequences of breaking those links.

1.12   **Excess Omega Six intake**–Trials link excessive Omega Six and lack of Omega Three to lower intelligence, higher aggressiveness, impulsiveness, obesity, and sex hormones. The list goes on. Evolutionary design seeks to achieve survival advantage within nature's supply levels of raw materials. We have broken the supply rules and do not know it. We oversupply our body with Omega 6, upsetting a long held fundamental dietary parameter, with dire consequences.

1.13   **Global emotional balance–Yin and Yang**–A balance of generosity of spirit, cooperation, reserve, intelligence, aggression, selfishness, and impulsiveness, by design or evolution, is fundamental to our survival.

These are the most fundamental human characteristics. Yin (Omega Three, passive feminine and responds to the night) and Yang (Omega Six, active masculine and corresponds to day) are surprisingly applicable to Omega Three and Omega Six, as will become evident through this book.

A seesaw of opposites. What is the consequence if the 'emotional balance' of the species is changed? If our leaders and we become more selfish, more aggressive, and less intelligent, what will be the outcome? If we lose the more feminine virtues, and tip the balance to the more male characteristics, what is our future?

Are we already seeing a glimpse of the future, in our changing behaviour patterns, and those of our children? Are we seeing the first consequences of excess Omega Six, the Devil's Fat, in our current world? I think we may be.

Society is becoming more self-centred and acquisitive. It is strongly arguable that Omega Six is a part of this. Are we becoming the ultimate selfish territorial settlers and consumers? What will be the consequences when the resources run short?

1.14   Cigarettes–a changed perspective–You are probably thinking this is a bit far fetched. Tarry a while, I beg. Cigarettes, and more recently trans fats, were originally promised and promoted as healthy.

1.15   You cannot make mother Omega Six–Ultimately, Omega Six can only be got from diet. We cannot make it. We can upgrade it to varying extents to make longer chains fats of the same family. However clever we are, our bodies cannot naturally make Omega Six (or Three) mother fats.

1.16   Seasonal mating and food availability–Timing of sexual mating and behaviour in mammals is very often seasonal. Breeding is timed and triggered by availability of food, which itself reflects the seasons.

Food reflects the earth's fecundity. If flowers are setting seed, conditions are productive. The food chain including prey will be plentiful. Water will be available. Seeds and nuts are the key source of Omega 6. It is an agent external to the body. Omega 6 links us to nature. It controls our hormone production. Without it, or when it is in short supply, we cannot breed.

1.17   Ultimate hormone controller–The body makes testosterone and oestrogen indirectly via Omega Six. The level of Omega Six available in the body stores and diet, controls the sex hormone levels. Excess body fat = excess hormone levels (both oestrogen and testosterone). Hormones are made in the fat tissue as well as the reproductive organs. Omega Six is essential to manufacture of hormones at all locations.

Oestrogen pushes up DHA production. Oestrogen, with DHA, endows the female characteristics of nurture, sharing, restraint, smaller size, and greater neuron density. AA, through testosterone, endows the male characteristics of aggression, acquisitiveness, and impulsiveness.

Omega Three and Omega Six act out a push-me pull-you hormone dance. By ingesting too much Omega Six, and too little Three, and we are operating outside design limits.

Excess Omega Six increases levels of all hormones, and disturbs the hormone cycle. Increased levels of DHA reduce the long chain Omega 6 hormone and steroid production. To make DHA you need sufficient Omega 3 in the diet. Often DHA in the diet is insufficient.

We are tampering with our fertility. We are risking our health. Increased hormones levels, due to increased Omega Six in the fat reserves, higher Omega Six chemicals, and lack of DHA give rise to hormonal disturbance and changes, which are leading to a rise in fertility related conditions.

1.18   **Conflict and the fertility cycle**—Omega 3 and 6 conduct a dance that controls sex hormones and steroids levels. Steroids include cortisol, and corticosterone [23.11.b]. Hormones and steroids, are made from cholesterol.

They are all made in the same chemical tree, that starts with cholesterol, as its exclusive raw material. The chemicals pass through a number of enzyme production lines, as they are made into steroids and hormones. [Fig 23.11 b]

There is competition for these production lines. So there is a constant powerplay for dominance between various hormones and steroids. The whole cholesterol, sex hormone, and steroid product range, looks as if it may have a monthly cycle in women. Hormones and steroids are in constant competition for raw materials, so if hormones cycle, steroids are likely to as well.

It is observed hormones, and steroids, do have seasonal, monthly, and daily cycles. The adrenal gland products including aldosterone have been observed to follow the monthly cycle[iii].

PGE2, a product of Omega Six, has significant control over the activity, of at least a number of the enzyme production lines, for steroids and hormones.

[PGE2 can only be made from the Omega 6 product AA through the COX2 enzyme. COX2 follows the monthly cycle, and is highest mid cycle.

Omega Six and Omega Three are truly external agents, only available through diet. They link us to the fecundity of the environment. They are ultimately the hormone controllers.

Omega Six, through the products of its chemical pathway via PGE2, is essential to hormone and steroid production, and fertility [See 23.11]. Both DHA and AA have been shown in animals to down regulate progesterone[iv].

---

iii   Effects of the menstrual cycle on mood, neurocognitive and neuroendocrine function in healthy premenopausal women Psychological Medicine (2004), 34: 93-102 Cambridge University Press C.S. Symonds, P Gallagher, J.M. Thompson and A.H. Young Psychobiology Research Group, School of Neurology, Neurobiology and Psychiatry, University of Newcastle upon Tyne

iv   Long chain polyunsaturated fatty acids and bovine luteal cell function Biology of reproduction (Biol. reprod.) 1996, vol. 55, no2, pp. 445-449 (38 ref.) Hinckely T. SR; Clark R. M. ; Bushmich S. L. ; Milvae R. A. Department of Animal Science, University of Connecticut, Storrs, Connecticut 06269-4040, ETATS-UNIS.

It is complex and multifaceted, but Omega Three and Omega Six are the key external variables. Excess of Omega Six, leads to excess of testosterone and oestrogen, through higher PGE2. Testosterone may push the body to make more long chain Omega Six, AA, and so PGE2, thus self-fuelling.

Higher oestrogen in women is the catalyst for women to make long chain Omega Three, DHA, and Omega Six, AA. (Women convert 10% of ALA the mother Omega 3 to long chain DHA. Men convert under 1 per cent.) So DHA and AA production will both follow and control oestrogen levels through the cycle.

DHA blocks the body making the AA, and so PGE2, thus turning down both oestrogen and testosterone. A foetus requires high levels of DHA to grow. The utilisation of DHA for growth by the baby, stops an excess of DHA developing. DHA is also likely to be required to build the additional cells to thicken the lining of the uterus. It could be in the monthly cycle, that the commencement of the thickening of the uterus, uses up the available DHA and most of the AA.

The cessation of thickening of the uterus walls and egg development, would allow a sudden increase of DHA levels. Excess DHA would turn down the production of AA. Reduced AA would result in falling hormone production reducing oestrogen, and bringing the monthly cycle to a end.

High AA equates to high sex hormone levels. If the egg is fertilised, rising DHA levels are used by the baby. AA production likely exceeds usage by the baby allowing the growing placenta to utilise the AA to keep hormone levels rising.

Rising oestrogen promotes greater fat conversion to DHA and AA . The DHA is used to grow the placenta and baby so creating a self fuelling cycle. This, I suggest, may be the foundation of the female fertility and birth cycle.]

Omega Three — Six imbalance leads to a whole host of reproductive problems. Large amounts of body fat in the West, generally equals large reserves of Omega Six. Low intake of Omega Three, combined with low storage by the body, equals a lack of DHA.

If adequate DHA is not available, because of supply shortage or conversion blockage, then the body will be unable to balance, and fully modulate, the monthly sex hormone and steroid cycle.

In the absence of DHA, the natural hormone balances and cycles are disturbed, leading to fertility problems, uterine conditions, PCOS, hirsuteness, osteoporosis, an increased risk of a host of illnesses and of certain cancers.

1.19 **Aggressive inflammatory chemicals** — [*Fig 1.19 See following pages*] From Omega Six, the body makes a huge family of very sophisticated chemicals, that control a vast range of body functions, including the fundamental ability to carry babies internally.

Omega 6 is the exclusive raw material of Arachidonic Acid [referred to in this book as AA]. From AA exclusively the body makes a huge array of chemicals.

To give an idea of the complexity and extent of the chemical cascades made from AA a chart [Fig.1.19] follows by kind permission of Cayman Chemical.

The detail is beyond this book and me. The point is to graphically illustrate how far reaching and influential the fats are.

Similar cascades will exist for the Omega 3s. This family of 20 long carbon chain chemicals are called the eicosanoids. These chemicals are involved in inflammatory reaction, tissue destruction and creation, repair, and the immune system, etc.

These chemicals interlink with probably all body functions in one way or another. The ability to manufacture these chemicals is based on the available supply of raw material to the cell membranes.

Supply of the raw material, Omega Six, to the cell membrane is based on dietary intake, and stored Omega Six. Cell membrane content is biased towards Omega Six, rather than Omega Three, by a number of factors.

We eat far more Omega Six than Omega Three. The body has instructions to burn Omega Three, in preference to Omega Six. The body has instructions to store Omega Six, and does so.

Omega 6 LA in body fat was in single figures in the 60s and 70s, and now ranges between about 10 per cent and 25 per cent. Stored Omega Three is often very low and rises to about two per cent, but is generally very much lower.

1.20 **Deflammatory chemicals**–Omega Three counterbalances Omega Six. More Omega Threes, and particularly DHA and EPA, stop the inflammatory Omega Six chemical products being produced. Omega Threes are essentially anti-inflammatory by a number of mechanisms.

More Omega Three raw material means more protective Omega Three chemicals. So, it is a double positive, less bad Omega Six products and more good Omega Three products [Because they need to be in balance].

More Omega Three and less Six in the cell membranes, will moderate inflammatory conditions in the body. This fact is fundamental to a huge range of processes.

DHA has been reported as being a more powerful Cox blocker than many drugs. Omega Three produces protective products called protectins and resolvins. Fish oil reduces the production of Omega Six inflammatory chemicals such as prostaglandin E_2 and thromboxane A_2.

Omega Three or Six chemical production is in a sense self-fuelling. DHA produces higher levels of oxidation in the mitochondria than Omega Six. Higher availability of DHA and more consequent oxidation, allows more Omega Three products to be made. More Omega Three raw material is available including the DHA, so the products will be Omega Three based, which will damp down inflammation.

If Omega 6 predominates, oxidation rates will be lower, but as Omega 6 reactions need less energy, and the Omega 6 cascades self fuel by producing oxidants, products will be Omega 6 based. Inflammation pressures will increase.

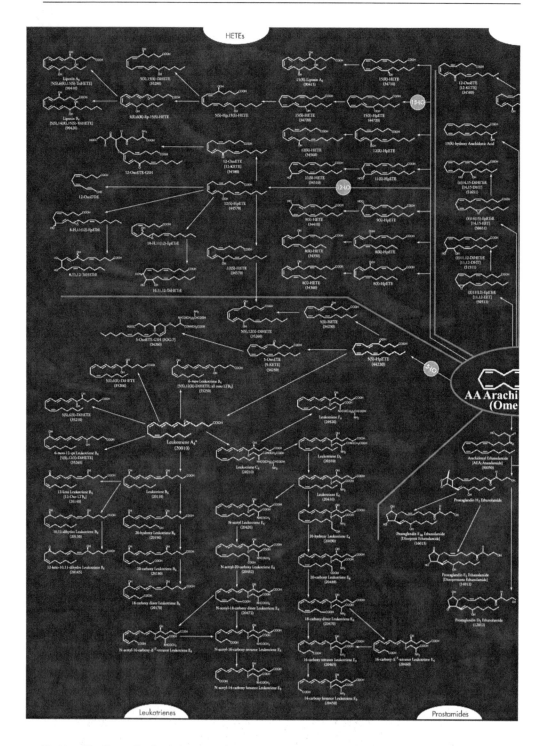

Fig. I.19   The Omega Six , Arachidonic Acid Chemical Cascade – An Influential Family.
Many Thanks to The Cayman Chemical Company for permission to use this wonderful chart.

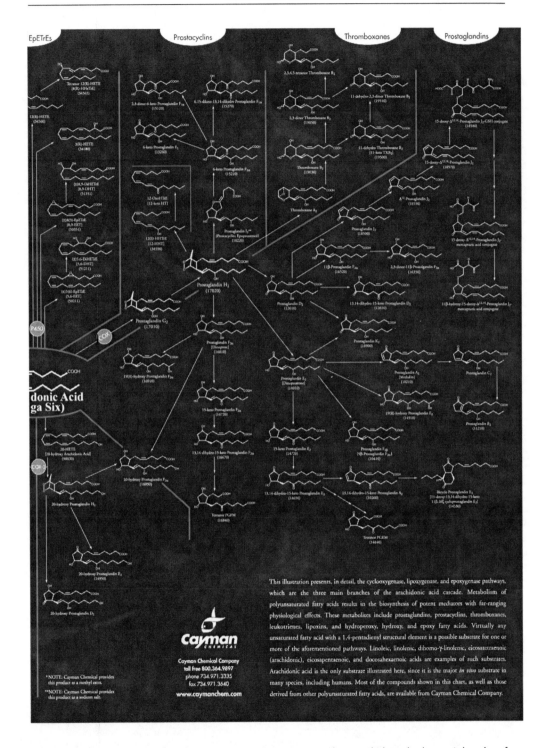

"This illustration presents, in detail, the cyclooxygenase, and epoxygenase pathways, which are the three main branches of the arachidonic cascade. Metabolism of polyunsaturated fatty acids results in the biosynthesis of potent mediators with far ranging physiological effects. These metabolites include prostaglandins, prostacyclins, thromboxanes, leukotrienes, lipoxins, and hydroperoxy, hydroxy, and epoxy fatty acids" [Caymanchem.com (For original full colour chart - see their web site)].

Newly discovered Omega Three family chemicals, the resolvins and protectins, are protective products. They shut down inflammatory reactions. Interestingly, aspirin helps the formation of these products, which are also produced naturally.

Even more fascinating and curious, aspirin is reported as enhancing the conversion of EPA to DHA and onward products.[v] This could suggest the mechanisms of aspirin are more complex than a simple COX blocker.

Resolvins and protectins, have dramatically reduced inflammatory pressures, including in liver function. [vi] They also mediate immune function.

DHA in trials was more effective than some COX blocking drugs.

Overall, balancing the Omega Threes and Omega Sixes, and ensuring a supply of the long chain Omega Threes, is an anti-inflammatory strategy through a variety of mechanisms.

1.21   **'Western' diseases of wealth**—Steep excess of Omega Six intake above natural levels, combined with a lack of Omega Three, is arguably responsible for much of the vast increase in our diseases of 'wealth! These conditions include obesity, decline in fertility, diabetes, depression, suicide, heart disease, osteoporosis, and macular degeneration. The list goes depressingly on. 'Western' diseases are diseases of affluence. There was historically a sharp divide between those who have disease of poverty, and diseases of affluence.

1.22   **Killing ourselves with excess of vegetable oil**—Omega Six in nature, is a scarce generally seasonal resource. It is only found in quantity in seeds and nuts. They have a limited seasonal time frame and are not easy to gather in quantity. There is competition. They need energy to find and gather.

Omega Six and sugars pre-packed in berries were the original super food. They were a truly scarce, treasured, essential nutritional requirement. We now imbibe Omega Six by the bottle.

We eat it in crisps, bread, bakery products, sauces, chips, biscuits, margarines, and the list goes on. We pass it through all sorts of chemical processes. We adulterate fat last to longer, or spread better.

We embrace with gusto—`polyunsaturated vegetable fat good, saturated fat bad'—an Orwellian consumer and food industry mantra—and we are gulping it down in quantity and it is killing us.

We truly and honestly believe based on what we read, that we are being healthy. The truth is, we are killing ourselves with kindness as we follow our genetic instruction code.

---

v   Scottish Crop Research (and Mylnefield Lipid Analysis) Invergowrie, Scotland. Resolvins and Protectins chemistry and biology. W W Christie.

vi   Novel Endogenous Lipid Compounds, Resolvins and Protectins, Protect Kidneys From Acute Renal Failure Brigham and Women's Hospital Harvard Medical School.

Excess Omega 6 and lack of 3 in our diets puts our very survival at risk. We need to be at our very best, most cooperative, and intelligent, to meet the global challenges of population resources and energy.

1.23   **Unknown recipe for conflict?**—Higher levels of aggression in men and women [4] have been associated with excessive levels of Omega Six.

This alone, and when combined with increasing consumption of alcohol [5] in some societies, might explain widespread changes in social behaviour in the young. Alcohol uses stores of DHA in the brain.

Low DHA has been linked with poorer brain function. Diet in mothers may link to aggression, depression, bipolar disorder, and increased risk of alcoholism in offspring. [6] [7] [8]

In situations of DHA deficit and excess Omega Six, DHA is replaced by the very second rate Omega Six substitute, DPA 22:5 n6. Symptoms of depression have been improved with EPA. [9]

Students supplemented with DHA exhibited lower stress and aggression during examinations. [10] Capuchin monkeys on a high Omega Six diet deteriorated so badly that by the age of two, they were showing self-mutilation behaviour.

A study of violent offenders in the prison system showed that fatty acid abnormalities were common. Blood measurements revealed very low DHA in violent antisocial men.

Resource conflict, global warming, religious and ethnic and economic divides, will demand the best from us if we are to survive. By putting high Omega Six on the menu, are we unconsciously and innocently setting the supper table for a more conflicted world? Kosher and Halal foods are both high in vegetable fats. [11] [12]

Omega Three and fish in contrast is long associated in many cultures with peace and wellbeing. (See section on Mistress of Fats-God's fat).

1.24   **Deficit of Omega Three**—The opposing yet symbiotic sibling of Omega Six is Omega Three. Long chain Omega Three, DHA, and EPA levels in humans in the West have dropped dramatically.

We have stopped eating oily fish. We have decreased the Omega Three content of the animals we farm. We have decreased the Omega Three content of the vegetables we grow.

We have increased the Omega Six levels of farmed animals dramatically. This includes, particularly, farmed fish.

Increased intake of the mother Omega Six linoleic acid, C18:2 n6, drastically reduces our innate ability to make long chain Omega Threes. Sugar, trans fats, high levels of alcohol, mineral deficiencies, age, and other dietary factors stop us from making DHA as well [11.13].

We eat less Omega Three mother fat. We eat less long chain fat EPA and DHA. We make less long chain Omega Three from the mother fat. In general, we are suffering from Omega Three deficit. Omega Three deficit is the other half of this human disaster in the making.

1.25   **Omega Three damps down inflammation**—Omega Three assists in long-term repair and maintenance of the body. It acts as a counter balance at the most fundamental and basic cellular levels [1.36], including controlling hormone levels [23.11.b].

It helps shut our system down at night, facilitating sleep and repair. The huge Omega Three chemical family is just as fundamental as Omega Six. It is in a constant power struggle with the Omega Six chemical family. It resists the inflammatory tendencies of Omega Six.

Too much 6 and lack of 3 and the body is out of balance, promoting ill-health, and lower brain function. It makes us lesser more aggressive human beings, who are less equipped to achieve their full potential.

1.26   **Eyes, brain, and reproductive organs** —The eyes, brain, and reproductive organs do not function properly without adequate long chain Omega Three, EPA and DHA.

It is a chemical and mechanical fact that these organs cannot function to full potential without adequate Omega Three. A lack of Omega Three means we are seeing less well, thinking less well, and breeding less well.

We are seeing increased cognitive dysfunction in statistics on depression, suicide, macular degeneration, Alzheimer's, and a host of brain conditions.

1.27   **Disaster for humanity** —A lack of long chain Omega Threes, combined with huge excesses of Omega Six, is a disaster for humanity. Unchanged, this dietary trend may prejudice our future survival.

Every year, global consumption of high 6 vegetable oils increases. Every year, 'western' disease is rising. It arguably puts the West at social and economic disadvantage to the East. We are exporting our 'western' ill-health to the world. Big rises are seen in China and India. Being more selfish acquisitive impulsive and less intelligent, will arguably not help the species survive in a resource pressured world.

With refined vegetable oils and western diet, the West is arguably spreading a more acquisitive, less intelligent, more impulsive, less cooperative human model. It is not a choice. The body is designed to act in response to Omega Six excess, and the consequential chemical products in defined ways. We have just broken the rules in the body operating manual, we have not yet written.

Through diet, we are altering the ethos, behaviour, and outlook of the world. Masculine traits are being exaggerated. More feminine attributes of cooperation, sharing, consideration and compliance are diminished.

WE ARE PUSHED TOWARDS THE SEVEN DEADLY SINS. EXCESS OMEGA 6 AND LACK OF OMEGA 3 IS A DEVIL'S BREW INDEED.

1.28   **Paedophilia**—Trials have linked high Omega 6 or low Omega 3 intakes to aggression, impulsivity, suicide, sleep disturbance, and crime including paedophilia.

1.29   **'Homosexualisation' in the womb**—Imbalance caused by the intervention of drugs in the Omega Six fats pathways, given whilst rat were infants in the womb has been linked with cross genderisation ('homosexualisation') of the brain, with the unequivocal reversal of gender behaviour to that of the opposite physical sex status. [See 24.29]

The drugs you take, could influence your child's gender outlook. This is serious stuff and warrants wider consideration. As usual, it acknowledged that more research is required.

1.30   **Alcohol** – Increasing alcohol consumption is the straw in parts of the West that may for some, break the camel's back. Alcohol has access to all cells in the body. The body system uses up DHA to deal with alcohol.

Alcohol processing depletes the body of DHA and Omega Threes. The largest repositories of DHA, the brain eyes and reproductive organs, will be the worst affected. Excessive alcohol blocks the conversion pathways.

Small to moderate amounts of alcohol will increase conversion rates, of the Omega Three and Omega Six mother fats, to the long chain fats. But if the body does not have the Omega Three raw materials, it cannot produce Omega Three long chain fats.

It is likely that low consumption of alcohol continues to increase long chain Omega 6 production in the absence of Omega Three. Theoretically, this would exacerbate the Omega Six excesses and consequent problems and issues.

In trials, animals consuming moderate to high amounts of alcohol (1.2 and 2.6g kg per day), that do not have an adequate supply of Omega 3s, develop liver conditions. Those who had an adequate supply of Omega 3s, despite equivalent medium to high alcohol consumption, did not develop liver disease.

Alcohol poses huge health risks in those who do not have an adequate intake of Omega Threes. This risk may extend even to low alcohol consumption where Omega Three supply is seriously inadequate.

1.31   **Sleep and fats** —The body's systems all interlink. Poor sleep is associated with 'western' conditions such as obesity, fertility and inflammation.

During good sleep, the body closes down the Omega Six inflammatory chemical manufacturing capacity. DHA is fundamental to the sleep close down process. Melatonin promotes DHA. Melatonin shuts down the Omega Six series two pathways, and not the series one pathway.

The body alert status is reduced. The body switches up long-term repair. The fat balance in the body is a fundamental part of this process. The Omega Six supply from the fat cells is turned down at night.

The Omega 6 COX2 pathway is switched down by DHA and melatonin, reducing the capacity to make inflammatory chemicals. A lack of Omega 3 means insufficient raw material for repair and moderation of inflammatory chemicals.

If you have excess Omega Six and low Omega Three, you are likely to suffer from poorer sleep quality. The body is simply unable to switch down the Omega Six processes that enable sleep.

Poorer sleep means the body does not shut down properly to repair. Lack of sleep, inflammatory conditions, fat intake, body fat stores, and brain chemicals all inextricably link. Improving the Omega 3:6 balance will assist with sleep.

The body stores high levels of Omega Six so changing the profiles of fats is a long-term process. But some results should be seen quite quickly.

Reis and Hibbeln quote Pen Tsao by Shen Nung "Father of Chinese Medicine" who said some 3000 years ago "The able doctor first attends to sleep and diet before resorting to drugs".

1.32   **Original elements**– I set out with a degree of trepidation theories as to the role of Omega 3 and 6 in, metabolic syndrome, puberty, the fertility cycle, sleep, and Omega 6 as an environmental controller with to links to fertility and behaviour. I have not seen these suggestions put together, viewed from the Omega 3–6 perspective, by anyone else. The bits of the jigsaw are the work of others. I have attempted to put parts of the jigsaw together.

I am sure others are likely to have considered such matters, but I have not seen them, if they exist in print.

1.33   **Mostly work of others** – I have tried to make this as understandable as possible, yet provide sufficient detail, with references for those who want to know more, or see the original trials I cite. The content brings together and draws on the work of others. The content is to the best of my limited comprehension and effort, firmly rooted in trials, and the extensive work and writings of others. The knowledge base is diffuse, but there is a great deal of it. This book would not have happened without the very excellent work of the specialists in lipids.

1.34   **No career to lose**–I can afford a few leaps of logic and faith, as I have no reputation, job, or career, in the world of lipids to lose. I do not claim to be right at every level. Much of this book is on the edges of 'new' science and knowledge is constantly updated. A glimpse through the fog would be enough.

I have skimmed vast areas of many lifetimes' work, in very many specialist areas. I do not begin to understand them all. I simply seek to sketch a wood in outline. It is for the real experts, to tell us about the trees and life in the wood.

1.35   **Much to be learnt**–Much is still to be learnt. I do not claim to have got it all right, but if only a portion is correct, the evidence for the potential health benefits of balancing the Omega 3s and 6s is still for me conclusive, urgent, and overwhelming. Thank you for taking the time to read this, and hopefully participating in the debate. I hope you feel more informed for having read it.

1.36   Late News-

☞ **Cholesterol in the cell membrane has an aversion for DHA and likes OA-**At a very simplistic level more DHA and less OA in the membrane may mean less accessible cholesterol. DHA makes disordered membrane areas outside lipid rafts, and encourages cholesterol and trans fats to gather in rafts. This may have significant implications for control of body 'chemical' activity through protein signalling by fats. [vii][viii]

☞ **Vegetarians had lower Omega 3 levels than omnivores-**A trial in Austria stated "To ensure physical, mental and neurological health vegetarians have to reduce the n-6/n-3 ratio with an additional intake of direct sources of EPA and DHA, regardless of age and gender". [ix]

☞ **DHA significantly improves Dsylexia-**Over 20 weeks following treatment with DHA and evening primrose 17 of 20 children improved reading speed by 60 per cent. "Significant improvements were observed in reading speed and motor-perceptual velocity. Thirteen of 17 children had a significant improvement on the word-chain test". [x]

☞ **Omega 3 reduces anger and anxiety in substance abusers-**A trial showed with strong correlation, EPA reduced anxiety, and DHA reduced aggression, "ensuring adequate n-3 PUFA intake via supplementation benefits substance abusers by reducing their anger and anxiety levels [xi]".

☞ **Formula fed babies have lower DHA in the brain-**Autopsies from bottle fed infants who died of non brain related conditions had 10 to 30 per cent lower DHA in the brain than breast fed infants. [xii]

---

vii Docosahexaenoic Acid Enhances Segregation of Lipids between Raft and Non-Raft Domains: 2H NMR Study. - Biophys J. 2008 Mar 13 - Soni SP, Locascio DS, Liu Y, Williams JA, Bittman R, Stillwell W, Wassall SR. PubMed 18339742.

viii Mechanisms by which docosahexaenoic acid and related fatty acids reduce colon cancer risk and inflammatory disorders of the intestine. - 2008 Mar 4 - Chapkin RS, Seo J, McMurray DN, Lupton JR. - Center for Environmental and Rural Health, United States; Faculty of Nutrition, Texas A&M University, USA.

ix Very Low n-3 Long-Chain Polyunsaturated Fatty Acid Status in Austrian Vegetarians and Vegans. - Ann Nutr Metab. 2008 Feb 28;52(1):37-47 - Kornsteiner M, Singer I, Elmadfa I. - Department of Nutritional Sciences, Faculty of Life Sciences, University of Vienna, Vienna, Austria.

x A 5-Month Open Study with Long-Chain Polyunsaturated Fatty Acids in Dyslexia - Lars Lindmark, Peter Clough. - Journal of Medicinal Food. - December 1, 2007, 10(4): 662-666. doi:10.1089/jmf.2006.399.

xi Associations between increases in plasma n-3 polyunsaturated fatty acids following supplementation and decreases in anger and anxiety in substance abusers - doi: 10.10 16/j.physletb.2003.10.071 - Laure Buydens-Branchey, Marc Branchey and Joseph R. Hibbeln Psychiatry Service, DVA New York Harbor Healthcare System, Brooklyn, NY, National Institute on Alcohol Abuse and Alcoholism, Bethesda, MD, USA

xii The influence of dietary docosahexaenoic acid and arachidonic acid on central nervous system polyunsaturated fatty acid composition. - Prostaglandins Leukot Essent Fatty Acids. 2007 Nov-Dec;77(5-6):247-50. Epub 2007 Nov 26 - Brenna JT, Diau GY. - Division of Nutritional Sciences, Cornell University, Ithaca, NY, USA.

2

DISEASE OF PROSPERITY

2.1   **Death rate steady at 100 per cent**—[Abbreviations listed at 1.1] As Campbell notes in *The China Study*, death and disease are certain. The aim is to stay as healthy as possible, as long as possible, to enjoy the time we have. There will always be a very welcome place for medical drugs.

But are there not enough medical conditions to cure, without increasing existing conditions such as vascular disease, and creating new conditions like ADHD, as early as childhood, through lack of dietary awareness?

It is widely accepted that a significant portion of western conditions are based in dietary habits. Are the drugs industry almost ignoring prevention options, in the quest for the market created by increasing levels of 'western' illnesses?

Is it just human nature, that western illnesses, are inevitably viewed as an economic market opportunity, and as a driver for research funds? Would we not be better looking for parallel ways to fund and encourage research, which do not rely solely on illness having an economic treatment value?

2.2   **Huge amount of research**—Over 15,000 articles and trials were found by a search on a medical database (NCBI) in June 2006 for fish oil, Omega Three, docosahexaenoic, eicosapentaenoic, etc. [13] It is a diffuse and complex subject. The number of trials indicates the depth of research into the subject. Most recommendations that promising trials be followed remain unfulfilled.

2.3   **'Western' conditions, a list**—*The China Study* labelled the following, as diseases of affluence; cancer (of the colon, lung, breast, leukaemia, stomach, liver, and brain), diabetes, and coronary heart disease. He also lists diseases of poverty. The book highlights a clear division between the diseases of poverty and prosperity. His staggering observations from China, include that between 1973 and 1975, not one among 246,000 men in Guizhou County died of coronary heart disease (CHD) before the age of 64. (There has been a huge increase in vegetable fats consumption in China in the last 30 years).

In England, CHD was reported on the Department of Health website as killing 110,000 every year. Breast cancer in the U.S. was reported as five times higher than in rural China. Excess Omega Six, lack of Omega Threes, fat imbalances, and blocking of conversion pathways, are 'western' traits, which are reflected to varying extents in 'western conditions'.

Many of these conditions cause great suffering to individuals, their families, and carers. The cost to nations in terms of medical care, and wider social and economic cost, must be truly staggering.

The diseases listed below have been shown as potentially benefiting from increased Omega Threes. Most are 'western' inflammatory conditions. A few are inherited, but have been included, as trials have shown response to Omega Three. Trials tend to concentrate on Omega Three rather than Omega Six, but the two are inextricably linked.

TABLE OF 'WESTERN' CONDITIONS WHICH HAVE BEEN REPORTED IN TRIALS TO SHOW SOME IMPROVEMENT WITH ADMINISTRATION OF OMEGA THREES / LINKS TO OMEGA THREES / SIXES (See Chapter 29)		
Acute renal failure Acne vulgaris ADHD Alzheimer's Arrhythmia Asthma Atopic eczema Atherosclerosis	Bone density Breast cancer	Cardiovascular Cognitive function Colon cancer Crohn's disease
Dementias Depression Diabetes Type 1 Diabetes Type 2 Dry eye Dyslexia	Eczema	Foetal development
Gliomas Hypertension	Inflammatory bowel disease Ischemia	Lupus
Macular degeneration Manic depression Melanoma Metabolic syndrome Migraine headaches Multiple sclerosis	Nephropathy IgA Neuropsychiatric Obesity Osteoporosis	Periodontal disease Pneumonia PCOS Postnatal depression Pre-eclampsia Pre-term birth Prostate cancer Psoriasis

Rheumatoid arthritis	Schizophrenia	Thrombosis
	Sepsis	Toxemia
	Systemic lupus erythematosus	Ulcerative colitis
	Sinusitis	
	Sjogren's syndrome	
	Suicide	Non-'western'
		Cystic fibrosis
		Macular dystrophy
		Sickle cell

2.4   **Drug development**–Drug development is a technological marvel. It is wondrous and a huge achievement. It must be continued. The development of drugs provides a window to the working of the body, and much needed 'here and now' relief for many conditions.

But, 'western' conditions are in large part due to factors in the way we live, and the response of the body to those factors. The starting point must be prevention. We are currently turning a blind eye to looking at cause, because ill people create a market for drugs.

Drugs create profits, jobs, employment, and research. Research is sexy. Discovery and achievement are thrilling, and in some cases have very positive impact. No researcher in a pharmaceutical company got promoted for saying, if we just changed this in people's diet we might not need this drug.

There is a mounting inability on cost resource grounds, to fulfil public expectation of access to all potential treatments. The socioeconomic cost, and the personal cost of 'western' disease is mind-boggling. At some not so distant point, we will be forced to look for cause and prevention as a primary step.

The foremost nations of the future will be those that recognise that prevention is the starting point. Those nations will have healthier, happier, more intelligent, and more cost-effective populations.

If we have a problem with the fuel for our car, we get the fuel problem fixed. We do not add all sorts of "make do and mend" bolt-ons on the engine. We do not try and overcome an operating condition that an engine was never designed for. That is what we are doing by ignoring prevention.

Autoimmune and inflammatory conditions are like a river in flood. Block it or divert it, and it will at some point, in a single flood or trickles, emerge somewhere else. To stop the flooding, you have to find the causes like removing water-absorbing landscape, and so it is with the body.

Treatment of immensely complex interlinked and sophisticated pathways underlying 'western' conditions, will never be a substitute for the determination and removal of the cause, so far as that is possible. Even after the best prevention, there will be a lot left to treat and improve. Medicine will not be redundant. It will just have to redirect some resources and skills.

2.5   **General diet**—Fat intake, the subject of this book cannot be divorced or taken out of the context of the principles of good diet. Sections are included on general dietary principles [See chapter 13].

Fats are arguably the most influential of foods, about which we are almost totally ignorant. They were a scarce commodity. They are now everywhere. Excess consumption of fats threatens our very survival.

We are programmed to lust after them and store them, and particularly Omega Six and fructose. Omega Six in the natural world is the most precious. It comes pre-packed with sugar in fruits and berries.

The lust for Omega Six and fructose does not have an 'off' switch. In the past, there was never a need to invent one. But now our admirable farming skills honed over generations, have, by divorcing us from nature, opened up Pandora's Box. The consequences of unbridled excess of Omega Six, which was a very scarce resource in the natural world, and to a lesser extent sugar, are mind-bending.

2.6   **A truth that puts smoking in the shade**—This book is about pragmatism and not perfection. Balance your Omega Threes and Sixes, ensure adequate long chain Omega Threes, and try not to block the fat conversion pathways. That's it in a nutshell. The easiest health and weight diet recommendation ever.

Excess Omega Six is arguably a killer. Enough is essential. Excess Omega Six is arguably worse than cigarettes for the reasons given in this book. You do not encourage your children to smoke '40 a day'. But you do feed yourselves (mothers) and children lots of something much worse, excess Omega Six. Many vegetable oils are the main source. This book takes the perspective, that most people have excess Omega Six intake.

Omega 6 is key to health, a balance not absence, is the target.

As a general rule, avoid all high Omega Six vegetable oils. Check the content of vegetable oils (see chart p.291). *Nutritiondata.com* is a useful resource, which lists fat content of foods and other food data. Flax, and perilla are useful high Omega 3 sources [30.31]. Virgin olive oil is low in Omega Six and high in Omega Nines, and has other benefits as well but is low in Omega Three [P. 287].

Some suggest that poor processing and extraction of oils, adds to the problem, by introducing toxic isomers into heavily processed oils. So, cold pressed where possible, is prudent. Oily fish, is desirable. A little coconut (milk or cream) and butter, as sources of short chain saturate fats may assist in weight loss. [See 11.31]. Get some long chain Omega 3s through oily fish, fish oil or vegetarian equivalents. Watch your nut and seed intake, as they are generally high in Omega 6—not more than maybe a palmful a day.

Get lots of greens, coloured fruit and vegetables, beans, etc. As wide a variety as possible is good. Avoid processed ingredients, refined flour, sugar, etc. Become an avid label reader, if you use any pre-prepared foods, and most of us do.

Avoid trans fats. Many commercial food products claiming dietary benefit are double-edged. The beneficial elements, are partnered with undesirables like sugar, salt, and vegetable oils.

I am pragmatic. We lead busy lives. Not everybody in the world has a garden. The work patterns and economics of families have changed. If we shift our buying patterns, and sue once or twice, manufacturers will alter prepared food content. Let us try by consumer choice to put pressure on manufacturers to make processed food healthier.

If your digestion is better, you will eat and need less food. If you eat less, there is more in the budget for more expensive, less intensively farmed food. The basics are set out in the Key Wider Dietary Rules and the Dietary Basics below.

2.7   **Work of others**–This book is based on literature, articles, and trials of others. I have just tried to explain how it is possible, that such humble common Omega 3 and 6 fats, could be of such enormous consequence.

My theories on Omega Six being nature's fundamental control element in the hormone cycles, our breeding, fertility, and survival tactics in famine, are largely a leap in the dark. I have not seen this theory proposed elsewhere, which is not to say it has not been proposed elsewhere. I just haven't seen it.

The suggestions as to Omega Three and Omega Six having a large part in sleep, puberty, metabolic x, basal metabolic rate, and the fertility cycle are also leaps into the unknown. I have not seen these gathered by anybody else.

I have read and Googled widely, gathered, ordered and extrapolated, for a wider audience. The Internet, Google, and particularly NCBI, have made this book possible.

The operation and interaction of lipids (fats) in the human body is many lifetimes' work for an army or researchers. It is totally beyond one person, let alone a part-time amateur, to understand how all of it works. But we drive cars successfully without taking an exam first, as to the exact science behind how it all works. I claim to see the hazy but unmistakable outline of the woods, and try to bring that image to you.

2.8   **Little motivation for preventive research**– Often, there is a recommendation, that a preventive diet-based finding in a trial, should be followed up. I have seen little evidence that promising areas are generally followed up by the necessary trials. This is presumably due to lack of governmental funding, and central organisation on an international level.

It is self-evident and understandable, that profit driven corporations, are highly unlikely to engage in unprofitable work, that might adversely impact on existing and future markets, by making people better.

How it feels to be screaming to yourself in a research lab, when you have made a non-commercial, fundamental dietary discovery, that would lead to a guaranteed dismissal and no re-employment prospects, I can only imagine.

2.9 Cause and effect—Is it not time to be pragmatic, and take the simple course? Just look at cause and effect. Correct the dietary imbalance, and monitor the outcome on 'western' conditions in patients, and worry about why later. The science behind fats and their utilisation is, despite popular impressions, only crudely understood at best.

One trial said, "Our current maps of these molecular events remain crude given the reductionist approaches required to study such complex events.[14]" Despite amazing advances in the understanding of the subject, a great deal is not yet understood or known. The subject is immensely subtle, interlinked, and complex. Every door opens out to a new door.

Absolute answers will take a very long time. We cannot afford to wait that long. Governments, in the absence of other sources, will have to invest heavily in some basic, long-term, preventive research. There are those that argue that government funding is not the best model. But who else will provide for research that does not lead to bottom-line profits for themselves?

There is a bottom-line saving for healthy nations at many levels, so arguably it is a matter for government consideration. Fats arguably have more of an effect on our lives, than almost any issue that a Government acts in.

This is a matter of consequence to nations. Increased levels of illness, reduction of cognitive skills, and higher aggression, in the population, is a fundamental worry for a nation.

2.10 Technical, convincing the health professionals—If I cannot convince you, and your doctor, that this book raises serious issues, it is a huge lost opportunity. It is not the fault of the doctors. They have huge workloads.

Dietary training for doctors is reported as limited. The ones I have spoken to, reported that nutritional training conventionally takes up less than a week, even just a couple of days. The emphasis of the medical industry is simply not on dietary prevention.

2.11 Format of the book—The book tries to be both readable and offer enough authoritative material to be of interest to professionals in the field. References are given in summary only. The list of references with web links will hopefully be available for download on the web at *www.omegasixthedevilsfat. com* or possibly available for order on CD in the future.

2.12 Counter arguments—The counter argument is "not proven", or trials are inconclusive. Much is unknown. Perspectives change continuously as new discoveries are made. It is hard to prove the effect of a single food agent on humans. The body is highly sensitive to small amounts of fats. Many fats are hidden.

Trials rarely take into account Omega Six intake, and even more rarely stored fat. High levels of Omega Six intake distort the body's fat conversion abilities. 'What did you eat' trials are of limited use. Body fat takes several years to fully reflect dietary change.

Government bodies are often perceived as being made up of industry representatives, be it food or alcohol. Therefore, given human nature, it is not surprising if the perspective of industry dominates. Some foods undoubtedly have particular properties, but so do a lot that are not represented by growers groups.

Low dosages of Omega Three are often of little use as the body stores of Omega Six dwarf them. Tiny amounts of Omega Three versus huge amounts of Omega Six, is a little like being tied up with a peashooter, and set against a tank.

'Hidden fats' in processed foods represent a huge challenge to quantify. Intake of Omega Three and Omega Six in diet is difficult to measure as it occurs in nuts, greens and seeds, processed foods etc.

It is going to take considerable long-term funding and determination to get absolute answers, but with a will it is possible. In the meantime, for me the 'writing on the wall' is bold and underlined.

BALANCE THE OMEGA THREES AND SIXES

2.13   **Comparative health care costs**–A 2005 trial from the Kansas University of Missouri on bipolar disorder included the following quote: "The United States (US) accounts for more than 51 per cent of the 430.3 billion dollar expended on pharmaceutical products worldwide each year". [15] The health care costs per capita in Japan are reported as being half those in the US.

3
THE ELEPHANT IN THE ROOM—STARK TRUTHS

3.1   **Not another book on diet**—[Abbreviations listed at 1.1] Not another book on diet, you cry. Miracle food—Eat this, don't eat that! 'What am I meant to eat this week' syndrome? It's good for you. It's bad for you. You don't know what to believe. You have a friend who was super fit, and diet conscious, who got cancer, heart disease, etc.

You are cynical about diet benefits. Why should you read this book? Because the Omega 3 and Omega 6 fats are central to life, and were in the game at kickoff. Because they are fundamental to the way the body works at many levels. Because there is a massive amount of evidence that you have not been told about.

It is the unheard story. It is 'painless' and easily and realistically achievable. Balancing the Omega Threes and Omega Sixes provides us with an ability to:

☞ Change and improve national health.
☞ Reduce the risk and incidence of 'western' conditions.
☞ Reduce our increasing trend towards aggression.
☞ Increase our national intellect.
☞ Reduce the cost burden on health services.
☞ Save heartache and pain for individuals and carers.
☞ Lead more fulfilled lives.

3.2   **Myth; Fat is bad**—Fat is *not* bad. It is a question of <u>what</u> fat, in *what balance* and *how much*.

3.3   **The Devil's Brew and the seven deadly sins**—Aggression, impulsiveness, self-interest, less cooperative behaviour, less intelligence, and more illness, are all factors that can be attributed at some level to Omega Six.

If the Devil, (real, or life essential construct, I leave to you) had to design a simple method, of unobtrusively and effectively manipulating our behaviour, to promote the seven sins and voluntary self-destruction, he or she could not have done a much better job.

3.4   Omega Six and whole body inflammation–Omega Six instructs the body to store fat. Excess Omega Six promotes low-level whole-body inflammation, and control hormones, steroids, and is an agent and copartner of immune function, and is key to cell membrane structure and function.

Here we look at inflammation. Inflammation as a process is key to body protection, tissue destruction, and rebuilding, including the creation of life. [16] Low-level whole-body inflammation, sets the body on permanent intruder alert. The body becomes permanently on edge and susceptible to allergies, inflammatory conditions, autoimmune disorders, and a host of 'western' conditions.

Obesity equates to subclinical inflammation of adipose tissue and chronic activation of the innate immune system. [17] [18] This is fundamental. Omega Six is the key ingredient of inflammatory chemicals. Omega Six promotes obesity.

Fatty tissue is the Omega Six store. The fatty tissue, and supporting matrix, is a significant source production unit of inflammatory chemicals made from Omega Six. Omega Six is conveniently stored to hand. Stress aggravates inflammation through the same pathways. [19]

Omega Three moderates the process. Many diets today, lack adequate Omega Three. Excess Omega Six, and lack of Omega Three, destroys a fundamental and long-standing balance between inflammatory Omega Six AA and moderating Omega Three EPA. The Omega Three-Six EPA : AA balance is a critical operating parameter. The consequence of the imbalance is a disaster for human health and happiness.

3.5   Omega Three inflammation and repair–Omega Three moderates inflammation and promotes repair. The Omega Three chemicals are far less aggressive than those of the Omega Six family. Omega Three ties in with melatonin, and the sleep and repair pathways.

Omega Three is in constant flux and cycle with Omega Six, controlling many aspects of the body's functions, through a variety of mechanisms. More Omega 3 cuts down production of Omega 6 chemicals, by filling a bigger share of the cell membrane, and competing for the enzymes to make the chemicals.

The Omega Three family produces protective chemicals, called resolvins, and protectins, which help shut down and moderate inflammatory reactions. Omega 3s reduce the inflammatory aspects of the immune response.[i] A lack of long chain Omega 3 is half the problem, the other half is excess Omega 6.

---

i   Immunomodulation by omega-3 fatty acids. Calder PC. : Prostaglandins Leukot Essent Fatty Acids. 2007 Nov 19 Institute of Human Nutrition and School of Medicine, University of Southampton, Tremona Road, Southampton SO16 6YD, UK.

3.6   **In the beginning**–In the beginning there were fats. Fats are petrol in tanks. Fats are stored energy. Without energy storage, the most basic life is not possible. No storage means constant energy acquisition. Constant eating is required to survive. Even sunlight is a cyclical energy source.

Fats are ubiquitous in all living things, including bacteria, algae, garden flowers, trees, spiders and bedbugs. Bacteria, algae, trees, and bedbugs can manage without ginseng, grape seed, green tea, and vitamin tablets. They all do contain and depend on essential fatty acids the EFAs Omega 3 and 6.

Fats cannot be compared to individual supplements. This is not soy, grape seed or green tea. Soy, grape and tea arrived very many evolutionary generations after fats. We rely on and are made of fats. Eat a blade of grass, a carrot, a piece

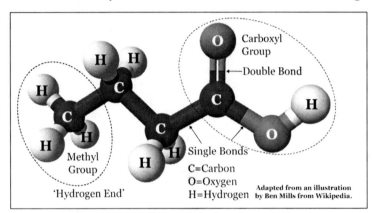

Fig. 3.6 Butyric Acid makes about 4% of the butter. When released it has a rancid smell.

Carboxyl Group
←—Double Bond
Methyl Group
Single Bonds
'Hydrogen End'
C=Carbon
O=Oxygen
H=Hydrogen
Adapted from an illustration by Ben Mills from Wikipedia.

of broccoli, an apple, a caterpillar, and you are ingesting fats. Fats are a key building blocks of cell membranes.

Fats play crucial and multiple roles in the body's most fundamental processes. Without Omega Three and Omega Six, your body cannot function. No fats = no energy, no immune system, no babies, no vision, no brain.

The list of fats is a huge. This is butyric acid (see diagram), which makes about four per cent of butter. It has four carbons that make the chain, with some hydrogen and two oxygen, attached to the sticky-out bits (the bonds). Omega Three and Omega Six are just longer chains, and have some double bonds.

Fats almost certainly were present by design or evolution from the beginning. Some suggest that fats rank with carbon and oxygen, in fundamental importance to the creation of life. [20] Omega 3 and Omega 6 are fundamental to us.

Male and female fertility are linked to Omega 3 and 6. Time of puberty is linked to Omega 6. The whole female reproductive cycle, is linked to the availability of the long chain Omega 3s, DHA and EPA, and Omega Six, AA.

Excess Omega Six with a lack of Omega Three is making our children, and us more depressed, aggressive, and stupid. Excess Omega Six contributes to the autoimmune conditions, atopic illness, asthma, diabetes, infertility, osteoporosis, and the huge long list above [2.3], in one way or another.

3.7   **Doh! It's your brain**—Omega 3s, and particularly DHA and EPA, are not stored in a significant amount in our body fat "adipose" reserves. [21][22] Omega Threes need to be replenished on a constant basis. This has huge consequences for body metabolism and function.

DHA is only held in quantity in some body parts, as part of the structure. The body is reluctant to give up substances that are part of the body's structure, the cell membranes, and essential to health and cell function. But in an emergency, the body raids the eyes, brains, and reproductive organs, which need and use high levels of DHA in the their cell membrane structure to function.

Babies, in pregnant women with a DHA deficit, rob their mother's brains. Women's brains can and do shrink in pregnancy. This is an explanation for postnatal depression. [23.35] Worse news, alcohol robs our DHA stores.

Alcohol has an all areas pass, which includes the brain cells. The body deals with alcohol by oxidising it. DHA is the best available oxidant in the brain. Alcohol likely causes DHA reduction when not replaced, due to inadequate resupply of the mother Omega 3, or conversion blockages to the long chain fats.

Lack of regular intake/manufacture of DHA is a problem for all, and particularly pregnant women. In the absence of adequate Omega Three, alcohol is a triple whammy, as it removes DHA, alters conversion pathways, and will eventually damage the fat factory—the liver.

Low to moderate level alcohol consumption, _where Omega Three intake is sufficient,_ may be an exception [1.30][3.28]. (Excluding pregnancy etc.). So it is important to ensure regular supply of the Omega Threes.

3.8   **Yo-yo diets**—Omega Threes are used for fuel (oxidised) in the body, in preference to the Omega Six of equivalent chain length. In a society that is constantly going on diets, the risk of a lack of Omega Three increases.

There is limited suggestion that yo-yo dieting, is linked to conditions related to deficiency of Omega Three. Yo-yo diets are a cycle of eating far more Omega Six than Omega Three, storing more new Omega Six and not much Omega Three, compounded by the lack of Omega Three in the diet, and then burning off what little Omega Threes you have [23], leading to increasing deficits.

Omega Three deficits could be increased in diets that rely on ketosis, as what little Omega Three there is, may be burnt in preference to Omega Six. Omega Three-deficient 'low fat' weight loss diets, likely present significant long term potential health risks.

Most Omega Three is used, as against stored by the body. "Complete oxidation of dietary 18:3n-3 [Mother Omega 3] to CO_2 accounts for about 25% of 18:3n-3 in the first 24 h, reaching 60% by 7 days." Most of the rest is turned into other fats. Very little is stored as mother Omega 3.[25] Omega Three is oxidised in preference to Omega Six. The moral of which is to review Omega Three intake on a regular basis, particularly when you are on a diet. [See Chapter 25]

3.9 Skin needs mother Omega 3–Skin has a high demand for 18:3n-3, the mother Omega Three Lino<u>lenic</u> Acid ALA. The body uses fats for fuels and the raw material for chemical defences.

The skin is a defence barrier. The skin requires constant renewal. The mother Omega 3, ALA, in the diet protects the skin against UVB radiation.

ALA protects against damage (sun burn), by reducing PGE2 and other Omega 6 inflammatory products. [24] Fats are a structural element in the skin.

3.10 Low fat diets deficit–People who have a low fat diet are equally, if not more, at risk of fat imbalances. It is essentially a question of balance. You may use 'healthy' oils but if you have no Omega Three sources, and excess Omega Six, you have a problem.

For instance, virgin olive oil has quite a poor Three-Six balance (about 1:10) In virgin olive oil about 10 per cent is Omega Six, BUT in 'processed' olive oil this may go up to 50 per cent. Processing carries a risk of removing or hydrogenating the Omega 3 content so further reducing the Omega 3 levels.

Significant chemical processing also will remove protective natural antioxidants. Udo Erasmus examines the processing of oils in *Fats That Heal, Fats that Kill*. In the absence of other fat sources, olive oil would result in accumulation of Omega Six, and low Omega Three.

If you do not eat Omega Three, you do not have it in your system. Safflower has no Omega Three, grape seed almost none, [See p.287].

One can envisage a situation where the 'healthy' oils chosen provided virtually no Omega Three. The small amount consumed would be at risk of prior oxidation, inhibited conversion, and factors such as alcohol washout. So, pay particular attention to balancing your Omega 3s, and Omega 6s, if you are on a low fat diet.

It is important to look at the Omega Three-Six content, of the oils you are consuming. *Check labels of all processed foods, for included vegetable oils. Omega Six gets everywhere.*

Industrial chicken can contain more Omega Six than you would think. Animals like us are what they eat. A high Omega 6 feed will produce a high Omega 6 chicken.

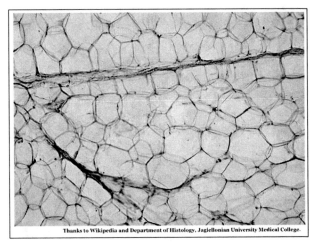

Thanks to Wikipedia and Department of Histology, Jagiellonian University Medical College.

Fig. 3.10 Yellow adipose tissue in paraffin section – Lipids washed out – You can see the cells which look like bubbles, and the connecting blood vessels.

The balance in your cell membranes, will reflect the balance of Omega Three and Omega Six you eat, in your low fat diet. Unknowingly, you could have a worse balance than somebody who is much less careful about his or her diet. A diet based round industrial chicken, salad, and olive oil would leave you with an Omega Three : Six imbalance.

3.11   **Omega Six storage and obesity**—Fat is stored in little bubbles—adipocytes—which expand and contract as needed. There are blood vessels, and nerves, in the supporting fat cell tissue matrix.

Omega 6 encourages bigger fat cells, and new ones to come on stream. Omega 3 encourages smaller fat cells. Omega 6 activates an automatic store instruction.

Historically concentrated Omega Six came in the seeds, and nuts and pips of fruit. The flesh of fruits, and berries, contains fruit sugars including fructose. Fructose is used to make the chemical fat storage racks for Omega Six.

So it's a double whammy; store the Omega Six, and the sugar that comes with it. Why is Omega Six and fruit sugar a problem? Because Omega Six was a scarce resource for the last 200,000+ years.

Is there a stop storage mechanism—Fat Park full? NO. That is the problem. Eat high levels of Omega Six and fructose, and you are priming the body processes to put on weight. I emphasise, I am not suggesting that consumption of whole fruit is not a good idea.

The problem primarily is with extracted fructose sweeteners, and concentrated fruit sugars, in drinks and processed foods. Some fruits now have much higher sugar levels, so look at fruit sugar content, avoid excessive dried fruit and high consumption of sweet fruit juices. Fructose sweeteners are found in baby foods.

3.12   **Subcutaneous and visceral**— Subcutaneous fat is found under the skin. Visceral fat is found around the essential organs, the heart, kidneys, and liver.

Internal fat is unseen and can be a big problem. Fat insulates and cushions. Problems with internal fats will not necessarily show as external fat, but may be evident through conditions such as fatty liver. You can be thin, and have a fat liver. Omega Sixes are stored in fat.

Human fat tissue contains about 87 per cent lipids. [26] Omega Sixes form 5–25 per cent of fats stored, depending on dietary intake. [27]

Omega Threes are only stored in body fat in small quantities, 0.02–2 per cent no matter how much is eaten.

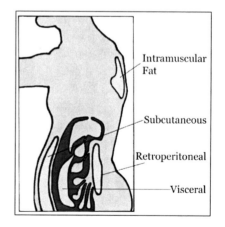

Fig. 3.12 Fat Storage Types

3.13 **Triglycerides**—Fats are stored in chemicals called triglycerides. A triglyceride is a backbone with three fats attached. Imagine a toast rack for three bits of toast. The fats are the toast. Glycerol is the rack. The three fats in each toast rack (a triglyceride) can all be the same, or all different.

It is the mix of Omegas, mono, and saturated fats, [toast type], which give complex fats [toast and rack together] their particular properties, and melting points.

The fats stored are most commonly 16, 18, and 20 carbons long. These triglycerides are stored in little balloons, which are fat cells. The fat cells connect into the body's other systems. Triglycerides are not used in the cell membranes.

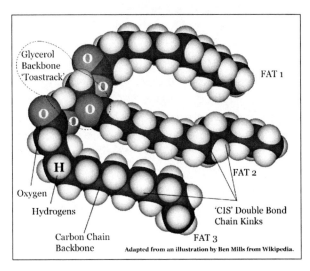

Fig. 3.13 A Triglyceride

3.14 **Cell membranes**—Cell membranes, are the skin to the bubble, that contains the mini factories found in a cell. A membrane is like two tiny concentric soap bubbles, one just inside the other. The main raw material is fats. Fats have a water loving and water hating end. [28]

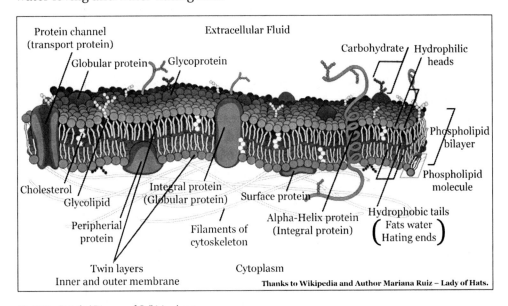

Fig. 3.14 Detailed Diagram of Cell Membrane

The water loving ends are found on the outside of the membrane, and the water hating bits on the inside. It is a natural process. The water hating ends hang out together, and so do the water lovers. It is the same principle as a drop of fat in water, an oil film, or soap bubble.

The membrane is selectively permeable–magic windows let things in and out. Fats are held in pairs including phospholipids, and glycolipids. *(Triglycerides fats held in threes, are used for storage and transport, and not structure)*. Cholesterol, and steroids also form part of the cell membrane.

Cholesterol is used to make hormones and steroids. The fat content of the cell membrane effects function [1.36]. The fact that different raw materials are used for storage and construction of the membranes, means that the body has more flexibility to decide how to make the membranes from the materials available [28].

The materials used by the body are self-evidently restricted to what you have put in it, or it can make from what you put in it. Far more Omega Six is stored than Omega Three.

Fat imbalance will influence membrane compositions. Fats are taken from the membrane to make the 20 carbon long [eicosanoid] Omega 3 and 6 chemicals [Fig 1.19]. This include fat store cell membrane walls.

➢   **Glycolipids**–Glycolipids are fats attached to carbohydrates. They are a large and complex family. Glycolipids in adipose cell membranes, must logically reflect the fat content of the cells. What the impact of glycolipids containing higher proportions of Omega Six is, on subsequent products, I have no idea. It would be reasonable to assume that an imbalance in structure or type, outside operating parameters, will have some sort of unexpected impact. I do not pretend to even begin to understand the implications, but given that glycolipids include antigens, it looks like pretty fundamental territory we are messing with, through of our 'western' eating habits. Look up glycolipids on Google. It is complex! I opened the door, saw it was a massive topic, and closed it. [29]

➢   **Cardiolipin**–The mitochondria have their own cell membranes. The inner membrane includes high levels, 20 per cent and more, of a chemical with four fats in the toast rack. It is fat called cardiolipin. Cardiolipin has an important role, and is very sensitive to diet. The cardiolipin toast rack has high levels of DHA. DHA is crucial to mitochondrial oxidation, and cellular quality control. Good mitochondrial function is key to the healthy operations of the body, and a subject this book returns to often. Mitochondria are highly sophisticated chemical factories, and power plants. [See 21.7].

3.15   **Metabolism**–Fats turn your genes on and off. The genetic disposition to store fat will vary. But a much bigger influence, is what you eat, and how much.

Omega Six encourages storage, and switches down the metabolism. Omega Three discourages storage, and switches up the metabolism.

So, more Omega 3 and less 6 will push the body away from fat storage.

3.16   **Food instructs genes**–Excess Omega Six is arguably the key factor in the increase in a huge range of 'western' diseases. Omega Three and Omega Six alter the way you turn your genes on and off. A complete set of genes is held in each cell.

Like light bulbs, they only respond if they are switched on. Copies of genes that are switched on are 'expressed'. The number of genes that are switched on, alters cell function. The fat content of the cell membranes alters the way your body functions [1.36]. So, the balance of fats in the diet determines body function, and you can alter your gene expression profile through the fats in your diet.

You have a certain amount of choice to turn genes on or off through diet. You are in charge of the food gene switches. DNA micro array studies show clearly that Omega Threes, usually provided as fish oil, alter the expression of a number of genes with a wide range of functions, such as "DNA binding, transcriptional regulation, transport, cell adhesion, cell proliferation, and membrane localization which may significantly modify cell function and development". [30]

Food is a hotline to your instruct genes. You may have been given your genes, but you have a say in the way they work, through what you eat, and put on your skin.

3.17   **Fundamental, deep reaching, pervasive, influential**–Fats, despite appearance after frying, are fundamental, deep reaching, pervasive, influential substances. Cells all over the body, including the brain, can make most fats.

The main fat factory is the liver. Fats are delivered by various mechanisms including the lymphatic system. Even your skin is part fat, which is why it is sort of waterproof. Plankton, plants, possums, petunia, pines, pets, all living things need fats to function and reproduce.

For example the body uses these 20 long carbon chain fats as the exclusive raw material to make families of influential chemicals the eicosanoids [Fig 1.19]. There are several families. Some are very powerful, and connect to Western illness. [e.g. Leukotrienes LTC4 LTD 4 and LTE4, connected to inflammatory reaction and asthma, are reported as a thousand times more powerful than histamine. [31]]

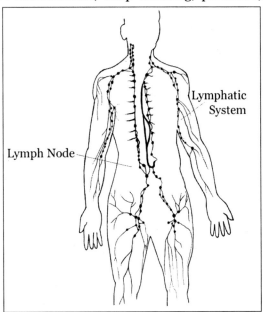

Fig. 3.17   A Simplistic Diagram of the Lymph System which Transports the Long chain fats from the Digestive System to the Blood Stream

The Omega Six chemicals are used in body repair, including wound and burn healing, [32] and immune system. They are involved with the control of hormones, and steroids. Omega 6 chemicals help modulate sleep. All that is for starters. Science is making big advances, but is a long way from understanding the full mechanisms. Fats are used in the body as:

☞ Key structural elements of all cell membranes, magic bricks.

☞ Hormones.

☞ Regulators of gene expression.

☞ Fuel for energy.

☞ A mechanism for energy storage.

☞ Lubricants to cells, joints and eyes.

☞ Regulators of cell division.

☞ Raw materials for many chemicals.

☞ Chemicals in the immune system.

☞ Controllers of the reproductive cycles.

☞ Enablers of sleep and sleep regulation.

☞ Fundamental structural elements of the brain.

☞ Reactive chemicals that enable you to see.

☞ Regulators of energy use and storage.

☞ Chemicals to induce delivery of babies. [33]

☞ Chemical messengers.

☞ Essential skin components.

☞ Controllers of inflammatory conditions.

☞ Baby food.

3.18   **Omega Six sensitises the body**–I believe that excess Omega Six, and lack of Omega Three, is likely to be the biggest factor, in explaining increasing 'western' inflammatory related conditions.

Excess Omega Six puts the body on permanent inflammatory, and immune alert. Like any system on permanent alert, this is likely to stress the system, and cause an overreaction. Obesity is an inflammatory condition.

The increased sensitivity to inflammatory agents, caused by excess Omega Six, is likely to reduce the ability of the body to cope with other environmental stresses. This may make us more open to allergens.

This would explain increasing pollen and nut allergies, reactivity to foods including dairy products, and susceptibility to agents that utilise the inflammatory pathways. It would explain increasing asthma, and might contribute to setting the body up for the occurrence of autoimmune conditions, such as diabetes 1. [Diabetes 1 may be triggered by external agents like milk.]

Other countries (Japan), with similar environmental stress, but a better Omega 3:6 balance, have a lower levels of 'western' conditions than the West.

Excess Omega Six primes the inflammatory and immune systems, impacts negatively on melatonin and sleep, disturbs hormone and steroid cycles, and reduces male and female fertility.

3.19 **Other factors**–There are of course many other environmental factors. Chemicals and minerals are having new and unforeseen impacts on our body function. For instance, the body sees cadmium, common in batteries, as a type of oestrogen. It was once very rare. Now cadmium, through a variety of mechanisms like fertilisers, batteries, cigarette papers, etc., is getting in greater quantity into the food chain and us. Weed killers, pesticides, heavy metals, dioxins, artificial hormones, and drugs, are all reaching the environment. We are increasingly using cosmetic products, which are directly absorbed.

3.20 **Health warning; Death and disease in a bottle**–Bottles of high Omega Six content seed, nut, and vegetable oils should arguably carry a 'health warning' like cigarettes. For instance;

EXCESS OMEGA SIX LINOLEIC ACID, MAY SERIOUSLY DAMAGE YOUR HEALTH, and could contribute to a wide range of long-term debilitating diseases, some of which are terminal. It may reduce your fertility and your child's intelligence. This bottle contains grams of Omega Six–and Omega Three–per teaspoon.

Amounts of Omega Sixes and Threes should also be listed where added to food. Even better, high Omega Six polyunsaturates should be excluded from processed foods, and people allowed to include them at serving if required.

It may even be justifiable to supplement foods with Omega Threes. Almost everybody in every age group is exposed. The negative outcomes are far more widespread and fundamental than smoking. Fifty years or so, was the time it took for recognition that smoking is a serious health risk.

Viewed in human terms, and the misery inflicted by of many of these conditions, declining national health, increasing aggression, and declining intelligence, this cannot wait another 30 years. Again this is more serious than smoking, the arguably higher risk of western conditions due to excess Omega 6 is an issue from the womb to the grave for everybody, not just a few for a while.

3.21 **Politics and economics; Drugs industry**–The short-term corporate benefits, for drugs companies in improving the fat intake profile of a nation, are minimal. Huge parts of existing and forecast markets for current treatments might decline considerably over a generation.

Many of the common drugs for 'western' conditions target the Omega Six downstream pathways, directly, or indirectly. A drug that successfully blocks a pathway will not magically redress the Omega Three-Six imbalance. These pathways are so fundamental, that the chance of long-term negative effects from drugs intervention, is high.

What research employee is going to say to his boss, this dietary change could significantly improve health in this area, but remove a significant part of our market, and our jobs?

The only other sources of funds are charities and government. If they do not fund prevention research, who will? Government committees have been reported in the media as often being populated by industry representatives. I do not question integrity or motivation, but viewpoint cannot but be coloured by specialisation, the vastness of the field of research, and limited hours in the day.

3.22 **Politics and economics; Farming industry**–Many food sources high in Omega Six are staple crops for the agricultural industry. A significant change in dietary habit will affect farmers. Current crops include sunflower, palm oil, and soy.

There are alternatives. Biofuel from oilseed is becoming competitive, if controversial, due to the impact on world food supplies and prices. High Omega Three seed oil crops like flax and perilla could be grown in greater quantity. Reservations as yet undetermined, exist for Canola and Hemp [26.5].

The improved living standards, and changing eating habits, of Eastern and some African countries, will give rise to new food markets, and greater demand for high Omega Three crops.

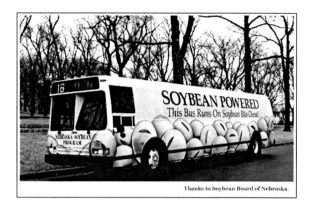

Fig. 3.22 Soybean Powered Bus that runs on Soybean Biodiesel

If a capital changeover subsidy is required, it will be well spent, and probably a small amount in comparison of the health costs of doing nothing.

3.23 **Research funding and direction**–Is it time for a look at how research is funded and directed? More emphasis needs to be put into preventive research, reward and recognition for preventive strategies.

Do Governments need to provide funding? Let's get real, who else can or will? Drugs research is lifesaving, allows us to understand body function, is very necessary, wondrous, and a great credit to researchers. But should a cycle be set, that ignores the search for simple preventive solutions to 'western' conditions?

Ignoring simple solutions creates a need, and a market, for drugs. Long-term side effects, and secondary issues, create a further market. Lack of attention to prevention, is a consequence of the reward mechanism, and human nature. A great benefit of research is the understanding of body mechanisms. The negative is research is funded in part, by diet reducible, early onset of western illnesses.

People do their very best, but do we not need a redefinition of goals, and emphasis on prevention? Are there not enough medical goals including, aging, tropical diseases, AIDS, genetic conditions, etc., without creating, enhancing, and perpetuating unnecessary suffering by failing to invest in prevention?

This is not a criticism of the individual. This is an observation upon the thousands of knee-jerk reactions that make the whole, and are the inevitable consequence of almost sole reliance on market mechanisms for prevention.

Market mechanisms are often a very effective solution, but I do not see how they can be usefully applied to prevention.

3.24   **National economies health competitive cost**—This is a competitive world. The health of a nation, is a serious factor, in assessing national competitiveness, and long term national economic competitiveness. Financial savings from prevention not needed for immediate health-care, are freed for other uses, be that research provision, or something else entirely.

Some countries have taken greater steps than others.

Japan has a higher level of supplementation of foodstuff with Omega Three, and higher fish intake. Japan's health costs per capita, are half those of the U.S. Japan has one of the highest IQ rates. Australia has started a policy of funding examination of prevention as well as treatment.

Nations are competitive. The potential implications of excess Omega Six, to the national interest, is a matter politicians should be seized of. Inaction will make their nations sicker, less intelligent, less socially adept, and burdened by, a greater health cost, educational issues, employment issues, and a less productive work force.

Inaction on prevention, and research funding for prevention, will result in poorer quality of life for many citizens, and their wider family network. The implications are truly global. Some factors are so basic that they are unavoidable.

Brains and eyes do not work properly without adequate DHA. It is an accepted fact, that increased Omega Three intake, reduces the risk of cardiac disease. Those facts alone should be enough to prompt people to action.

Billions of people are likely to be affected by excess Omega Six. We are exporting our dietary habits, including the high consumption of vegetable oil. Consumption of vegetable oils in China has increased by about 50 per cent, between 1991 and 1994. China is taking a lead and looking at taxing vegetable oil intake, according to an article in *Scientific American* in September 2007.

3.25   **Threat to the species**—The costs of wrong decisions are likely to be enormous. It is no exaggeration, to say that the consequences of a world full of more aggressive and selfish individuals, could be the decline or eradication of the human species.

Omega 3 and Omega 6 programme our behaviour. In a world of inherently more aggressive, more selfish, dumber individuals, the total outcome, is the sum of knee-jerk reactions of all of us. Our leaders and civil servants are subject to exactly the same dietary modified behaviour patterns as the rest of us.

'Industrial' eggs in Washington, and any other centre of administration, have the same poor Omega 3:6 profile, as those on your supermarket shelf.

This is not a voluntary matter, or one within our mental control. Our behaviour is being programmed by the food we eat. We can only moderate our response, by moderating our diets, and balancing the Omega Threes and Sixes.

3.26 **Increasing consumption of vegetable oil**–Vegetable oil consumption is increasing in China and the "Third World". Vegetable oil consumption in the developing world has grown dramatically since the 1960s. It is predicted to continue to rise. Those nations that use more high Omega 6 oils [p. 287], are likely to be more vulnerable to increases in 'western' conditions. Further, raised Omega 6 intake, combined with the increased usage of sugars and excess alcohol, adds to the problem by blocking the fat conversion pathways. The fat conversion pathways are part of the body's regulatory mechanisms.

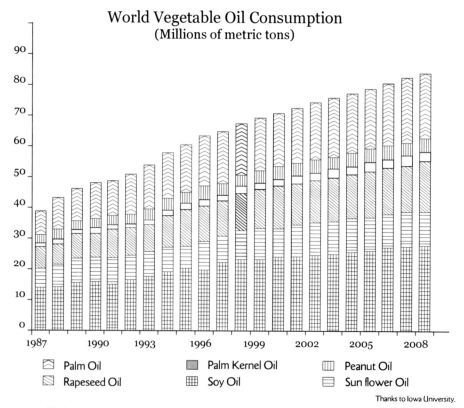

Thanks to Iowa University.

Fig. 3.26 World oil consumption figures are rising [Figures vary according to source]

Many of the oils in the graph are high in Omega 6. With current consumption patterns, the world is heading towards the ever-increasing levels of 'western' illness, and the changing behaviour patterns, that occur with significant Omega 3:6 intake imbalances.

3.27   **Lifestyle illness, who can afford it?**–Even if we could totally cure these conditions with drugs, without any side effect risks, which is extremely unlikely, can we afford the bill? Palliatives will become ever more costly and complex, and only be available to the rich.

In these hugely complex 'western' conditions, cure requires dealing with cause. The fat pathways responsible for these conditions, are so inextricably linked with almost every aspect of the body's function, that intervention will almost certainly have side effects.

Processes in the fat pathways are long term. Side effects of drug intervention, may not be evident, or understood for sometime. The pathways are so fundamental, on the balance of probabilities some consequences will be serious.

An Orwellian future of lifestyle illness for all, at the point of consumption, faces us. We are unknowingly creating a vast economic market of illnesses, for partial solutions complete with side effects, at huge social and economic cost. The benefit is advancement of understanding. Why not make the people better as far as possible by prevention, and spend savings on illness we cannot prevent.

3.28   **Alcohol**–Alcohol as social drink comes in a 'package', in many cases with nutrients from its source (e.g. grape). The benefits of the accompanying nutrients, should not be confused with the impact of the alcohol, good or bad. This comment is restricted to the alcohol part of alcoholic drinks, called ethanol. Dress alcohol up in the undoubted nutritional benefits of hops or grape skins, it is still alcohol. Alcohol is intimately linked to the body fats in a multilayered relationship.

- ☞ Alcohol can pass into all cells in the body including the brain, so the brain barrier does not protect the brain from the effect of alcohol.
- ☞ The body is reported to use DHA to breakdown alcohol by oxidation. DHA is the body's favourite fat to metabolise alcohol.
- ☞ The body uses structural DHA from the brain, and, likely, eyes and testes and the rest of the body to metabolise alcohol. [34] (Bleary eyes and fuzzy brains with a hangover? You likely have been removing working structures of your eyes and brain, to metabolise the alcohol).
- ☞ The body does not store much Omega Three.
- ☞ Unless Omega 3s/DHA are replaced continuously in diet, or by conversion from the mother Omega 3, a deficiency will develop.
- ☞ Moderate to high alcohol, and low intake of Omega Three, leads to liver damage in rats. Adequate Omega Three intake, gave protection against liver damage in rats.

☞ Liver damage is likely to impede conversion and manufacture of fats.

☞ Alcohol dissolves fat. This might provide a mechanism to liberate DHA from the brain, eye, etc., to the rest of the body, and for usage in the brain for neurochemicals, but it depletes the DHA content of the structural membranes of essential organs including the brain. Could the release of scarce fats for the production of neurochemicals give rise to an emotional high that drives drinking habits? DHA is closely tied to, and required for, dopamine and serotonin production. Low levels of dopamine and serotonin are linked to aggression and mental issues. [1.36]

☞ An equivalent Omega Six DPA, or Omega Nine, which are very much second-rate substitutes at best, will replace the missing DHA. DPA n6 is associated with loss in nervous system function, loss of brain function, and degradation in eyesight [38] [39] in animals.

☞ *The only good news is lab based animal research suggests adequate Omega Three intake may protect the liver in the face of moderate alcohol intake. So the message has to be, if you drink even moderate amounts, ensure you get a regular and adequate supply of Omega Threes, mother and long chain fats, or increase the risk of liver disease.*

Alcohol quickly permeates cells including those of the brain. Studies in animals suggest that moderate to high consumption of alcohol (1.2 and 2.6g per kg per day), where adequate Omega 3 and 6 is available, if anything enhances long chain fats conversion. [35]

Higher DHA may account for trials that report benefit of low alcohol intake, on heart disease for instance. But where the Omega 3 intake was low, the trial in animals showed marked liver damage at 1.2 and 2.6g/kg day. [36] Alcohol uses up DHA and other Omega 3s. [37] Omega 3s are oxidised in preference to Omega 6s. Organs of the body high in DHA, may be drained of DHA by alcohol.

Increased fat conversion and Omega 3 oxidation with low-level alcohol consumption, may denude the body of Omega 3s, and push the body to convert the mother Omega Six, to Omega 6 AA inflammatory chemicals. This would put the body in an inflammatory state, and replace structural DHA with DPA n6.

The body's protection system when DHA gets low is to stop using DHA, and use Omega Six DPA and then Omega 9 instead. [40] Does alcohol bypass this safety mechanism by allowing the preferential utilisation of DHA?

Alcohol consumption at any level, where Omega 3 supplies are insufficient, may pose health risks based on animal trials. Where Omega 3 supply is adequate, low alcohol intake may result in improved conversion to long chain fats, which might compensate for greater oxidation, by resupplying the necessary DHA.

If you enjoy an occasional drink consider if you have an adequate supply of Omega 3 to reduce the risk of liver damage, and discuss with your Doctor, as we are all different, and some may not be able to tolerate alcohol.

4

HOW I CAME TO THIS,
AND MY BACKGROUND

4.1   **How I came to this, and my background**—In early 2005, my knowledge on the subject was almost zero. I came upon the enormous importance of Omega Three and Omega Six by accident, whilst researching breast cancer. I kept finding links to fat metabolism, and suggestions Omega 3 was protective, and Omega 6 increased risks.

Everything pointed to these fats having a central role in a whole range of conditions. I had previously seen the articles about Omega Three in the newspapers. I mentally filed them with all the other seesaw dietary tips. They were filed alongside blueberries, ginseng, green tea, and the latest 'fad'. They were desirable, but no more than that. After all, I got a reasonably varied diet, didn't I? I juiced, took supplements, etc.

I had read some health literature. I had no inkling that to balance Omega Three and Omega Six mother fats, and ensure an adequate supply of the long chain Omega 3 fats, DHA and EPA, was truly a preventive health imperative. When I saw how far my own Omega Three:Six balance was out, I was shocked by the implications.

I had irritable digestion, minor skin problems, and poor fat digestion. I did not have the energy I used to, but did not connect it to Omega 3 and 6. Feta in sunflower oil—healthy polyunsaturates I thought. I made sure I did not waste the 'healthy' high Six sunflower oil that came with the feta cheese in oil. A little meat, non-oily fish, no sugar in the house; the usual recommendations; a healthy diet I thought, but my Omega 3:6 balance must have been 20:1, if not much higher.

I was a big fan of polyunsaturated oils high in 6 and low in 3, like grapeseed and sunflower; the lighter and more polyunsaturated the better. I was entranced by the message we were all getting through the media, which I suppose reflected some sort of medical 'groupthink'. I changed my Omega 3:6 profile swiftly.

I saw several benefits over the first year, greatly improved digestion, more fitness, I was calmer, my gums improved, fatty liver symptoms returned to normal (as determined by long running periodic fats blood tests) and the list goes on.

I was shocked by the wider implications for society. As I read more, the journey went from an interest, to a feeling of indignation, to a point of almost a desperate obsession. I needed to try and explain to all and sundry why, this was so important to their health, and well-being. I was once likened to a visiting Jehovah's Witness for the intensity of my communication.

This book is my journey from virtually no knowledge about the importance of the Omega Three–Six balance, to a point where I believe it is arguably the most fundamental aspect of diet. My only knowledge at the starting point was an A level in chemistry, and some background reading of a few health books. This process has taken about three years of consistent and extensive reading, researching, cross checking and cross linking.

I have just followed, where the subjects and questions took me. I had a great advantage of time, and no restrictions or constraints in my web and book wanders. It has involved a lot of burning of the midnight oil. It has been time-consuming, pushed aside other necessary activities like the garden, maintenance and socialising, and been life absorbing. (A nerd I think is the description "lacking social skill and boringly studious", [Oxford Dictionary] but I do not accept that nerds are foolish or contemptible. They are simply different.). But, it has been fascinating.

The body is enormously complicated, and I have only skimmed the surface. I am made aware of how very little I know each time I go on a Web search, or browse a specialist book. It has been a journey. I see another piece fitting into the jigsaw almost every day. Today, it was a comment on *Radio Four* (BBC) that males in American schools, from puberty to the end of college, lose ground in intelligence terms [compared with girls and other nations] [See 27.17 and Chapter 24].

The book started almost by accident, and has almost 'happened' and matured by a series of fortuitous events that combined and conspired to provide the time and motivation for me to complete it.

I hope I am able to make a difference by communicating the importance of Omega Three, and the implications of excess Omega Six, in the diet.

5
THE FAMILIES, THE EFAS, THE MATRIARCHS

5   **The Families, the EFAs, The Matriarchs**—The Omega Three and Six families are both essential to the function of the body. They are inextricably linked. They are in a constant dance of opposites. They are in constant tension. They pull in opposite directions struggling for dominance. Each separate member of each fat family has distinct and different functions in the body. There is one mother fat for each family. Only plants can make the mother fats.

Omega 3 and 6 mother fats are in constant competition for the common conversion resources, the desaturase and COX enzymes, to make their particular families of fats and chemicals. Desaturase enzymes are used to make longer fats from the shorter mother fats. COX2 enzymes are used to make the chemical families, from the Omega 6 AA, and Omega 3 EPA fats [Page 286].

In simple terms, 20 carbon long fats Omega 3 EPA and Omega 6 AA compete for usage of the same fat and chemical production lines, support teams and mechanics; arguments over the photocopier and phone if you like.

There is one *fat* production line manager for each process. There is one *chemical* production line manager for each process. This competition for production line managers, controls whether inflammatory or repair chemicals are made. Omega 3 and 6 fats have different strategies and means of achieving their objectives. The body has always worked on the basis that the Omega 3 and 6 mother fats were available in more or less equal quantities.

Long chain Omega 3s, DHA and EPA, block the Omega Six 6 AA chemical cascade. EPA is reported as working competitively against Omega AA, with the intent of producing chemicals in its own pathway. It is reported that Omega 6 AA, effectively has preference in the conversion process over Omega 3 EPA. Omega 6 production requires less energy to start than Omega 3 production and once started self fuels by producing the necessary oxidants. [See Chapter 22].

If the balance between Omega 3 and Omega 6, is heavily distorted by excess Omega 6, Omega 6 gains dominance, and body system start to break down.

DHA [22 carbons long], blocks Omega 6 [20 carbon] eicosanoid chemicals production, but does not result in the Omega 3 eicosanoid chemicals.

In evolutionary terms, it would make sense to give preference to Omega Six, as the Omega Sixes were arguably scarcer than the Omega Threes, and fundamental to a number of the body's functions including reproduction. It therefore becomes a big whammy when there is excess Omega Six.

Omega Six can produce Omega Six inflammatory chemicals, both because there is more Omega 6, and because it has preferential access to the necessary desaturase enzymes. It is acknowledged by those that work in the lipids research that a very great deal is still unknown. Whilst I have searched, I have not found very much material on the action of DHA and EPA in the membrane.

The above were based on an online lecture by William L. Smith, Ph.D., Professor and Chairman of Biochemistry, Michigan State http://efaeducation.nih.gov/sig/video.html and the Lands' book. The key is both DHA and EPA have a role to play in determining eicosanoid chemical products.

5.1   **The EFAs, The Matriarchs, Omega Six** – The Omega Six 'mother' fat, linol**eic** acid LA 'The Devil's Fat', ***CANNOT BE MADE IN THE BODY***. Omega Six is more male in characteristics than female, but for the purposes of this book has been treated as female, simply because that was my initial start point. Mother Omega 6 cannot be made in the body, and must be got from diet.

The Omega Sixes are the heavies. They attend the initial emergency call, create clotting, inflammation, defence, start building new blood vessels, encourage cell migration, control hormones, break down tissue, and open pathways to new life. LA is found at high levels in many vegetable oils, 50–70 per cent in sunflower, soy, safflower, corn oil, etc. [Page 287] These oils are commonly and extensively used in processed foods.

The body can take the mother fat, and add carbons and double bonds to make the daughter fats. In general terms, long chain Omega Six shortages, are not likely, but may be an issue for some.

AA is the raw material for the Omega Six, COX2, cascade of chemicals. GLA is the raw material of the Omega Six, COX1, cascade of chemicals. Much is still unknown and conversion is complex.

LA Matriarch	(Omega Six)	18:2 n6	Linol**eic**
GLA Child	(Omega Six)	18.3 n6	Gamma linolenic
AA Senior child	(Omega Six)	20:4n6	Arachidonic
AD Senior child	(Omega Six)	22:4n6	Adrenic
DPA Substitute	(Omega Six)	22:5n6	Docosapentaenoic

The first number is the number of carbons in the chain. The second is the number of double bonds. The third 'n' number is the number of carbons from the hydrogen end that the first double bond occurs.

You can get the same number of carbons and double bonds for an Omega 3 and 6, but in different positions, which gives rise to different shapes e.g. there is an Omega Six 18:3 GLA and an Omega Three 18:3 ALA but the double bonds are in different places which, makes them behave differently at a chemical level.

DPA n6 is used in the absence of DHA as a substitute in the eyes and brain. It is a very poor second, and leads to degradation in neural and retinal function.

Fat testing in the only way to determine an individual's fat status.

5.2 **The EFAs, The Matriarchs, Omega Three**–The mother Omega Three, Alpha Lino**lenic**, ALA, 'God's Fat', *CANNOT BE MADE IN THE BODY*. Omega Threes are the moderators–they attend after the initial emergency call, calm things down, organise and clear up, and talk the Omega 6 heavies down and send them home.

Mother 3s are found in quantity in a limited number of foods, like flax, perilla, and chia [30.31]. Longer chain fats are found in oily fish. These oils are not used much in prepared food due to shelf life issues. You will know an Omega 3 because it has the first double bond three carbons from the hydrogen end. [30.10]

The body can make the daughters from the mother fat, but the paths are easily blocked. Shortages of the daughter fats in the West, may simply be because our western diet blocks the pathways. Or it may be because we are not getting enough of the mother fats, and daughters, in our diet, or a combination. Trials suggest that supplementation with the mother fat alone will not bring DHA levels up to those of Japanese or Inuit fish eaters. [41]

Western diet is full of conversion blockers, [13.11] and so for many Westerners, fish oil, or a vegan equivalent supplement, and long chain Omega 3 food sources are required.

ALA	Matriarch	(Omega Three)	18:3 n3	Linol**enic**
EPA	Senior child	(Omega Three)	20:5 n3	Eicosapentaenoic +
DPA		(Omega Three)	22:5 n3	Docosapentaenoic*
DHA	Senior child	(Omega Three)	22:6 n3	Docosahexaenoic

[*NOTE there is a docosapentaenoic DPA for both Omega Six and Omega Three. DPA n6 (the Omega Six fat) features quite frequently in trials. Less attention seems to be given to the Omega Three version. DPA Omega Six is used by the body as a substitute for the Omega Three DHA.

The fact the first carbon in Omega Three starts at 3 rather than 6 carbons from the hydrogen end, gives it space for one more double bond than an Omega 6 in a chain of the same length. The number of double bonds and positions in chains of the same length defines the different shapes and character of the Omega Threes and Omega Sixes. [30.10, 30.20]]

6

WHY EXCESS OMEGA SIX MATTERS

6.1   A dumber, sicker, more aggressive nation?–[Abbreviations listed at 1.1] Significant excess of Omega Six over Omega Three, is linked with greater incidence of 'western' diseases [See 2.3 and Ch. 29], increased aggression, early puberty, sleep issues, obesity, behaviour modification and poorer brain function. Links have been shown to cardiovascular conditions, cancer, depression, obesity, suicide, infertility, diabetes, asthma, osteoporosis, the long list goes on.

Diet is one of the most powerful forces there is in safeguarding health. Omega 3 and Omega 6 have multiple roles. Omega Three and Omega Six act at very many key levels in the body, and through multiple mechanisms such as cell membrane function and structure, hormone messengers, and chemical pathways.

6.2   Incidence of chronic 'western' disease–We are seeing rapid increases in many 'western' diseases, diabetes, asthma, cardiac, and obesity related conditions. They are often inflammatory, and relate to immune regulation.

It may even be that these conditions are not degenerative diseases, but diseases of inflammation, eicosanoid, hormone, steroid, and immune system imbalances, arising from excess of Omega Six AA and lack of Omega Three EPA in the cell membranes. Excess inflammation is a chemical consequence of excess Omega Six, and lack of balance with Omega Three.

The potential future cost of these conditions, in financial and social terms, at individual, and national level, is enormous. A paper in the *American Journal of Clinical Nutrition* in 2005 included the following figures in respect to the U.S.–65 per cent of adults (20 or under) are either overweight or obese–estimated deaths from obesity was 280,184 per year–64 million plus have heart disease–38.5 per cent of deaths are from heart disease–11 million have type 2 diabetes–7.2 per cent of post menopausal women have osteoporosis, and 39.6 per cent have osteopenia–Cancer accounts for 25 per cent of deaths.... [42]

6.3 **Impact on the family**–With the wisdom of age, or experience of illness, comes an appreciation of the fundamental importance of health. Illness has a huge quality of life price to the individual. Illness come with a high emotional and support burden for families and carers.

Those hardest hit are the young. We are visiting the children of the world with a long list of diseases. Diseases in the young include behavioural problems, ADHD, diabetes, asthma, impaired cognitive function, possible poorer vision, and vascular disease. It appears to be getting worse in the newest generations.

The state of the mother's nutrition moderates the infant's immune system, and fats in membranes including the eyes and brain. Young infants are reported as not being able to make the long chain fats well. This continues until weaning and beyond.

Trials suggest that early infant nutrition, and the mother's nutritional status, may increase the risk of obesity in the child in later life. High Omega Six in processed food, higher vegetable oil intake, and lack of Omega Three, in the infant's diet, or in the mother's milk, may be factors [25.33].

Excess Omega Six, and lack of Omega Three, could set the scenario for permanent low-level inflammation, and consequent greater sensitivity to antigen based conditions such as diabetes 1 and asthma [29.29].

6.4 **Cost to the nation**–A sicker nation is less effective and less competitive in a global market. A sicker nation spends a greater proportion of its GDP on maintaining basic health, and related care and support costs. Money spent on maintaining basic health is unavailable for other things. Increasing illness lowers a nation's potential productivity.

6.5 **Health access a socially divisive issue**–The citizen's expectation of healthcare is increasing. People will want access to the best treatment options reflecting the latest research. Costs are rising dramatically.

Western conditions are increasing. The reality is that there will come a point where resources have to be restricted. Resource restriction leads to feelings of inequity, powerlessness, and social division. Protection of family is one of the strongest, most emotive, human drivers.

Nothing is likely to be more divisive, or open to emotive marketing exploitation, than a sense of inequality of access to healthcare, particularly where life itself is at stake.

A sense of injustice and inequality, as to right to life, through accessibility to medicine, will lead to a more uneasy, divided, and less cohesive society. Prevention that reduces treatment need, would result in a more effective, balanced, and happier society.

6.6 **An aggressive society**–Omega Three and Omega Six are highly influential mind-altering substances. They alter the chemistry that controls behaviour in humans.

Fats act through many pathways, including as hormone and chemical messengers, by alteration of cell membrane properties, electrical potentials, calcium transport, etc.

Omega Six promotes aggression. DHA reduces aggression. Omega Six, and Omega Three, both act on the sex hormone and steroid pathways, and through serotonin, dopamine, melatonin, and norepinephrine production. We seem to be facing a greater culture of aggression. We have become a less gentle, and a more self-centered society.

Increased propensity to aggression in individuals, could have wider global impacts, for the stability of our world. Excess Omega Six has been linked, in several trials, with increased aggression. [43] DHA pre-birth deficit, has been linked to impaired cognitive function, elevated anxiety, aggression, and depression in animals. [44] Omega Six results in higher testosterone levels. Testosterone levels are linked with aggression. Low levels of DHA are linked with low levels of serotonin. Lack of serotonin is linked with impulsiveness.

6.7   **Aggression**—Omega Six derivatives of PGE2, testosterone and the steroids, and the Omega 3 DHA with serotonin, are players in a dance which controls behaviour. [See 23.11b]

The steroids like cortisol, corticosterone, produced from cholesterol are also directly, or indirectly, controlled or influenced through PGE2. There is competition for the cholesterol enzymes between hormones and steroids. The level of the stress related hormone norepinephrine is reduced by DHA. Steroid and hormone imbalance has been linked to aggression.

6.8   **Serotonin**—Aggression, impulsiveness disturbed behaviour, etc., has been linked with lack of serotonin. Serotonin manufacture is enabled by DHA. DHA deficiency in early development has been linked with anxiety, depression, aggression, and ADHD. [45]

Serotonin can be regarded as the master-control neurotransmitter with at least 14 receptor subtypes. Testosterone has an inverse relationship with serotonin. [46][47] Increased testosterone reduces serotonin levels.

High Omega Six increases the Omega Six chemicals including PGE2. PGE2 controls aromatase, which controls the hormones. Increased PGE2 will lead to higher testosterone and oestrogen. Oestrogen increases DHA. DHA will turn down the production of PGE2.

So, here we have a fat responsive control loop. Omega Six will push down DHA and push up testosterone. Both higher testosterone and lower DHA will jointly and individually reduce serotonin levels thus increasing aggression, etc.

DHA intake conversely will increase DHA, and reduce testosterone, both of which will increase serotonin thus decreasing aggression.

The absence or low levels of Omega Threes, predisposes the body to aggression, and a likelihood that a rise in testosterone will give rise to an aggressive incident.

If there is no Omega 3 material to make DHA, the body has no way to moderate increased testosterone and reduced serotonin, and so reduce aggression.

Basal hormone production levels of oestrogen and testosterone, could in part account for the different aggression profiles of men and women, by differently modulating the fats and interlinking hormone pathways.

Western women convert about 10 per cent of the mother Omega Three, ALA, into DHA. Men convert under 1 per cent to DHA, and trials suggest some men convert only a fraction of one per cent. DHA promotes serotonin production. Lack of serotonin, is associated with an inability to control behaviour, and impulses of all sorts including violence, and anger.

6.9   **Testosterone**—Testosterone is controlled by aromatase. Aromatase is controlled by PGE2. PGE2 is a product of Omega Six. Excess Omega Six and lack of Omega Three alters hormone production. Higher DHA, downgrades the production of arachidonic acid, and thus testosterone. The primary effects of testosterone occur after aromatisation (PGE2 is required for aromatisation). Testosterone has an inverse relationship with serotonin. [48][49] Excess Omega Six and lack of long chain Omega Three would arguably increase aromatase, leading to increased testosterone (and oestrogen). Increased testosterone and lower DHA would independently and jointly result in serotonin reduction, leading to aggression and impulsiveness.

Higher testosterone and lower serotonin has been linked with delinquency, aggression, substance abuse, violent and sexual crime, antisocial behaviour, alcoholism, and high risk behaviour, particularly in more financially disadvantaged groups. Testosterone has been linked with dominance, and low serotonin with aggression. Aggressive and impulsive behaviour, may be the result of triggering both low serotonin and high testosterone together. High testosterone alone is not generally sufficient to trigger aggression.

It may be that such behaviour is the result of the coming together of high testosterone, low DHA, and low serotonin, and all being exacerbated by the dietary factors of low Omega Three and high Omega Six.

6.10   **Monthly aggression in women**—In women, increasing oestrogen increases DHA levels. Increased DHA would normally moderate aromatase, as oestrogen levels rose. Increased DHA would increase serotonin thus damping down the aggression cycle. If DHA, or the necessary Omega Threes to make DHA, are not available, the moderating pathway is blocked. Lower DHA would also result in disturbances of the steroid balances (cortisol etc.), and stress hormones. The creation of cells to thicken the uterus lining, and create the follicle may require high levels of DHA, and have a priority call on the body's supplies.

All of these factors could lead to lower DHA, lower serotonin, higher testosterone, and disturbance of steroid balances, leading to greater aggression, and may explain mood swings in PMT.

6.11   **Aggression and alcohol**–Alcohol will oxidise DHA, and possibly liberate fats of all sorts from the brain. If the brain already is high in AA, and low in DHA, this could result in more AA than DHA being released by alcohol, which is likely to exacerbate inflammation and aggression, as observed in reality. Lower DHA will result in lower serotonin. Higher Omega Six may lead to higher testosterone and hormone levels.

Lack of DHA in the brain has been linked to impaired neural performance. Missing structural DHA is substituted by DPA n6, the nearest Omega Six. DPA is a poor substitute. Degradation of neural function leading to impaired performance may well aggravate hormonal effects of additional testosterone. To reduce aggression, ensure that intake of Omega Three and Omega Six are balanced and intake of long chain Omega Threes are adequate.

6.12   **Brains are fat**–Your brain is over 60 per cent fats. A significant portion of that fat is Omega Threes and Sixes. Not enough DHA, and your brain does not function properly. If you don't eat the mother Omega 3 fat (greens, flax seed, etc.) and make DHA (blocked by sugar, trans fats, too much Omega 6 fat), or get DHA in food (primarily oily fish), you may well be short.

DHA is unique and special. DHA has very particular bioelectrical and mechanical properties. DHA is part of the cell membranes. It acts as a messenger, a source of important chemicals, controls electrical function and more. If DHA is not available, the body will use the nearest Omega Six DPA or in rare cases, Omega Nine as a substitute.

The consequence is poorer brain performance. It is a bit like putting oil from the fryer straight into your diesel. It simply will not work as well. If pathways are blocked, Omega Six fats could be affected as well. AA and AD are also plentiful in the brain and crucial to brain function.

Different genetic tendencies may also affect individual ability to make and use fats. It is all about ensuring, as far as possible, that the body has the raw material it needs, and that the processes are not blocked from happening. Our 'western', highly refined diet, disturbs the body's mechanisms, and does not provide adequate raw materials in the proper proportions.

If brains do not have an adequate supply of DHA, they do not function properly. It is that simple.

6.13   **Depression, suicide, ADHD, . . .**–We are seeing increasing rates of depression, suicide, mental conditions, and dementia. The brain is 60 per cent or more fat. If the brain does not have a balance of Omega Three and Omega Six, it does not function properly. Adequate DHA is essential to neural function. It is that simple.

All animal brains in the wild, have a ratio of one Omega Three to one Omega Six. I have not found data on the fat distribution in the human brain. (See chapter 24 on the brain for more detail).

6.14   **IBS and digestive disturbances**—The processes in the body are so intertwined, that there are considerable wider consequences of fat imbalance. Higher Omega Six leads to greater risk of inflammation.

Inflammation is a factor and trigger of irritable bowel syndrome, IBS. IBS leads to poor conversion of food and ingestion of fats. A lack of nutrients in the diet is exacerbated.

Undigested food results in unfriendly bacteria, wind, etc. Inflammation leads to a layer of mucus. Mucus prevents proper contact of the food, with the cells that do the work. Fat intake may be impaired.

Impaired fat intake could exacerbate low levels of Omega Three in the diet. Omega Six intake combined with high fat stores, fuels the inflammation cycle. Omega Three is required to calm things down, and help repair.

The absence of Omega 3s further worsens the situation, as there is then a lack of the Omega 3 raw material, in the cell membrane to make the substances to dampen down the inflammation. Omega Three and Six are key components of cell membrane structure.

Compromised bowel cell membranes, allow leakage of foreign products into the bloodstream, which leads to further problems. My experience was that increased Omega Three in flax seed, and fish oil combined with highly restricted sugar intake (in my case restricted fruit juice intake) slowly but significantly normalised bowel function.

6.15   **Cell walls are fat**—Imagine a double skinned soap bubble, with lots of tiny factories, and a raw material store inside.

You have just imagined a cell. The primary constituent of your cell walls is fat. This includes the essential fatty acids, EFAs, Omega Three and Omega Six. It also includes saturated and monosaturated fats like Omega Seven and Nine.

Long chain or short, they all have a role and place. Fats have different shapes. Fats with no double bonds are little zigzags in a straight line. Each double bond introduces a small bend.

Six double bonds creates an almost circular shape. Saturated fats fit together like soldiers in rank. Highly unsaturated fats are more like a bag of marbles. Saturated fats make inflexible membranes. Unsaturated fats make very flexible membranes. A mix gives you something in between [30.10, 30.24].

The fats in the cell membranes are attracted to each other but not locked. The fats in the membrane are in constant motion. Fats in the cell membrane are in pairs. The compound that clasps the pairs of fats together, has a liking for water, and so is always on the outside. The free ends of the fat have a hatred for water, and create a water-free zone between the two skins of the membrane. [30.27]

The fats you eat influence the flexibility and qualities of membranes, including the cell membranes that are your skin. Fats have been called magic bricks; they link to other chemicals, act as gatekeepers, and pass things in and out of the cells. Their individual shapes and structures give them particular and special roles.

They form little gangs for special projects. If they do not have the right members of the gang all in attendance, they do not work properly. The right fats are essential to the gang for proper function.

Fats are not interchangeable. If you have more Omega Six, than Three, in the cell membrane wall, which is the raw material store of long chain fats, the body makes more inflammatory Omega Six chemicals. This is why it is important to have the right balance of Omega Three, and Omega Six, in the cell membrane walls. [1.36]

6.16   The body cannot tell Omega Three from Omega Six–*The balance in which fats are present in the cell membranes alters the chemistry of the body. When selecting long chain Omega Threes, and Sixes, from the cell membranes, the body has no programme to choose an Omega Three or a Six.*

It only knows what chain length it wants. The body is not fussy. The body takes the fats from the cell walls, as it needs them. If it needs a long chain 20 or 22 carbon fat, it takes one.

The body does not care if it is an Omega 3 or Omega 6. It is blind to whether the fat is an Omega 3 or 6. So even if your membranes have an excess of Omega Six, the body is not aware of that.

It has no mechanism to select between an Omega Three and Omega Six of a particular chain length. There was never any need at an evolutionary level to have a mechanism to select between Omega Three and Omega Six. Omega Threes and Sixes, in primary food sources, were always more or less in balance.

Since food is the only source of Omega 3s and 6s, there would never be a long-term imbalance. The seasonal change in balance of Omega Threes and Sixes in the diet, provided a link that allowed body function to be manipulated automatically, to best meet environmental conditions, and follow the seasons.

Excess Omega Six was scarce and seasonal. If any fat HISTORICALLY was likely to be available in excess, it was Omega Three not Omega Six. Shore feeders would have had access to high levels of Omega Three.

Diet alters body function through the ratio of Omega Six (highly inflammatory) and Omega Three (moderating) chemicals. Human behaviour changed according to season, food supply and Omega Six intake, because of the consequent changes in the balances of hormones, steroids, fats and chemicals in the brain.

If the body had a way to choose an Omega 3 or 6 from the cell membrane, the body would not respond automatically to food supply in the environment.

6.17   Local repair crew–The chemical derivatives of the Omega Six pathways, are key to emergency repair or invasion response. We need an instant initial response to injury, or invasion, to help us survive.

The body has systems of local emergency repair crews. Raw materials, are kept to hand and accessible for immediate use, by storing them in the walls of the cell membranes. This includes stores of Omega Three, and Omega Six.

It is like having hundreds of miniature ambulances and fire crews, with supplies, built into the wall of your house, everywhere and anywhere you might need them at a moments notice.

The raw materials the fire crews draw, are those available in the cell membranes. So if you have a lot of Omega Six in the cell membrane, the crew will use a lot of Omega Six. The Omega Six fat content of your cell membrane depends on how much Omega Six and Omega Three you eat, and the amount of Omega Six in your fat reserves.

Emergency messengers are sent to the main depot, the fat reserves and liver, for back up. The balance of Omega Three, and Omega Six, in your diet will shape your immune responses, and many other body processes as well, through the fat balance of the cell membranes.

6.18   **Central store, the body fat**–When there is an emergency in the body, the nearest local cells will send messengers out asking for backup. One major source of backup, is chemicals from the fat cells, and supporting matrix. The amount of inflammatory chemicals, the body can produce, is dependent on the factory cell capacity, and the stores of raw material available.

Omega Six is the raw material. It is held in bubbles in your fat cells. [Fig 3.10] It is accessed through the membrane of the bubble surface, with reception at one end, and dispatch at the other.

The amount of raw material available depends on the amount of Omega Six per cell, and number of cells. The more fat you carry, the more Omega Six that may be available.

Proportions of Omega Six in body fat vary from 5–25 per cent. It takes at least __two years__ to change the make up of half of your stored fat. The total Omega Six available in the cell membranes for immediate usage, will depend on a mix of your intake levels, circulating fats, and body fat stores.

Historically, it is likely we did not carry high levels of fat. Omega nine, and other fats, will also be stored, and reflect diet too. Wild animals have relatively low cyclical fat stores.

Excess body fat equates to high levels of stored Omega 6–a multiple of total fat and percentage [5-25 per cent] of Omega 6 in the body fat.

6.19   **Innate and learned immune systems**–The local cellular emergency service is called the innate immune system. It has a range of weapons and applies basic universal responses. The longer term learned immune system is more cumbersome, but more effective and follows up the innate system.

6.20   **Steroids and hormones**–Omega Three, and Omega Six, are the exclusive raw materials at the top of two very complex and influential cascades of chemicals. [Fig 1.20] They are called the eicosanoid pathways. The chemicals control the inflammation, repair, and reproductive pathways.

Omega Six downstream chemical products, interact and control enzymes that make key hormones and steroids, so altering the amounts available [Fig. 23.11b] The steroids and hormones interact with the pituitary gland, hypothalamus, and adrenal gland.

The hypothalamus is a region at the front lower centre of the brain, which interacts with the nervous system. The pituitary is at the bottom of the brain, and secretes body controlling hormones. The adrenal glands, sit on top of the kidneys, and respond to stress by producing steroids such as cortisone, from cholesterol.

The three are known as the HPA axis and viewed as being a close working team, important to many body functions. Omega Six controls immune function in a number of ways, through its control of the steroid/hormone manufacture enzymes. Omega Three controls and moderates Omega Six production, so also moderating steroids, hormones, and immune function. Omega Three also produces its own chemicals that are anti-inflammatory. The Omega Three– Six balance is truly fundamental to the way the body operates.

6.21   The battle DHA, EPA and Omega Six–DHA has profound effects on the damping down of the Omega Six eicosanoid pathway. PGE2, a product of Omega Six, is closely connected to inflammation. PGE2 production was significantly reduced by DHA.

This is truly fundamental. PGE2 is indirectly a precursor for the sex hormones. DHA controls hormones levels by limiting Omega 6 products AA and PGE2. Increased DHA reduces PGE2.

[For the technical six grams of DHA a day, fed to young men over 90 days, increased DHA concentration from 2.3 to 7.4 wt. per cent in blood cells [PBMNC] total lipids, and decreased arachidonic acid concentration from 19.8 to 10.7 wt. per cent. It also lowered prostaglandin E2 (PGE2) and leukotriene B4 (LTB4) production, in response to lipopolysaccharide, by 60–75 per cent.]

6.22   Stem cell activation–Omega Six, in vastly over stimulating repair processes, could be facilitating the opening of the stem cell processes. The innate body repair system, has some communality with the creation of new life. Some consider cancer is in part an activation of those processes.

It is suggested that some cells in early pregnancy are little different from highly malignant cancer cells. Inflammatory processes are being linked as a factor in cancer. [50]

6.23   Cancer–A number of studies have suggested that excess Omega Six is connected with progression, and associated with higher risk factors for cancer. The Omega Three family has been connected with reduction of risk.

There are a number of potential mechanisms by which the fats may influence cancer progression, including the fat pathways, hormone levels, inflammatory factors, steroids, sleep deprivation, stressed immune function, oxidation quality, DNA protection, and cell death.

Cancers trialled with Omega 3 include breast, prostate, melanoma, and lung. There are a significant number of trials looking at Omega Threes, particularly DHA and cancer. One trial on breast cancer, suggested risk reduction factors as high as 70 per cent, between the highest and lowest levels of DHA and EPA in breast tissue.

A thought provoking interesting article reported a single lung cancer incident, that was professionally followed. A very elderly patient was recorded as choosing to balance his Omega Threes and Sixes, rather than undergo chemo. His progress was followed through with scans. Tumours of significant size very substantially regressed over some years; a thought provoking result even if isolated. [51]

A number of trials have also implicated oleic acid and DGLA, in moderating the PGE2 products of Omega Six. [52] The impact of Omega 3 and 6 on cancer, is very much work in progress, and debated among specialists.

6.24   **Sleep**–The Omega Three and Omega Six pathways, are intimately involved in the process that allows sleep. The Omega Six inflammatory pathway activity is turned down in sleep. The supply of Omega Six fat from body fat stores is switched down in sleep. Omega Three pathways that reduce Omega Six activities are upgraded. Higher Omega Three activity is linked with body repair.

Melatonin also triggers production of DHA, which shuts down the Omega Six pathways. Melatonin self fuels by increasing DHA production. DHA is used to allow serotonin to be made. Increased serotonin increases melatonin. Melatonin shuts down the Omega 6 COX2 pathways.

Melatonin is also an antioxidant. This mechanism of higher DHA assisting with sleep, and DHA being increased by melatonin, would be consistent with the need of children for sleep for brain growth, and growth taking place in sleep. Melatonin normalises and increases REM sleep in the elderly[i].

DHA is fundamental to brain formation. Children produce more melatonin. Higher melatonin results in higher DHA.

The Omega Three–Six sleep cycle, provides a mechanism for the body alert level to be dampened down, allowing sleep and repair. (See chapter on melatonin and sleep for more detail). Omega Three and Omega Six also provide links to regulate the sex hormone, and energy pathways, in sleep.

6.25   **Fertility cycle controlled by fats?**–The fertility issues are dealt with in a separate chapter – The Omega Six pathway is a primary route, to trigger the cellular processes that make new life. Successful reproduction is tied to the ability of the wider environment to support new life.

---

i   Melatonin in Patients with Reduced REM Sleep Duration: Two Randomized Controlled Trials The Journal of Clinical Endocrinology & Metabolism Vol. 89, No. 1 128-134 Dieter Kunz, Richard Mahlberg, Cordula Müller, Amely Tilmann and Frederik Bes Department of Psychiatry and Psychotherapy (D.K., R.M., C.M., A.T.), Charité Campus Mitte-Universitätsmedizin Berlin, 10117 Berlin, Germany; and Medcare Automation (F.B.), Amsterdam, The Netherlands.

Omega Six is the measure of fecundity of the environment. If seeds and nuts are plentiful, the world is fruitful, and likely to successfully support new offspring. Omega Three is the essential partner.

If there is excessively more Omega Six than Three in the diet, the outcome is higher oestrogens, and higher testosterone or androgens. The body is on permanent time to breed code red alert. The body lacks the supplies of Omega 3s it needs. Hormones are out of balance. Fats are out of balance. Control systems are disrupted.

The Omega Three–Six pathways provide the basis for hormone cycling and the control of the fertility cycle. Lack of shutdown and proper regulation of the menstrual cycle leads to fertility issues and fibrosis, amongst others.

Oestrogen increases DHA production. When a baby is conceived, it has a high consumption of the long chain fats, and particularly DHA. Removal of DHA from the mothers system allows hormone production to remain high. If there is no conception, DHA levels rise, and shut down the Omega Six PGE2 pathways, and so hormone production.

This system works optimally with certain fat levels and Omega Three–Six stores. High levels of fat lead to high stores of Omega Six. Higher stores of Omega Six lead to higher hormone levels. The problem is the lack of DHA, and excess Omega 6.

In the absence of Omega Threes, the body has no raw materials to damp the cycle down. *DHA is essential to hormone balance.* Higher testosterone levels in women lead to PCOS, hirsuteness, and failure to shut down the monthly cycle. Omega Sixes and pregnancy are dealt with in the chapter 23.[53][54]

It is a key sexual difference that men are very poor at making DHA. Men make less than one per cent according to trials. Women can make more than nine per cent [55]. Omega Six is, in a sense, male, and DHA female, in the attributes it confers. The balance of the fats is another part in the complex jigsaw that defines our behavioural and gender characteristics. (See chapters 23 and 28).

6.26   **Omega Six at the core**–After reading fairly widely on the subject over a three-year period, I believe it is unavoidable that excess Omega 6 and lack of Omega 3 is a core factor in the vast increase in 'western' health conditions.

7
SOME OMEGA THREE AND OMEGA SIX BASICS

7.1   So influential—[Abbreviations listed at 1.1] If you don't eat them, Omega Three and Six, you don't have them. There are no other natural, commonly ingested, external agents, that are part of our diet:

- ☞ That are so central to the body's structure and function.
- ☞ That are so universal to all the body's processes.
- ☞ That have such global usage.
- ☞ Whose intake levels have changed so hugely in the last 100 years.
- ☞ That can biologically account for all these conditions.
- ☞ That connect us directly to the fecundity of our environment.

7.2   Critical to life—Omega 3 and 6 are called essential fatty acids, EFAs. They are called that because they are essential to life. This includes the whole family, the mother fats and children. Each fat has a different and distinct role.

Omega 6 and 3 are separate families. They are not interchangeable. They cannot be made from each other, in animals, or man. Plants can make the mother Omega Six, into the mother Omega Three. Plants cannot naturally make the long chain fats. We get mother EFAs directly or indirectly from plants.

As a last resort, if there is insufficient Omega 3 in the diet, the body uses the nearest equivalent Omega 6 or 9. Omega 6s and 9s have different shapes and structures, and do not function in the body in the same way. They are very much second rate emergency substitutes.

7.3   Differences between men and women—Women make about 10 per cent DHA, and 20 per cent EPA, from the mother Omega 3 ALA. Conversion figures are based on western subjects, with western diets. Conversion rates in those with low levels of Omega Six intake, could be well be higher.

Many men make very little DHA, under one per cent, with two per cent as a maximum. The difference in the ability between the sexes, to convert the mother Omega 3 fat to long chain fats, may explain a number of physical, mental, and functional differences between men and women.

Excess of Omega 6 over 3 links to the male characteristics in both men and women. Omega 6 confers largely male characteristics (aggression, impulsiveness, acquisitiveness), and Omega 3 largely female characteristics (softness, more cooperative, more restrained).

Higher levels of Omega 6 metabolism inherently carry a price of greater stress due to higher oxidation. DHA may reduce stress from oxidation. Lower oxidative stress, combined with higher DHA, might link to longevity.

For women, the DHA demands of the reproductive cycle, and greater functional need for DHA, including more neurons in a smaller brain, leads to greater risk of alcoholism, osteoporosis, fertility related issues, depression, neurological decline in old age, and other conditions.

7.4   A little worse each generation–Limited trials suggest that degradation of brain function due to lack of essential fats including Omega 3, may become cumulatively a little worse each generation.

There is limited evidence that as well as being what you eat, you are what your mother ate. There is no reason why this should not work in the other direction. We can influence our genes with diet. Separated identical twins often experience very different health outcomes.

7.5   We cannot make the mother fats–The mother Omega Three and Omega Six fats cannot be made in the body. All other fats can be made in the body. Mother Omega Three and Omega Six can only be obtained in food. [Mother fats;Omega Six–18:2 n6–Linoleic Acid; Omega Three–18:3 n3–Linolenic Acid]

7.6   Making long chain fats–The children of the mother fat linolenic acid include DHA and EPA (see section 5 for names). Long chain Omega Sixes include AA and DPA. The basic Omega Three/Six chain is 18 carbons long.

The body can amazingly add up to another six carbons, making the daisy chain up to 24 carbons long. This is done by a series of chemical reactions. Double bonds are added by further reactions.

Elongation is adding more carbons. Desaturisation is the creation of double bonds. The desaturisation enzymes for Omega Three and Omega Six are called desaturase five and six [p.292].

Other desaturases exist for making other fats. The desaturase process is quite sensitive to a range of factors set out below [11.13]. Blocking of one desaturase, but not another, will change the balance of fats.

Factors that block the desaturase functions, and so our ability to make long chain fats, include sugar, trans fats, and high intake of Omega Six.

Desaturases behave differently at different concentrations of fat in the body. Higher levels of DHA or AA will switch down the creation of long chain fats. High levels of the mother Omega 6 push the system to make Omega 6 long chain fats.

It is very complex and interdependent. Factors such as fat levels, in the blood, fat tissue and brain, may all influence conversion. Some people may have a poorer genetic ability to make long chain fats, but this is not yet clear.

If you cannot make them, you must eat them. Consumption of food sources high in DHA, EPA, etc., is a good insurance to secure an adequate supply of long chain fats, in case you cannot convert the mother fats. Animal food sources like fish, eggs, etc., contain a range of long chain fats, not just DHA and EPA[56].

Clearly if you do not have the mother Omega Three and Six fats in the diet, you will not be able to convert them to the long chain fats, even if your conversion function is AAA rated.

7.7   EPA conversion to DHA–Dr Michael Simpson, Nu-Mega Ingredients Pty, asks if EPA in supplement form is converted to DHA. DHA is to some extent retro-converted to EPA.

7.8   Infants do not make EPA and DHA well–A trial suggested that infants could convert some mother Omega Three to the long chain DHA and EPA, others suggest conversion in infants is very poor. There is considerable variation in outcome and opinion.[57] Factors in the mother's diet, milk formulas, or early foods, may lead to conversion blockages in infants. It may be babies simply do not convert the mother fats, to the long chain children very well.

Quite simply, much is not known. So it seems prudent for a mother to ensure an adequate intake of long chain Omega Threes. Where children are not breastfed, and formula feeds are used, consider the formula content, balance of Omega 3 and 6 mother fats, and long chain fats and short saturated fats. The ratio of fats is very important to infants at many levels (See chapter 23, 23.26, 23.27).

7.9   DHA poor replacement options–

This is applicable to your brain, your heart, yours eyes, your reproductive organs, your skin, and everything else...

The body has second and third redundancy options. In the absence of Omega 3, the body uses the nearest Omega 6, or Omega 9.

These are second grade materials in the context they are used. Like any machine, running on second grade fuel or unsuitable spares, the body will start to go wrong. The more make do and mend, the greater the risk of breakdown.

The substitution of Omega Six DPA for DHA leads to memory function loss, learning disabilities, impaired visual acuity[58], and other losses of neural performance. [If the body lacks DHA, long chain Omega 3 22:6 n3, it will replace it first with the nearest Omega 6, DPA, docosapentaenoic acid, long chain Omega 6 22:5 n6]. Almost all of the DPA information is based on animal trials.

As the body simply selects on chain length, it is logical that alternates of the same chain length will be used. For example for DHA 22 carbons, this would be DPA Omega 3 or 6, both 22 carbons long. If Omega 3s were low, then DPA Omega 6 is second choice available.

In absence, or deficiency of Omega Six, the body will use an Omega 9, with just one double bond [30.34]. The body can make the Omega Nine family from carbohydrates, so this would be the ultimate reserve in times of famine.

7.10   **A load of poo?**–If your digestion is poor, fat is not properly absorbed. Precious Omega Threes could be wasted. This also applies to other nutrients essential to body function, available in the diet in very limited amounts.

YOU ARE WHAT YOU DIGEST.

Undigested expensive nutritious food, or supplements, have no more trouble going down the lavatory pan, than any other sort of food. If your poo is loose, floaty, and greasy, you are likely not absorbing fats properly, not to mention other nutrients. (See also 25.41, 42, 43).

Without adequate Omega Three, you are likely to have inflammation in the gut, so your digestion will be poor. Permanent low-level inflammation leaves the body's repair system on constant standby.

This stresses the body. It could make you more sensitive to minor insults, allergens, hay fever, etc., as well as making you more prone to inflammatory conditions such as arthritis.

Intestinal inflammation can lead to a coating of mucus. Mucus may accompany stools. Excess mucus stops food contact with the gut lining.

Multiple mega whammy. The downward spiral is self-reinforcing. As inflammation gets worse, digestion gets worse. Fat absorption suffers. The Omega Threes and Omega Sixes become more imbalanced. This imbalance leads to greater inflammation.

For those taking fat absorption blockers or similar products, it may be multiple mega whammy, plus compounding the problem. If fat absorption products block the intake of essential Omega Threes, and they are already at low levels in the diet, the consequences could very damaging on a long term basis. Indications that your digestion may not be working include:

- ☞ Foul-smelling faeces
- ☞ Pale stool
- ☞ Loose stool
- ☞ Greasy stool [60]

Fat blockers have been linked with digestive problems. [59] I raise the issue; I don't know the answers as to the impact of fat blockers on digestion of Omega 3. If you have problems talk to your doctor, and discuss digestion with him or her.

7.11   Why industry and we love fats—

☞ We are programmed to seek them out and have an inbuilt taste for them.

☞ A myth has been built up that polyunsaturates are good for you, no matter in what proportion type or quantity. Until recently the myth included trans fats (Hydrogenated margarines, etc.).

☞ They are cheap.

☞ They have become a staple market agricultural product. They have commercial momentum behind them.

☞ The food industry will give us what it perceives we want.

☞ They 'improve' the texture of food.

☞ Fats can be chosen to extend shelf life.

☞ Omega Six has a better shelf life than Omega Three.

☞ Trans fats extend shelf life thus simplifying distribution, production, scheduling, and decreasing wastage.

7.12   Rising fat intake—Fat intake has substantially risen in the last 100 years. It has also changed significantly in the last 50 years. Vegetable oil consumption is rising globally, including in poorer Nations [3.26].

Many common vegetable oils are high in Omega Six, and generally very low in Omega Three. Some have fairly low Omega Six e.g. virgin olive and palm oil but almost no Omega Three. Some like soy have some Omega Three [p287]. A diet based on olive oil but low in Omega Three, could still give rise to an Omega Three : Six imbalance.

It is not denied that excess saturated fat is an issue. Our ancestors had never seen artificial saturated fat. Animal fats of wild grazers were lower in quantity and more balanced than fats of grain raised farm stock.

7.13   Low-level whole body inflammation—Permanent low-level, all body inflammation has been suggested as a condition. Obesity has been described as an inflammatory condition. Fat stores, and the supporting cellular matrix, are a major source of inflammatory cytokines, including IL6 and CRP. Cytokines are connected with immune response.

An effective immune response is essential to health. A system that is on high alert for too long is likely to be less effective, and respond disproportionately. Omega 6 puts the immune system on permanent alert. Cytokines, signalling compounds [30.7] appear to recruit prostaglandins (the Omega Six products)[i].

---

i   Demonstration of a novel technique to quantitatively assess inflammatory mediators and cells in rat knee joints. J Inflamm (Lond). 2007 Jun 13;4:13 Barton NJ, Stevens DA, Hughes JP, Rossi AG, Chessell IP, Reeve AJ, McQueen DS. Division of Neuroscience, University of Edinburgh, Medical College, 1 George Sq, Edinburgh.

The immune system cytokines, and others agents, are linked with a wide range of conditions associated with obesity, and are well-known risk factors for diabetes, hypertension, heart disease, osteoarthritis, hyperlipidemia, stroke, sleep apnea syndrome, and some types of cancer.

Heart diseases in the industrial world account for 40 per cent of deaths. Markers of inflammation, IL6 and CRP, are strongly related to waist circumference, and waist hip measurement in women [61]. Other conditions reported as having raised IL6 and CRP include:

☞ Dementia, "the combination of high CRP and high IL6 was associated with risk of vascular dementia". [62]

☞ Hypertension. [63]

☞ Arthritis [64] [IL6 IL10].

☞ Cardiovascular disease. [65]

☞ Gestational diabetes. [66]

☞ Melanoma [67] [IL6 and IL12].

☞ Prostrate cancer. [68]

☞ Lung cancer. [69]

☞ Breast cancer. [70]

☞ Several chronic inflammatory autoimmune diseases. [71]

☞ Inflammatory bowel disease, peritonitis, rheumatoid arthritis, asthma, and colon cancer, progression can be interrupted in animals by interfering with IL6. [72][73]

☞ A search for IL6 on NCBI/PubMed (an online medical trials database) produced 1500+ reference and links to trials

Omega Three and Omega Six are yin and yang. Omega Three "yin" is linked with peace and tranquillity. Omega Six "yang" is linked with aggression. You can't have one without the other, for the body to be in harmony.

Too much Omega Six in fat storage and circulation, and not enough Omega Three to shut it down, combined with a condition the body regards as inflammatory, like arthritis, IBS or vascular disease, or obesity, and you have low inflammation that does not switch off. You have created a self-fuelling cycle.

The system is on constant alert, like an engine out of control, which will in the long-term cause degradation and breakdown. Our cells are no different.

Cell stress results in leaky cell walls, degraded immune response, damage, and finally genetic damage and terminal breakdown. The off-switches are the long chain Omega Three Fats, DHA and EPA, which block Omega Six Activity.

If you cannot make the inflammatory Omega 6 off-switches, EPA and DHA, or do not have them in your diet, you have no off-switches. A house full of lights you cannot switch off.

7.14   **Prevention is better than cure**–In health terms, prevention has to be better than cure. Drugs and medical developments are truly wondrous. I do not in any way wish to denigrate the ethos of those in the industry. But for the complex inflammatory conditions, single target agents have a very long way to go before they match the body's complexity of interlinking pathways.

We are increasingly seeing unexpected long-term effects of some medications. I am a great respecter of modern medicine, deeply grateful to those that give their lives to it, and very highly appreciative of it. However, I am saddened that prevention for western conditions is not given more weight, as being the first step.

The increasing costs of medical intervention and a finite public budget, will result in rationing on some basis, be it financial, seriousness of case or personal circumstances. The prospect of rationing, and future restriction, reinforces the importance of prevention, and personal responsibility for health.

7.15   **Gene expression altered by foods**–Food environment, lifestyle, and toxin exposure alter gene expression. Diet is an environmental factor, with which we have regular and hugely intimate contact. Genes are trendy these days. The vision in the media is cure by gene.

It is important to understand the difference between gene expression and mutation. Inherited mutations are rare. We are all different but the genetic differences between us are relatively small, if at times very crucial.

Every cell carries a copy of your very long string of genes. Each individual gene codes instructions to the body, but only when switched on or expressed.

Many trials have mapped changes in gene expression by significant factors for different Omega Three and Six fat balances. Gene expression differences can be ten times and more for different diets. Genes subject to significant alteration of expression included BRAC and HER2.

The ability of our genes to alter the way the body functions, by switching on and off in response to things such as diet, enables us to adapt to changing environmental circumstances.

Response at a genetic level to food is arguably a basis for our evolutionary or design adaption, to changing circumstances, including food. Where environmental circumstances including diet are outside the body's traditional operating parameters, unusual outcomes can be expected in the form of body malfunction or disease.

7.16   **Provoking dietary facts**–Seventy-plus per cent of daily energy intake in the U.S. is comprised of processed dairy products, refined sugars, refined vegetable oils and alcohol–none of which our hunter gather ancestors would have had access to in significant quantity, or at all. Refined sugar intake in England increased from 6.8 kilos in 1815, to 54.5 kilos in 1970. Our ancestors may have consumed 2 kilos of honey a year.

8

EVOLUTION–OMEGA SIX, NATURE'S FERTILITY CONTROLLER

8   **Evolution**–Omega Six, nature's fertility controller– [Abbreviations listed at 1.1]. Everything is interlinked and interdependent, like a giant highly sophisticated cats cradle. It is all exceeding complex and intertwined, and I have only managed a misty overview, which I try to bring to you.

Every door opened leads on to more. Every tiny area is a specialism on its own. The point of this next section, and chapter 23, is not a need to understand every detail, as it does not alter the conclusion, but simply to see that everything is highly interdependent. Omega 6 is the lead external controller that cannot be made by the body, and reflects the environment.

The body's design and operating specifications, are constructed round a given, that Omega 3 and 6 will be supplied more or less in balance, or there will be more long chain Omega 3 from marine sources. Omega 6 is a measure nature's health in the environment. If there is Omega 6 there is food to eat, plants, and the animals that feed off them.

The Omega 6 mother fat is the primary control mechanism, because it cannot be got in any other way except through diet. Other products which are entirely necessary to life cannot be used as regulators of fertility because they;

☞   Have more than one source - E.g. Proteins can be obtained from both marine and land sources, so do not reflect the fertility of the land. Omega Three can be obtained in quantity from marine products.

☞   Can be made in the body - E.g. Many proteins can be made in the body

☞   Are not dependent on the state of the environment - E.g. The availability of minerals is not exclusively dependent on the fertility of the environment

Omega Six is nature's key controller of the body's fertility. Omega Six links us to the fecundity of the earth. High levels of Omega Six are found in seeds and nuts. Seeds and nuts are the consequence of a fertile environment, flourishing plants, and nourishment being available, for every level of the food chain.

Omega Six products, like PGE2, indirectly control some, if not all, of the enzymes, that convert pregnenolone, the exclusive raw material, into sex hormones, and steroids [23.11.b]. Cholesterol is made from pregnenolone. Omega 6 as a regulator makes sense as an evolutionary and survival strategy.

The availability of background hormones needed for fertility, is determined by the amount of stored Omega Six, and the amount of body fat. Obesity and anorexia are link to hormone imbalance. Fats cells make the same hormones for men and women. DHA is the moderator, and a hormone dimmer switch.

This is an Omega Six centric view of design evolution, and control of human fertility, based on Omega 6 being an external agent exclusively available in diet.

8.1   **Evolution - In the beginning**—It is likely that fats, at the simplest levels, were in the earliest primordial soup at the beginning. In evolutionary and design terms, fats do not come much behind carbon and oxygen in importance. The shortest fats are very simple carbon chains containing carbon, oxygen, and hydrogen. *They are far more fundamental in body structure and operation, than any food-based supplement like ginseng or purple berries*. Ginseng and purple berries came along far later than fats in evolutionary or design terms.

8.2   **Environmental human fertility controller**— Omega Six is the regulator, by the environment, over human fertility. The quantity of Omega Six in the diet, influences adipose and visceral fat depositions. Adipose and visceral fat deposition controls background hormones levels.

Rates of manufacture of hormones in fat tissues appear to be sex independent [74]. In a high Omega 6 diet, more body fat = higher Omega 6 = higher hormone levels, and future hormone production reserves.

Stable fat reserves are required for pregnancy, and breastfeeding. Adequate general fat, as well as Omega Six, is essential to breeding too. Excess fat and Omega 6 stores, on a permanent basis, may increase the risk of a number of conditions. Animals do not carry high fat reserves on a year round basis.

All the sex hormones, including oestrogen progesterone and testosterone, are indirectly controlled by Omega Six. The system is complex, and inter links to other agents as well.

Leptin is a body fat sensing hormone. Leptin links into the hormone pathways too. Leptin is not an external agent as it is made by the body.

IF Omega Six levels were high in the environment, so were sugars in fruit and berries, carbohydrates in other plants, and fat from animal sources. To take advantage of scarce seasonal supplies, and the fecundity of the earth, Omega Six triggers and comes with a general 'store fat' instruction.

Carbohydrates are turned to fats, and saved with ingested fats. Fructose can be made into fat directly, bypassing control mechanisms. Omega Six sets the body to prepare for breeding.

When body fats fall to very low levels, fertility drastically falls. This was observed after World War II, and is observed in women with fat deficiencies. Excess Omega Six fat stores, on a long-term basis, are a new phenomenon.

8.3   No 'stop storing fat' button –

High Omega Six triggers the body to store fat. There is no off button. Nature never needed one.

Long-term Omega 6 dietary excess never happens in the natural world. Omega 6 has only been available in quantity since the intervention of man.

We alter the Omega 3:6 balance in the food we eat. We reduce Omega 3s and increase Omega 6s in food, by crop selection, feeding grains to animals, and industrial processing of foods and oils. We have vastly increased Omega 6 intake by industrial farming, extraction, and cheap high Omega 6 vegetable oils.

8.4   **Not a design issue** – The body was designed to function within a broad range of environmental conditions. Those environmental conditions never included permanent excess of Omega 6, and lack of Omega 3. Nature never produced vast levels of foods rich in Omega 6, (seeds and nuts or bottles of oil) year round, and year on year.

Our excess intake of Omega Six, takes us well outside our design operating criteria. Food alters gene expression. Absence of food can lead to genetic mutation[i]. Dietary change can lead to genetic mutation[ii]. For example in cattle rearing areas, like Europe, and East Africa, we adapted to digest dairy products.

This demonstrates genetic change is food responsive. In trials small dietary changes in a wider pattern over time, have produced genetic change in birds, and flies. *Excess Omega 6, and a deficit of Omega 3, are massive dietary changes, because of the very fundamental effects of them, on the body's operations.*

A host of factors, suggest that Omega Three and Omega Six in the diet, would have been reasonably balanced. Omega 3:6 ratios may have ranged between, at a guess, 1:4 to 4:1. Ratios now commonly seen, of 1:10 and up to 1:50, were never on the design drawing board.

Brains in all wild animals have a 1:1 Omega 3:6 ratio. Run anything well outside its design parameters, and sooner or later it will start to break down.

---

i   Adaptive divergence vs. environmental plasticity: tracing local genetic adaptation of metamorphosis traits in salamanders Molecular Ecology, Volume 13, Number 6, June 2004 , pp. 1665-1677(13).
     Authors: Weitere M. Tautz D. Neumann D. Steinfartz S.
ii   Nutritional and genetic adaptation of galliform birds: implications for hand-rearing and restocking Tuija Liukkonen-Anttila Department of Biology, University of Oulu, Finland.

We are breaking down. Is increasing illness a result of immune and inflammatory stress, and body systems breakdown, due to usage of Omega 3 and 6, outside specified design parameters?

The effects I guess are compounded by the body's efforts to circumvent the raw material shortage, develop new production processes and procedures, to take account of fast change in raw material supplies.

The body, in the absence of other options, may be making random directed attempts, to adapt to a new food supply. Unsuccessful attempts at adaptation might be manifested as 'diseases' of varying intensity.

8.5   Neural function and behaviour—Omega Six modifies behaviour, through mechanisms including, the hormone and steroid pathways, brain chemical levels, brain cell membrane structure, mitochondrial function, sleep disturbance, and increased inflammatory and immune function. Higher levels of Omega Six, and fat deposits, mean higher hormone levels.

Deficits of DHA have been linked to behavioural issues, lower cognitive function, lower intelligence, suicide, depression, aggression, impulsiveness, criminal activity including paedophilia, and possibly murder, etc. Omega Six deficit did not impact on sensory, and motor skills, in the same way.

The different roles of Omega 3 and 6 would add to the theory, that a balance of Omega 3 and 6 is the expected operating norm, and Omega 3 deficits, combined with excess Omega 6, have no place in body systems.

In the modern world, alcohol usage, in the absence of an adequate supply of Omega Threes, is a compounding factor in depleting DHA.

Your brain needs a balance of both AA and DHA to work properly. It is that simple.

8.6   Controls of the menstrual cycle—PGE2 is a product of Omega Six, which controls aromatase and similar enzymes, which control sex hormone production [Fig 23.11.b]. Omega Three limits hormone and steroid production, by limiting production of the enzyme raw material, Omega Six AA, and its products such as PGE2 and P450. Omega Three is part of a cyclical process. Higher background Omega Six, distorts sex hormone, and steroid levels.

During the fertility cycle oestrogen levels rise. In women, higher oestrogen produces higher DHA. Higher DHA shuts down the Omega Six AA production pathways, which shut down the source of PGE2. Lower PGE2 results in less aromatase, and thus oestrogen and androgen production.

I guess that the production of the egg, and thickening of the uterus, utilises high levels of DHA, to make the required cell membranes. This keeps hormone levels high, in the first and second half of the cycle.

When fertilisation does not take place, and the uterus no longer continues to thicken, levels of free DHA would rise, so shutting down PGE2 and related enzymes, and cutting the hormone levels.

Add time delays, and this is a possible basis of the monthly fertility cycle, controlled by an external agent, that reflects the fecundity of the earth; Omega 6.

The cycle is interrupted by pregnancy. The foetus has high DHA and lower AA demands, leaving a free excess of AA, so the fat elongation pathways, and PGE2 production remain upgraded, until the end of pregnancy.

The fertility cycle breaks down if adequate DHA is not available. I suggest from the body's perspective if there is inadequate DHA, the body thinks it is because DHA is being used to make cells for a new baby, and not because we have stopped eating it, and or blocked the pathways to make it.

If there is inadequate free DHA, the fertility cycle is incompletely shut down, possibly because the body thinks it is pregnant, or is confused as to its fertility status. (See chapter 23, where the subject is covered in more detail if required).

8.7   Omega Threes not significantly stored—Omega Threes are not significantly stored in the body. This would suggest that in evolutionary or design terms, we were accustomed to a regular supply. An adequate supply of greens [and low fat intake and no fat conversion blockers] may just supply adequate Omega Three and Omega Six. I prefer the idea, that the need for regular intake of Omega Three, is consistent with man developing as a shore dweller. Lack of storage of Omega Three is fundamental. It implies and requires constant replenishment of Omega 3 in diet, by marine sources, or vegetable sources and conversion.

8.8   A little history—Fats are considered to rank with oxygen in terms of developmental importance [75]—

☞ **Mitochondria**—At some point in time, some energy producing cells, got together with a fat producing or collecting organism, and came to a mutual understanding. Mitochondria supplied energy, and chemical factory facilities, in return for fats and a host. Mitochondria are the original symbiotes. They have their own DNA. We have 'alien' life forms in us. Mitochondria still have their own special unique lipid type Cardiolipin. [77] Cardiolipin is found in the inner leaf of the mitochondrial membrane. Cardiolipin is the most unsaturated fat in the body. Cardiolipin in normal circumstances contains high levels of Omega Three. DHA through cardiolipin is likely key to mitochondrial function, and cell death.[iii] Appropriate cell death and replacement is key to health. Mis-function of cellular controls have a function in cancers. Look after your mitochondria. Ensure they have enough DHA through diet, and melatonin antioxidant protection through quality sleep.

---

iii   Lipids, cardiolipin and apoptosis: a greasy licence to kill Cell Death and Differentiation (2002) 9, 234-236 M Degli EspostiCancer Research Campaign Molecular Pharmacology Group, School of Biological Sciences, University of Manchester, Oxford Road, Manchester M13 9PT, UK.

☞ **Algae**–Fats go back billions of years. "Marine microalgae, or phytoplankton, provide the food base which supports the entire animal population of the open sea. The microalgae are the primary source of EPA and DHA." [76] Bluegreen algae produced proteins, carbohydrates, Omega Three rich fatty acids, and oxygen. Once the oxygen level rose, life began to take off. The oceans were the primary repositories of life for a very long time. Life developed, or was designed, around the available food sources of Omega Three rich algae.

☞ **Demise of Dinosaurs**–Following the demise of the Dinosaurs, plants changed, and became flowering and seed bearing. This was the new land of Omega Six. [78] Much higher levels of Omega Six, allowed the development of new Omega Six dependent species, with on-board gestation. If you need to travel to follow food sources, the ability to carry your young is a significant advantage. At a practical level, the ability to carry young onboard allows longer gestation periods. Longer gestation allowed more sophisticated development or design. Protected gestation requires a hugely complex control system. Omega Six sits at the top of probably the body's most influential, and powerful, set of systems and control mechanisms.

☞ **Waterside gatherers**–There are some strong arguments that we evolved by lake and shore line. High levels of Omega Three would have been available to support increasing brain size. A constant source of Omega Three would complement our preferential usage of it as a fuel. It would also explain why we do not store Omega Three, to a significant degree beyond a minimal requirement. Highly nutritional foods could be easily gathered by all ages, without the need for highly specialised hunting skills (clams, worms, shore crabs, etc.). The evolution of fire, to extract nutrients like starches, was not an absolute necessity. Evidence of early H. Sapiens is also found around the Rift Valley lakes, and up the Nile Corridor into the Middle East. Recent evidence suggests man's ancestors had jaws less well equipped for vegetation, than some of his counterparts who did not survive in evolutionary or design terms. It is suggested that restriction of food sources, to land-based foods, as postulated by the savannah and other hypotheses, would have led to degeneration of the brain and vascular system, as happened without exception in all other land-based apes and mammals as they evolved larger bodies [79]

8.9   Fecundity of our environment – *Omega Six links us to the environment through food. Before supermarkets, the need for food determined our survival strategies, fertility, and breeding patterns. Food availability, and consequent territorial need, impacted on breeding, social interaction, cooperation and aggression.*

We have acquired a survival advantage, by automatically responding to our environment. We are inextricably linked to it. The body is designed to respond to what is going on about it. We can only get Omega Three and Omega Six by eating them. This means we need either a constant and plentiful supply of primary foods containing Omega 3 and 6, very large quantities of greens, or creatures that have concentrated them. Nuts and seeds would have been seasonal.

We were in the same basket, as all animals. It became an evolutionary and design advantage, not to breed when food and resources were scarce, and to go forth and multiply when times were fruitful. Nature chose as the main yardstick Omega Three and Omega Six. The mother Omega Six is only found in large quantities in seeds and nuts. Long chain Omega Threes are only primarily found in oily fish, and wild eggs. Omega Three in marine sources were probably more constant, and less weather sensitive, than Omega Six in seeds and nuts.

There are no seeds if the land is infertile, but Omega Three is still likely to be available in fish. Seeds were time consuming and energy demanding to gather, as well as being seasonal and rare. Seeds reflect the fecundity of nature. So by design or selection, Omega Six became the biofeedback link between the land and humans. We were programmed to breed when times were good, and go into economy mode when they were not.

Breeding age, puberty, the menstrual cycle, male and female fertility hormones are all linked to Omega Six. Responding to seasonal availability like other creatures of the earth, conferred further survival advantages. Limiting our number to those the land would support, and modifying our behaviour to each other, based on the fecundity of the land, was a good strategy.

When food was more plentiful, we had energy to spare, and ease rearing another generation. [80] As a survival strategy in good times, it would be an evolutionary advantage to be more aggressive, acquisitive, territorial, impulsive, selfish, and less cooperative. Excess Omega Six confers these characteristics.

In lean times, energy had to be conserved by humans to survive. In lean times, tentative cooperation was a better survival strategy than fighting. *Our diet moderated our behaviour without us having any say in the matter, to provide us with the best chance of survival. Nature presented enough challenges to survival without adding to them. We have broken our Omega Six link to nature. We have excessively overloaded Omega Six.*

Excess Omega Six pushes our hormone and chemical pathways to making us more aggressive, acquisitive, territorial, impulsive, selfish, and less cooperative. We see those behavioural characteristics in today's society.

8.10   Outside design parameters—We now have a situation the body has never seen before. We are massively oversupplied with Omega Six, well above and beyond the design parameters. We alter our behaviour automatically, and unconsciously, to this huge glut of Omega Six.

We are possibly, at an automatic functional level, altering our behaviour with excess Omega 6 fat stores, and becoming more aggressive, impulsive, and acquisitive.

Excess Omega Six brings about early puberty. We store fat. We make higher levels of sex hormones from our fat stores. We are simply responding to our built-in programme.

Our ancestral memory tells us this glut is certain not to last forever. Go breed whilst the going is good, it tells us. But the Omega Six gauge has gone beyond the red line, and well off the scale.

The body simply has no normal way to deal with this level of excess Omega 6, over 3. The body has no ancestral memory, or experience, of this much Omega 6.

Omega Six is the precursor of inflammatory repair systems, and related reproductive pathways. Chronic Omega Six oversupply, and vastly excessive body stores of Omega Six in our fat, pushes the body into a constant state of low-level inflammation. We are on permanent alert. Our sleep shutdown immune and repair systems, start to breakdown (melatonin indirectly requires DHA). Inflammatory conditions are more easily triggered. 'Western' diseases including arthritis, asthma, and diabetes proliferate.

A viscous cycle of low-level inflammation starts, vascular disease, IBS, asthma, and sleep degradation etc. Excess Omega 6 intake and fats stores, combined with a lack of the moderating Omega 3s, fuel the inflammatory cycle. The inflammation cycle never shuts down, because the Omega Three required is missing. Immune functions are stressed to the point of exhaustion, on permanent high alerts, due to excess Omega 6, but without related invaders to deal with.

This time we have inadvertently, with the best intentions, found a way to meddle in a fundamental evolutionary or design control mechanism. In addition to behaviour modification that threatens to undermine society, and the setting up of an inflammatory platform for 'western' disease, the body is being stressed.[iv]

Further, Omega Six may open the pathways to evolution, by activating stem cell mechanisms outside pregnancy, that could lead to random cell mutations and greater risk of cancers.

Animals show genetic mutation in response to captivity, food and environmental factors. It is only logical, that the body would respond at a genetic level, to a lack of arguably the most fundamental mitochondrial function fat, DHA, and excess of a key functional regulator, Omega 6. Stem cells and cancer are very much still areas of vigorous debate, in the research world.

Are dietary changes so rapid and significant the body simply cannot cope?

---

iv   Mechanisms for ovarian cycle disruption by immune/inflammatory stress. R Stress. 2002 Jun;5(2):101–12 Reproductive Sciences Program and Department of Physiology, University of Michigan, Ann Arbor, MI 48109, USA.

8.11   Redesign is not a short-term option—The inability of the body to manufacture Omega Three and Omega Six fats, has tremendous consequences. These fats are so deeply rooted in our past, and we are so long lived and complex, that redesign is not an option. The point is Omega Three and Omega Six predate broccoli, ginseng, gingko, vitamins, enzymes, drugs, and people.

Fats were in the daddy and mummy mix of nutritional factors. Fats are of fundamental importance, over and above almost all other dietary factors. In times past, the link to the environment provided a survival advantage. We now have developed ways to break our link with nature. But we have no mechanism to naturally modify and adapt our body design in such a short time [26.10].

We have to work out the rules, which lead to the creation design criteria. We have to learn to live within those rules. Our design rules are fundamental, in the same way as the instruction manual, telling you not to put diesel into a petrol engine car.

We have survived droughts, famines, and exoduses. We have adapted to an amazing range of lifestyles. We have survived and derived nutrition from everything, from old leather, to bark, insects, grass, and algae. Through the food chain, we are most likely connected to most living things on the planet. Animals utilise substances from their food for all sorts of exotic uses. Cats eating grass is an example. Why should we be different?

We retain a genetic memory of our adaptations. Many foods have very large numbers of active ingredients (40, 50). We have learned to use these and respond to them. We are unable to make the sort of changes our new western diet is demanding, in the time span of maybe 50 to 100 years. Evolution does not happen in a time span of 50 to 100 years. We are unable to cope with the excess Omega Six, and lack of Omega Three. We are maybe forcing the body to try random genetic mutation to adapt. The manifestation of poor adaption could be uncontrolled cell activity.

The current intake Omega 3:6 balance of 1:10, and above is totally outside our design parameters. You do not put fat straight out of the fryer, in your diesel car, because your car manual tells you not to. Why do we treat ourselves much worse, than we treat our cars?

8.12   Our ancestors' diet—Our hunter-gatherer ancestors would have had limited, and seasonal access, to seeds and nuts, and wild meat products. Domestication has given us access to grain and dairy products, to which we have 10,000–40,000 years to adapt. Some people have developed genes that assist; others struggle with these foods.

We have developed methods of preparation, that make grains and dairy products more digestible, such as fermentation, cooking and sprouting. Industrial vegetable oils production (excluding olive), refined grains, and sugars are totally new in the last 100 or so years.

We have stripped these food of their accompanying nutrients. We were not designed to run on these fuels. We cannot run on these refined foods any more than the average car can run on pure ethanol. We have no chance of developing genetic adaptations in 100 or so years.

8.13   Evolutionary discord–Omega Six was a scarce environmental resource. We have increased the availability and intake of Omega Six, beyond any previous experience. We have also substantially reduced our intake of Omega Threes. We have introduced other previously unseen refined foods, such as sugar, and trans fats, that block the body's pathways to make long chain fats.

Our genes are out of sync with our environment. Are 'Western' conditions diseases of genetic asynchronicity with the environment? In a sense, are we witnessing self imposed, evolutionary, pressure and consequence?

Are diseases of diet, our way of trying to adapt to a new environment, in the face of very rapid change? If so it is evidently easier to bring our diet back within our operating parameters, than suffer the dreadful consequences we are self-inflicting.

8.14   Shrinking brains, a real possibility–Brain size can actually permanently shrink, over several generations of Omega Three [DHA and EPA] deficiency. This has been observed in animals, including dogs with very large litters and inadequate nutrition.

It is argued the only way our ancestors could have had sufficient supply of DHA, over a very long term was by living as shore dwellers. It raises the spectre of the shrinking brain in the face of DHA deficit. [81] Women's brains are smaller but have more neurons. Reversible shrinkage is seen in pregnancy. Shrinkage is also seen in association with Alzheimer's, dementia, and diabetes.

8.15   Viruses and inflammation–Viruses can switch on production of the long chain Omega Six AA [82] to increase inflammation to serve their own ends. Sepsis and pneumonia have both been reported as showing beneficial results from Omega 3.

Is this mechanism more widely available to bacteria and viruses or cancers? High Omega Three lipid infusions benefit a number of medical conditions from cachexia to psoriasis, and have been demonstrated to reduce hospital and ICU stay duration. Response in psoriasis from infusion, was much greater than that by oral administration.

Infusion may provide possibilities for adjunctive treatment. Balancing the Omega Threes and Omega Sixes, may in the future be a factor in the control of some viral conditions such as the human papillomavirus HPV. Is excess Omega 6 a factor driving increases in susceptibility to hospital infections? [See *Omega Three in Clinical Nutrition*].

9
FOODS SOURCES OF
OMEGA THREE AND OMEGA SIX

9.1   Greens, roots, and fruits–[Abbreviations listed at 1.1] The Omega 3 and 6 **mother** fats, are found on average in equal quantity in greens plants, roots and fruit flesh, which we and animals eat. This might explain why we appear to work best, when the Omega 3 and 6 mother fats are more or less in balance.

Greens, and animals, would have been our staples as hunter-gatherers. When intakes of the mother fats are low, we convert a bigger proportion to long chain fats. *Animals contain some long chain fats, **plants nuts and seeds do not***.

Levels of Omega Three and Six mother fats are low in greens, approximately around 1 part in a 1,000. [Sprouts higher, cabbage lower] Some greens, roots and fruit flesh have more Omega 6, and some more Omega 3. On an average, it about evens out. Omega 3 in foods crops has fallen with selective cultivation. [83]

9.2   Nuts–Nuts and seeds do not contain long chain fats, only mother fats. Nuts are generally high in mother Omega Six. Very limited exceptions like walnuts contain significant mother Omega Three, about 10 per cent. But a walnut still has about five times as much Omega Six, as Omega Three [p287].

So to balance the high Omega Six in nuts, sources high in mother Omega Three would still be needed.

9.3   Seeds–Seeds and grains are seasonal. Grains contain 1–2 parts of mother fats per hundred. For instance, 192 grams of wheat, contains 1.7 grams of mother Omega Six, and almost no mother Omega Three.

Seeds contain more. 146 grams of sunflower seed for instance, contains 15 grams of mother Omega Six, and a fraction of a gram of mother Omega Three. Omega Six is by far the more common content in most seeds.

The seed exceptions with a higher Omega Three content, include flax perilla and others [30.31]. Soy has some Omega Three. Be aware seeds are generally high in Omega Six, when looking at your Omega 3:6 balance.

9.4   **Meat fat and offal**–[See 11.25 11.17 13.8 13.9] Herbivores like us, can change the mother fats into the longer chain children. An animal's fat profile depends like, us on what it has eaten. Meat would have been seasonal for many.

The long chain Omega Three and Six content of beef cuts is relatively low, between one and six parts per thousand. Total Omega Six in meat is about 1 part in 500, and total Omega Three about one part in 2,500. Offal has higher levels of EFAs.

Carnivores including your cat do not make long chain fats very well, which is why they choose offal first. They have essential need of long chain Omegas. [84]

High levels of corn oil, and absence of long chain Omega 3, result in a high level of stillbirths and deformities in felines. Low levels of corn oil allowed healthy litters [85]. Diabetes is increasing in cats [Check Labels].

The Omega Three:Six balances in animals like us depends on what they eat. Grains fed herbivores have a much lower Omega Three:Six ratios than grass-fed animals, which is visible in their milk. Grass fed animals, and their products contain more Omega 3, than grain fed animals.

Wild ranging chickens' eggs had 10 times as much Omega Three (17.7 mg per gram) as Washington DC supermarket eggs (1.7 mg per gram). The Omega 3:6 ratio of true free range eggs was 1:1.3, and of the Washington DC supermarket eggs was 1:19.9, and no doubt is little different in many other supermarkets. [86] Adequate supplies of Omega Threes are required for effective neural function.

9.5   **Fish - Fat energy and storage**–Fish and shellfish would have been relatively plentiful for our shore dwelling ancestors. Fish, shellfish, and marine animals contain high levels of Omega 3 and much less Omega 6. Sea food contains a mix of fats, mainly long chain but also some mother fats. A diet high in marine foods would have high levels of long chain Omega 3s and some Omega 6s. Mother fats in marine animals are quite low.

Omega Three encourages fat burn for warmth, which may be a mechanism to deal with excess supply over the body's minimal process and structural needs. Omega Six encourages storage. Fish do not make Omega Three and Omega Six. They harvest it and may convert it to longer fats.

Lean fish have a low percentage of fat, Cod one per cent, Flat fish one per cent, Sea Bass four per cent, Halibut seven per cent, and Plaice seven per cent, of which most is Omega Three. The oily fish like Mackerel have about 24 per cent fat. Omega Threes in wild fish are 10 to 12 times higher than Omega Sixes. Farmed fish have more fat, but a far worse Omega Three : Six ratio, 1:1 rather than 10:1 and contain much more Omega Six than wild fish.

9.6   **Fish - DHA and EPA**–100 grams of Mackerel will provide about three grams of Omega Three of which about a half is DHA (1500 mg. = 3tps cod liver oil approx.), where as Cod will only provide a 10th of that (150 mg.). Vegetarian DHA and EPA made from algae are available. The question of alternate sources, sustainability, fish farming, etc., is considered in chapter 26.

10

BEST OR WORST, IT'S NO QUICK FIX

10   Best or worst, it's no quick fix −[Abbreviations listed at 1.1] At the best or worse this is not a quick fix. Balancing the Omega Threes and Sixes will take time, and cannot be taken out of the context of a need for a varied diet, high in nutrient dense foods. [Chapter. 13]

There are several members of the Omega 3 and 6 families. They all have essential and different roles. [Chapter 5].

Excess Omega 6 LA takes body processes well outside our design specs. We actively store Omega Six [25.1]. Excess Omega 6 in our diet has taken body ratios from around 5 per cent 40 years ago to 10 to 25 per cent today.

Membranes are largely made of fat. The composition of the cell membranes controls many functions in the body. Fat in the cell membrane reflects diet and stored fat. High levels of stored Omega 6 in body fat result in a high content of Omega 6 in the cell membranes. Omega 3s balance the action of Omega 6.

The body evolved or was designed to work within specific operating parameters; to function optimally mother Omega 3 and 6 intake need to be near balanced.

FOR OMEGA 3 TO WORK FIRST YOU HAVE TO EAT IT

10.1   At the worst−If I and those I cite are wrong, it is still good news. Medical circles accept that Omega 3s improve your cardiovascular health.

10.2   At the best−At the best, there is significant evidence, balancing Omega 3s and 6s reduces your risk profile for, and postpones, a long list of conditions.

Balancing 3 and 6 will save families, and particularly the young, a great deal of suffering and heartache. It will save lots of money, to use for other conditions.

Balancing 3 and 6 will help us to be more caring, intelligent, and less aggressive individuals. It will improve digestion and so reduce food intake. It will allow the farming resources to be used for more nutrient dense healthier crops.

10.3   No quick fix—The half-life of adipose tissue is 600 + days—The impact of diet, on health, is long-term and insidious. It takes nearly two years to make a 50 per cent change in your body fat. [87]

The fat in the bloodstream will change quite rapidly, in response to dietary change, but continue to reflect underlying stored Omega 6. Much more Omega 6 than 3 is stored. Fat in breast tissue will take some months to reflect changes. Changes in fat content are still being observed at year five. Your fat is a reflection of your last few years' diet. The change is inversely exponential.

IBS can reduce fat absorption, which will take a while to correct. An Omega 3 splurge will help, but in absence of continuing supply will simply wash back out. The mother Omega 6 is stored, little Omega 3 is stored.

Balancing Omega 3 and 6 mother fats is key. Regular supply of long chain Omega 3s (which will come with some long chain Omega 6) is also essential.

10.4   We are all different—No absolute rules—We are all biologically different. We have different characteristics. But we cannot escape that what we have in common, binds us far more fundamentally than our differences.

Much is made of genes. Caution is needed. Pellagra is a condition originally believed to be genetic, but in fact is diet-based. Separated identical twins often exhibit very different disease profiles. Adopted children have been reported as having similar disease outcomes to their host families.

The increase in 'western' diseases is linked to lifestyles change. The rate of change is far too fast for 'western' disease to be due to genetic mutation. But change may be due in part to gene expression, the number of copies of a gene that are 'switched on' in each cell, by factors like diet or environment .

Different diets switch on different genes, or combinations of genes by different amounts. Food has significant effect on gene expression.

Within limits there are broad rules of life, except nobody has yet got around to writing a reliable operators' manual. Voluntary or unavoidable evasion of the design operating parameters, will result in us ceasing to function as efficiently as we should, or at all.

10.5   Personal responsibility—We have to take responsibility for developing the best health profile that we can. We are not averages. We are all different. Future treatment costs are likely to be unaffordable for many.

11

DIETARY BASICS OF OMEGAS THREE, SIX, NINE, AND OTHER FATS

11.1   **Balance**—[Abbreviations listed at 1.1] Diet is about variety, balance, and whole food sources. Excess of any product abstracted from its source may give rise to other issues. That applies even to fish oil and DHA products. The removal of some pollutants by molecular distillation is a counter argument in favour of fish oil as against whole fish. It is a matter of balance, and a reminder about the consequences of polluting our food sources.

11.2   **Danger Vegetable Oils**—*Treat high Six vegetable oils with extreme respect and care, like a very powerful medicine. Mother Omega Six is essential. But for most of us, avoiding it is the problem. It is everywhere. Check labels.*

In **excess**, I believe that mother Omega 6, linoleic acid, is the insidious hidden killer of our age. In excess it is also likely altering our behaviour for the worse, and reducing our intelligence. The optimal Omega 3:6 range is suggested to be around 1:1 or 1:2, but not more than four mother Omega 6 to one mother Omega 3 fat. [88] Vegetable oils contain the mother fats, but not the long chain fats [P.287]. Long chain fats can only be made by animals and aquatic organisms.

The biggest sources of Omega Six are processed vegetable oils. To make matters worse, vegetable oils are found in most processed food. Margarine is often vegetable fats. Be very aware of vegetable oils in processed foods.

Many vegetable oils are very high in Omega Six, and low in Omega Three. A number of vegetable oils have Omega 6:3 ratios of 50:1 and more, including Corn Sunflower, Safflower, and Sesame. [See chart p.287].

Do not forget that the seeds are the sources of the oil, and packed with all the necessary nutrients. So instead of a little vegetable oil how about a few seeds.

Double check the fat content of everything you eat, and look at it in terms of your Omega 3:6 mother fat balance. Eat more Omega Three high sources and less Six, try to balance the two mother fats, and get some long chain fats.

11.3   **Oils, moderate use**—Virgin olive, and flax, are better vegetable oil options but in strict moderation [p 287 and 30.31]. Some have reservations over hemp and canola [26.5]. You need to keep an eye on your intake and balance, as a *lot of a little Omega Six* (e.g. olive) is still a lot when compared with a very low Omega Three content. So you need to eat some high Omega Three sources to balance the mother Omega Six in olive.

Vegetable oils were available to our ancestors in very limited amounts. 'Processed' olive oil as against virgin oil can have up to 50 per cent Omega Six. Too much mother fat and particularly Omega Six (and Three which is less likely), will block production of EPA and DHA.

11.4   **Heat harms**—Remember that vegetable oils are very sensitive to prolonged or high heat. Many contain polyunsaturated fats [p.287]. They have double bonds, which makes them more flexible, and more chemically reactive. They are less chemically stable. It is their greater instability, inherent energy, and chemical flexibility, that makes them prone to degradation by heat.

For cooking it is better to use saturates e.g. butter or coconut, or monounsaturates, or add highly unsaturated oils at the end of cooking. Fat intake in cooking should be considered as a part of the overall fat intake in diet

Oils have their own antioxidants which can be damaged by heat. For example the antioxidants in olives keep the oils in olives on trees, from going rancid in hot summers and glorious sunlight. We benefit from these antioxidants. These antioxidants are part of the health giving factors in olive oil.

Heat destroys these natural protective anti oxidants to a certain extent. At a pragmatic level, it is again about moderation, personal choice and balance. Flax seeds, as against oil from flax, appear to be more resilient to baking.

11.5   **Bypass potential production blockages**—Omega Threes are a family. Linolenic 18:3 n3, is the mother Omega Three fat. EPA and DHA are longer chain children of which there are a number. DHA and EPA are found primarily in significant amount in oily fish. Omega Three eggs are a good source. Most commercially produced eggs generally are not.

The body can make EPA and DHA from the mother fat, but the pathways can be blocked. Try and get some DHA and some ALA every day - recommendations as to quantity vary. (American Heart Association recommends 2−4 grams DHA/ EPA per day for elevated triglycerides [89]). A trial shows optimal uptake in women drops off at about two grams of DHA a day (3−4 tsp. of fish oil typically). Women have a higher need.

DHA connects to oestrogen levels, fertility, the monthly cycle, and the more visible things like hair, nails etc. Men benefit too. DHA connects to male fertility, higher intelligence, and lower aggression. DHA has been shown to increase sperm activity and viability, and improve the swimming ability of sperm in animals. Higher levels of DHA are found in the testes.

11.6   **Fish oil**–Oily fish is a good source of DHA and EPA. The very best quality, molecularly distilled oils have virtually no taste and do not repeat. Fish oil comes in different types depending on the source, and method of extraction.

The amount of vitamin A and D in cod liver oil can be an issue for pregnant women. Fish oil made from the fish body tends to be lower in vitamin A and D. Good quality fish oil is distilled which reduces environmental pollutants like mercury found in fish. The number of pollutants in our food is growing so everything we eat carries risks.

The ratio of EPA to DHA, and amount, alters in fish oils, depending on the type of fish used as the source. DHA has a bigger role in the structure of the body. EPA may be more effective at blocking the inflammatory pathways.[90] I have not seen any trials that provide absolute answers to which EPA:DHA ratio is best.

For me, benefits of supplementing with quality fish oil products far outweigh the risks. Please consult with your doctor before taking fish oils, as they can cause blood thinning, and other issues, for a limited number of people.

11.7   **Fish and fish oil–Risks and issues–**

☞ **Bleeding times**–Trials on Omega Threes suggest increased intake does increase bleeding time, but by how much and for what dosages is the subject of debate.[91] So please talk to your doctor about supplementation, and ensure that you re-advise prior to any surgery, giving birth etc. Interestingly Eskimos living a fairly native life with high fish and Omega 3 intake did not show bleeding time differences from non-natives, but historically times were longer [*Fish, Omega-3 and Human Health.*]

☞ **Haemorrhagic stroke**–Haemorrhagic stroke, is vessel fracture in the brain and heart. There is a evidence that Omega Threes creates a greater risk in populations like the Inuit. Interestingly, drug treatment for CVD in Eskimos pushed up DHA levels and the EPA: AA ratio.[92]

☞ **Suppression (or enhancement) of the immune system**–The Omega Three–Six balance is closely tied to the inflammatory immune system through a number of mechanisms. Omega Three dampens inflammation down, and enhances long-term repair. DHA alters T cell expression. The immune system is a balancing of immediate 'shock and awe,' and a more long-term strategy. Omega Three may, reduce the length of time for shock and awe, assist in a more structured long-term strategy, and in ensuring system alert stand down. Does high Omega Three compromise the immune system? There may be conditions where a very strong initial reaction by the body and compromised follow-up, is better that a moderate initial response and better planned and resourced follow-up. It is very complex. Eskimos showed higher susceptibility to TB in times gone by. On the other hand the list of conditions for which Omega Three supplementation shows advantage is impressive, including AIDS and malaria, but as pointed out in the paper, very limited trials have been done on fats, and the immune system. [93] The book *Omega 3 Fatty Acids in Clinical Nutrition* notes that Omega 3s were linked to improved recovery in peritonitis, trauma, abdominal SIRS, sepsis and infectious complications in post operative patients. Hospital stay times including in ICU were significantly reduced.

☞ **Diabetes**–General suggestion seems to be that DHA and EPA may assist, but ALA may not due to possible difficulties in conversion (See chapter on obesity and metabolic syndrome, and sections on diabetes). Discuss dietary change with your medical advisor.

11.8   **Farmed fish**–It takes 3–5 tons of wild small oily fish to make one ton of farmed carnivorous fish, like salmon. They are what they eat. Feed farmed fish grain rather than marine food, and they develop a higher Omega Six profile, and possibly much higher AA content. For people with poor Omega 6 conversion as well, higher AA in farmed fish may be a bonus. A breakdown of fats in farmed fish is not easy to find. Much is not known.

Farmed fish may contain more fat, but have far more Omega Six, 25 to 50 per cent of the fat. Wild fish contain very little Omega Six, about a tenth. So farmed fish do help provide Omega Three but do not assist in cutting down Omega Six as much as wild fish, but may for some provide necessary AA. [26.2]

11.9   **Imbalance in the food chain**–Feeding our animals a high grain diet, distorts their fat profile in the same way as we distort our own. We may also be encouraging fat storage, and so breeding fatter animals.

Omega 6 pushes the body to store fat. Meat, eggs, and milk from grain-fed animals have higher Omega 6s and lower 3s, than their more naturally grass fed brethren. Sheep fed canola rapeseed [an Omega 3:6 ratio of 1:2] increased Omega 6 muscle content, but not the Omega 3 levels. [94]

Omega 3s are not stored well. Interestingly, plant strains selected for agriculture often have lower Omega 3 than their wild cousins do. [95]

11.10   **Trans fats–Why take the risk?**–Excess Omega Six is made worse by trans fats. A large proportion of trans fats will be Omega Six based. Trans fats block the ability of the body to make long chain fats like DHA. The body before has never seen most artificial trans fats.

You are participating in a giant medical experiment. Trans fats provide no known nutritional advantage. The body elongates trans fats. Elongated trans fats are to be found in the brain, retina, micro vessels, myelin, and probably lots of other places too. They have different electromechanical properties.

Trans fats have different shapes, are less bendy, and so cannot hug, and interact properly. Trans fats have been reported as causing problems with vision.

Those with brain and nervous system diseases, and learning, mood, and behaviour disorders, may be prudent to avoid trans fats. Similar concerns apply to those with age related and fertility conditions. American trans fats intake was approximately 38 grams a day (25 per cent of estimated daily fat intake of 145–258 grams per day). [96]

Potential areas of concern have been expressed for a long time, so why were exhaustive long-term trials not done? It is the good old human dynamic again. Without consumer or government pressure, or possible legal action, there is no commercial motive, and no funds for continuing research after approval.

Changes are starting some 40 years later. A case against trans fats was won in California with damages of several million dollars. Regrettably, it is often only consumer legal actions that focus corporate minds. Commercial pressures mitigate against lone voices being heard or funded.

Particularly vulnerable groups are pregnant mothers and young infants, because of the potential and the unknown implication of the inclusion of trans fats in fast growing brains. High levels of trans fats are found in breast milk (see 11.28-30 and 23.16 on breast milk).

Other manufactured fats called mono and diglycerides are also used as food additives. They are potentially alien to the body. The glycerides are not trans fats, but a WHO report in 1974 said, "The various fatty acids that may be present in preparations of di- and monoglycerides used as food additives are not necessarily absorbed and metabolised in the same way as those of the natural food fats and their nutritional significance may also differ." [97]

My question is if we don't know what they do, and they do not confer a clear dietary benefit, why take the risk?

11.11   **Cut out sugar**—It is full of empty calories. Sugar impacts on the body's fat control and manufacture mechanism. Sugar may block the ability of the body to make long chain Omega Three and Omega Six. Further, sugar pushes your body to make more fat.

11.12   **Alcohol and Omega Three**—High alcohol consumption is claimed to block the conversion pathways; although there is some evidence, that low to moderate consumption, may increase conversion rates.

There is not sufficient evidence to determine if this applies to all population groups, or just those that can metabolise alcohol. Most trials have been in animals which also means conclusions are less authoritative. Alcohol strips DHA from the brain.

Generally, the brain is reluctant to give up DHA, when it is in short supply in the body. Alcohol allows that protective mechanism to be bypassed.

Our evolutionary ancestors did not have off-licences and distilleries, even if they had limited access to very low levels of weak alcohol or vinegar.

A recent trial suggested that brain shrinkage, is seen to accompany moderate alcohol intake, in certain groups. These comments apply to moderate and excessive intake. I have seen no trials on low intake.

The issue of alcohol is worse for women [This makes sense as women have a greater need of DHA. A lack of DHA has greater consequences for women as essential to fertility, monthly cycles, and reproduction]. For women who do not eat oily fish, and rely on the body to make enough EPA and DHA, blocking the conversion pathway with high fats, excess sugar etc. is a double whammy.

If there is an adequate supply of the mother Omega Three in the diet, low alcohol intake may assist conversion of mother to long chain fats. A supply of long chain fats, by conversion, or supplementation, may balance the use of those same fats, to metabolise alcohol. In those who do not have adequate supplies of the mother Omega Three fat, consumption of moderate levels of alcohol leads to DHA depletion and liver damage (Based on animal trials).

In the absence of resupply of Omega Threes, the body has no ability to replace the Omega Threes it is using to metabolise alcohol. This may explain the increasing liver damage being seen even in low to moderate drinkers. Lack of Omega 3 and oxidation of DHA by alcohol, may explain why minority native populations (hunter-gatherers) who are likely to have low mother Omega Three fats might be so susceptible to alcohol. DHA deficit will also have all the other risks attached, as listed in this book.

The moral is if you drink moderately, ensure you have an adequate supply of both long chain and mother Omega Three fats. A supply of the mother fat may be sufficient but if you are failing to convert the mother fats, you may still have a deficit of DHA and EPA.

So the safest option would be to supplement the long chain DHA and EPA as well. A supply of the Omega Threes may protect your liver and brain. The increased ability of the body to convert fats due to low alcohol intake might explain the heart benefits for those who have adequate Omega Three intake.

11.13 Making AA, EPA, and DHA—[Conversion is blocked by: see next page.]

There are two key enzymes in the process by which the body makes long chain fats. They are called desaturase 5 and desaturase 6 enzymes. There is competition for usage of the pathways and the available desaturase products between Omega 3 and 6.

These reactions seem to be a sensitive bottleneck point. A recent Canadian trial suggested conversion rates of the mother Omega 3 ALA are low.[i]

---

i   Extremely limited synthesis of long chain polyunsaturates in adults: implications for their dietary essentiality and use as supplements. Plourde M, Cunnane SC. Appl Physiol Nutr Metab. 2007 Aug;32(4):619-34 Research Center on Aging, Departments of Medicine, and Physiology and Biophysics, Université de Sherbrooke, 1036 Belvedere St, South, Sherbrooke, QC J1H 4C4, Canada.

Conversion is blocked by:

☞ Getting older - Age in rats is a big factor in poorer conversion. There are many reasons for older people to supplement EPA and DHA [98].

☞ Too much Omega Six mother fat.

☞ Too much Omega Three mother or long chain fat (unlikely for most).

☞ Too much fat.

☞ Trans fats (which can include frying oils etc.).

☞ Sugar is reported to block conversion pathways. Sugar blocks release of fats from storage. Insulin increases conversion. It is complex 25.5).

☞ Deficiency of minerals–iron, zinc, selenium, manganese.

☞ Deficiency of vitamins–Biotin, E, B6, B12.

☞ Some drugs?

☞ Low alcohol levels assist conversion dependent on genetics, historic intake, and conversion ability, but in some may have a blocking effect. A trial on Inuit showed 1–4 drinks a day reduced DHA+EPA by about 20 per cent, and worsened the EPA : AA ratio by about 30 per cent. [99]

☞ High intake of carbohydrate.

☞ Other blocking factors I have seen cited included processed vegetable oils, viral infections, and diabetes.

☞ Possible genetic variation between various racial groups. It is suggested for example that Greenland Eskimos have lower conversion ability. [100]. A similar question has been raised in respect of 'Celts' as shore dwellers, but remains unanswered. [Usher's II [loss of vision and deafness] sufferers may have DHA conversion or absorption blockages - Dr DR Hoffman]

☞ Stress blocks conversion inhibiting the desaturase 5 and 6 conversion enzymes, and increases oxidation of long chain fats [325 -]

Conversion is increased by:

☞ Higher protein.

☞ Relatively low and balanced intakes of the mother fats.

11.14 Stop the craving–Within reasonable limits, in terms of fats intake, overall less is more. If you are getting adequate Omega Three, you may find your taste and craving for fatty foods declines, mine did.

Do we have an innate ability to sense the foods our bodies need? Are those on diet binges are simply trying to find nutrients they are lacking?

The problem may be, the food they are eating, does not contain the nutrients they seek. So they seek out more fatty food. Evolutionary programming says fatty food contains some Omega Three. A vicious circle. If they are seeking out Omega 3, they would crave fatty products, burgers, chips etc., only to find them selves in a never-ending cycle, as these foods probably contain little Omega 3.

11.15 **Read every label**—Look for vegetable fat, hydrogenated fats, monoglycerides, and diglycerides as food additives in processed foods. Ask if unsure e.g. olives in oil often means sunflower. Make no assumptions. If unsure look it up. A site, *nutritiondata.com* on the Web, gives the fat make-up and nutritional density etc. of foods.

In preprepared foods, the type of vegetable oil and quantity is often unspecified. You may wish to look for food products that do specify the fats used and the Omega 3 and 6 content. Bear in mind a table spoon of many vegetable oils contains a significant amount of Omega 6 and very little Omega 3.

Hopefully in time, in response to demand, manufacturers will list Omega Three and Omega Six content etc.

11.16 **Whole foods**—Try and eat a wide range of 'whole' foods. Include lots of greens, highly coloured fruit and vegetables, roots, a few nuts, some beans if you like, and quality protein including oily fish. All these contain fats at varying levels. All taken as part of a varied diet will give an acceptable balance.

Nuts have to be eaten in moderation, as they are generally much higher in Six than Three. Vegetable oils, as ever should be treated with caution as a general rule. The treatment and processing of oils, sometimes is suggested as creating trans fats.

Solvents used in extraction may result in the inclusion of unwelcome additives. So where available cold pressed is the first choice.

11.17 **Meat and eggs**—Remember, just as we are what we eat, so are the animals we raise. Grain is high in Omega Six. Grain feeding of animals results in the skewing of their fat profile. Our high grain-fed animals are likely to be suffering in many instances with high Omega Six too. This includes particularly chicken and eggs.

Grass fed and free range products are better options. High Omega Three eggs from hens, fed with high Omega Three food sources look like a promising dietary addition. Moderation in meat protein is probably the watchword.

The China Study, postulates a link between meat protein and 'western' diseases. Whether the reasons are animal fat, protein, products administered to animals, the way we farm animals, related foods or preparation factors, there is no question the disease differentials are striking, but what are the underlying reasons? There are risks and benefits. Grass fed organic animal products provide more balanced fats. Fats play a very important part in human health.

Our ancestors ate protein from animals, but the fat profile of grain fed hormone assisted animals is very different. Eskimos and fishermen had high fish protein intake but were healthy as were traditional Swiss dairy eating folk.

There are many questions, and some thought provoking facts. This book is about Omega Threes and Sixes and not protein. Fats are essential to human health. I leave the difficult issues of farming practices, and morals to you.

11.18   Pregnancy—Pregnant and nursing women, need to take special care, for themselves and their babies. We are not just what we eat but what our mothers ate too.

Brains need DHA. Babies' brains need DHA even more. Babies' brains are being wired for life in the womb and early months. Babies will even strip DHA from a mother's brain if needs be.

Trials have suggested DHA, and EPA may reduce pre-eclampsia, protect against early term, and help postnatal depression. Care has to be taken to consider the impact of the pollution of fish, in working out optimal fish intake, and the type and amount of fish oil supplementation.

On a separate note, trans fats in your food are expressed in your breast milk. (See chapter 23 on pregnancy and women's issues).

11.19   Saturated fats—Saturated fats are carbon chains with no double bonds. Single carbon to carbon bonds are more stable than double carbon to carbon bonds.

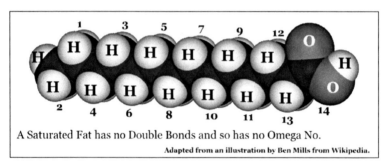

A Saturated Fat has no Double Bonds and so has no Omega No.

Adapted from an illustration by Ben Mills from Wikipedia.

Fig. 11.19   Myristic Acid–A Saturated Fat with 14 Carbons

Because saturated fats have no double bonds, they are more stable, and less susceptible to damage by heat. They are also more rigid. Each bond has a small ability to flex, but no ability to change overall shape.

The body uses saturated fats in the cell membranes to make the cells more rigid. For example, myelin nerve sheath has higher levels of saturated fat, giving it a more rigid structure.

Brain contains higher levels of unsaturated fat giving it a much softer and more flexible structure.

The body itself manufactures saturated fats. Saturated fats are entirely necessary to body function. They may have particular properties in the digestion system too [The digestion system is 'outside' the body].

Some saturated fats like lauric acid have antibacterial and anti viral properties [11.31]. It is as ever a question of balance, and moderation. Avoidance of saturated fats in the diet may well bring its own risks.

11.20   Absorption after digestion—The digestion of fats is complex. It requires the digestive system to be working properly. The digestive process is in a sense outside the body.

Long chain fats are turned into an emulsion called 'chyle' for processing. Digested products pass into the body through the digestive membranes.

After digestion short and medium chain fats of all types, are transported differently from long chain fats of all types. Short and medium fats can short cut the fats transport delivery processes, with a direct conveyor system to the liver. Long fats are a bit like a "heavy load" on the road system. They require to be sent by a different road network. They are too large, or it is in the design manual, that they are not to be sent on the direct conveyor to the liver. They have to take a motorway tour. They are loaded in packages called chylomicrons.

They take the lymphatic 'road' network. Lymphatic 'road' junctions directly join into the digestive network. Fats are sent through the lymphatic system [Fig 3.17] up to the neck. At the neck the 'loads' pass into the blood transport network system. The liver, and other cells, can pick up fat consignments from the bloodstream and unpack them for processing, for use or storage in the cells.

Fat cells unpack the loads and the repack them for storage. Some fats can be used as they are when they arrive. Some require reprocessing into other products. The liver is the main fat processing factory and production plant. Short and medium length chain fats are allowed on the conveyor direct to the liver. So short and medium chain fats are available in the liver more quickly for processing after eating. They also do not clog up the blood stream and lymphatic network with additional fat freight traffic.

One of the processes in the liver is oxidation. Oxidation of fats in the liver reduces hunger and consumption. Short and medium chain fats are more effective fuel than Omega Six [See 11.31,32,33 and 25.44 and Lauric acid]. So in theory, and it is observed in trials, short and medium chain fats will reduce hunger and consumption more effectively and quickly than polyunsaturates.

There are valid arguments as to how much saturated fat we should consume. Do we need biscuits and cakes in our diet? The reality is we like cookies and cakes. At a pragmatic level it is once again about moderation, and using whole-food quality ingredients. Saturated fats are produced by the body. Saturated fats are entirely necessary to life and health. Saturated fats are part of the body structure. Shorter saturated fats form an essential part of the body's defence mechanisms against viruses and infective agents.

We have always had limited access to saturated fats in the diet. Arguably saturated fats have only become a problem when consumed in excess, or where we have tampered with their composition. So the message is get a mix of natural saturated fats from a variety of sources but in moderation. Finally be aware that hydrogenated polyunsaturates, 'trans' fats manufactured by man, and used extensively in process foods, are in fact partial saturates. It is now accepted, some 30 or 40 years after serious concerns were first raised, that these artificial partial saturates are harmful to human health. We have been eating these harmful trans fats since the turn of the century.

11.21　**Fats and baking**—Dr Mary Enig's book "Know Your Fats", inspired me to add this section on saturated and 'trans' fats. Dr Enig passionately puts detailed and convincing arguments, that we should not be replacing natural saturated fats, with artificially partially saturated 'polyunsaturated' fats. Dr Enig explains why fats with the consistency of saturated fats are required for optimal commercial baking.

Flaky pastry apparently requires certain characteristics in fat. For reasons that are not entirely clear, a sensible message to moderate saturated fat intake, has been turned into an unreasoned deep-rooted public fear of saturated fats. The public has an equal and opposite unreasoned belief, that polyunsaturates are unequivocally healthy, no matter in what quantity or type.

The food industry understandably gives us what it perceives we want. *To meet public tastes in light flaky pastry, and the fashion for 'polyunsaturates', the food industry has taken polyunsaturated fats and turned them into partially saturated fats.* When this is achieved by hydrogenation it creates 'trans' fats.

Dr Enig points out these fats may taste and bake the same, but they do not function the same in the body. After long years of efforts by people such as Dr Enig there is finally a recognition that trans fats are on the balance of evidence, and based on the biology, likely to be significantly harmful to human health. These products were not created to fill a true need.

The reality is there are perfectly good natural, animal, and vegetable equivalents that have been used for varying extents for thousands of years like coconut, and butter. With the best of intentions and subtle market pressures to find uses for oils, the public has been convinced an artificial creation is better.

Unfortunately many of these substances are new to the body. The body does not have the appropriate mechanisms to properly process them. Trans fats are on the way out, but to fill the baking fat void, interesterification [30.19] is now on the way in. Should we really be embarking on another dietary adventure into the unknown, just as we are coming to realise the potential implication of the last?

Fats are fundamental as outlined. Consequences of errors could be significant. Why take such enormous health risks in areas such as fertility, diabetic and cardiac health, by using artificial fat creations, when there are natural vegetable and animal products to make flaky pastry and crunchy biscuits?

11.22　**Culture Belief and Ethics**—There are a large number of groups that consume only, or primarily, vegetable fat for a variety of reasons. They include Kashrut (Kosher) and Halal groups, Buddhists, Jains, Hindus, vegans, and vegetarians [1.36]. These groups are particularly vulnerable to the usage of trans or chemically altered fats, including spreads and baking fats. I have only seen trials on fat consumption, that relate to consumers of Halal and Kosher food, but trans fats are likely to be a factor, in the diet of the wider group. The impact of trans fats on metabolic body processes, and cell membrane structure, is in addition to that of excess Omega Six.

11.23   **Interestification**—Food manufacturers are replacing hydrogenated fats with interesterified fats. There are suggestions that interesterified fats may not be easily metabolised, or may have adverse consequences in the body. Interesterified fats can be used to prolong shelf life. Interesterification can also be used to change the physical properties of fats, for example to turn a fat, which is liquid at room temperature, into a semi-solid or solid. This is done by removing one leg of the triglyceride. A polyunsaturated fat is removed, and replaced by a saturated fat. In the diagram below are two triglycerides.

A triglyceride is a chemical rack that holds three fats. [See 30.19] There are consequences to making these substitutions, in addition to those described below. There are questions as to the health impact of these products.

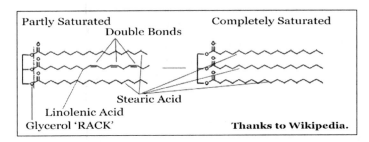

Fig. II.23 Interestification of A Triglyceride Linolenic acid is removed and replaced by Stearic Acid so saturating the Triglyceride

The resultant product would be more solid, have a longer shelf life, and make flaky pastry. The use of esterified fats is another leap into the void. Perfectly good natural alternatives exist, providing they are used sensibly and in moderation.

Concerns have been expressed about Interestification in recent trials. The lead researcher Dr K C Hayes who has 35 years experience in the field suggested that the rearranged triglycerides, placing saturated fats in a position in which they are not normally found may not be as easily processed by the body.

Concerns have been raised as to the impacts of interesterified fats on fat metabolism, and consequential effects. In one trial it was noted there were "differences in early metabolic processing and postprandial clearance, which may explain modulatory effects on atherogenecity and thrombogenecity".[ii][iii]

These are early days. There are more questions than answers. Like trans fats, history will probably tell if interesterified fats, will have a wider health implication. The health experiment will once again have been conducted on you, and your children.

I am puzzled why if the industry needs more solid fats with a longer life, it simply does not to use traditional vegetable and/or animal fats.

---

ii   Effects of stereospecific positioning of fatty acids in triacylglycerol structures in native and randomized fats: a review of their nutritional implications Nutr Metab (Lond). 2007; 4: 16.
       Tilakavati Karupaiah and Kalyana Sundram.

iii   Stearic acid-rich interesterified fat and trans-rich fat raise the LDL/HDL ratio and plasma glucose relative to palm olein in humans Nutr Metab (Lond). 2007; 4: 3.
       Kalyana Sundram, Tilakavati Karupaiah, and KC Hayes.

If the point is to convert non-saturated triglycerides to saturated triglycerides, why not use naturally more saturated triglycerides in the first place? (See 11.19)

So many questions. With rising fuel prices are there not alternate economic uses for vegetable oils that are surplus to consumption need, if that is an issue? I am not a Luddite, but have the risks of interesterified fats been fully assessed? If there are any risks why take them when natural alternatives are available?

11.24   Mono and Diglycerides—Mono and Diglycerides are found in natural products such as olive oil. The body also makes and uses them. 'Artificial' mono and diglycerides are made. I have searched and have found it difficult to find information on the health risks, if any, of 'artificial' mono and diglycerides.

A world health organisation report in the 1970s quoted the following "The various fatty acids that may be present in preparations of di- and monoglycerides used as food additives are not necessarily absorbed and metabolized in the same way as those of the natural food fats and their nutritional significance may also differ..." (Frazer, 1962). "The mono- and diglycerides most likely to cause unwanted effects are those containing long-chain saturated fatty acids, especially stearic acid."

11.25   Animal Fats—Animal fats are described as saturated fats. They are in fact a mixture of fats, as are margarine, or shortening. 'Saturated' animal fats contain a wide mix of saturated, mono, and polyunsaturated fats. Fat content reflects the animal's diets. Hydrogenated margarine, and shortening, are a manufactured mixture containing trans and saturated fats. A swap is being made.

Natural 'partially saturated' animal fats, which have been eaten for many thousands, if not hundred of thousands of years, are being swapped for unnatural partially saturated fats which the body regards as 'misfits', because it has no history of them in its processing manual. Vegetable alternative do exist as well .

Against animal fats, we feed some of our animals grain and restricted diets, and so distort their fat ratios. We then consume these distorted fats. Animals' fat may concentrate persistent organic pollutants we are putting into the atmosphere, and pass them back to us. Animal body fats contain few other nutrients.

Trials suggest that excess animal fat consumption carries significant health risks. To what extent is that due to how we keep the animals, what we feed the animals, how we medicate the animals, and persistent organic pollutants?

Some environmental pollutants, are resistant to degradation, bioaccumulate and biomagnify in food chains, have significant health impact, and end up in us and our environment. Animal fats can accumulate such agents, as can grains and most other foods, so you cannot get away from the pollution we make.

Do I still eat small amounts of meat and butter? – Yes. Swiss mountain folk survived very healthily prior to the arrival of western refined food, and had excellent teeth with decay in only .3 per cent of teeth. Their diet included bread slice sized pieces of cheese daily, and meat once a week. [*Weston Price*] Their cows had access to a much wider range of grazing than most modern cattle. Today's Swiss mountain grazed cattle have much better Omega 3:6 profiles.

We are not all the same. Some tolerate dairy products much better. Butter contains minerals, vitamins, and a mix of fats. This is evidence that there is a place for unadulterated quality dairy products and meat, at least for some if not all consumers.

Dr Price observed tooth decay and crowded teeth arrived with western refined foods, in a variety of cultures still on "primitive" diets . [*Nutrition and Physical Degeneration, Western A Price, 1939. Republished*] Many cultures prior to the introduction of refined foods were healthy on a wide range of diets, that included a variety of animal protein and fat.

11.26   **Vegetable fats**—If you want a solid fat for baking with, it has to be probably 40 per cent or more saturated. That provides three options. Palm oil, [52 per cent saturated] palm kernel, and coconut oil [92 per cent saturated] [Page 287], and mixing them with less saturated fats. Before you hold your hands up in horror, hard margarine is 80 percent saturated. Trans fats and artificial fats are in effect artificially saturated polyunsaturates.

Again I reiterate moderation. This is not an invitation to greatly increase your saturated fat intake, but to suggest there are better options than artificially partially saturated polyunsaturates, or engineered fats. In general terms less, closer to war time rations than supersize meals, is more, and variety is good. Some bake with monosaturates. Polyunsaturated oils are not good for baking.

Coconut is a bit of an oddity as it is mainly composed of medium to short chain triglycerides, which follow a different treatment process in the body to long chain fats. There is fierce debate over the impact of coconut intake and cardiac health. Dr Enig's thoughts and advice on coconut, may be found on the Westonaprice.org web site.

A trial suggested that those on traditional diets which are high in fish, that included a high intake of grated coconut or coconut milk, had no increased CHD[iv]. Native diets would not include manufactured saturated coconut fats.

Palm oil contains longer fats. Palm kernel oil has shorter fats [287]. There is fierce debate on the cardiac implications of palm *oil* fat as high in palmitic acid.

11.27   **What is a trans fat?**—Carbons have four attachment points they must use [Four elastic string connections]. Fats are chains of carbon atoms. The carbons may form one or two string attachments with the next door carbon. If it is a two string attachment, a double bond, you get two shapes depending which bits of string are attached to which carbons. The double bond is either more of less a straight line [Fig 30.37], or a significantly kinked [Fig 30.4]. Straight connections are called 'trans' bonds. Bent or kinked connections are called 'Cis' bonds. Chains containing 'trans' bonds are called 'trans' fats.

---

iv   Dietary intake and the risk of coronary heart disease among coconut-consuming Minangkabua in west Sumatra, Indoesia. Asia Pac J Clin Nutr 2004;13 (4):377–384 Nur I Lipoeto, Zulkardain Agus, Fadil Oenzil, Mark L Wahlqvist, Naiyana Wattanapenpaiboon.

Trans fat chains have different shapes, which alters their ability to interact with other chemicals. Shapes alter the properties of cell membranes. Trans bonds shapes look and behave more like saturated fats, so making membranes less flexible. Trans Fats make cooking fat solid, and your cell membranes including your brain more solid. 'Trans' fats are rare in nature, most bonds are 'Cis'.

11.28   Natural Trans Fats–Trans fats do occur naturally in the food chain, and mainly in the food from ruminants [Grass eaters]. These natural trans fats are different to many artificial trans fats. Natural trans bonds are found at specific locations on the carbon chain. This means they have shapes that are recognised in the body's instruction manual. In manufactured trans fats the trans bonds are may be found in locations on the carbon chain the body does not recognise. Meat fat, butter and milk from ruminants contain 2–5% trans fats.

The trans fat in ruminant products is called CLA, or Conjugated Linoleic Acid. There have been over 2000 trials looking at CLA, in its various forms.

A number of trials on CLA have shown benefits to metabolism, and possible reduction in cancer risks. The more beneficial natural trans fats are found in grass as against grain fed cattle[v]. We have been eating grazing animals for a very long time. We have been using their milk products, in various forms for a much shorter time, but still some tens of thousands of years.

The New York Times of March 7, 2007, reported that the FDA does not differentiate between natural trans fats ruminant CLAs, and artificial trans fats. Both are required to be included in the total trans fat figures for labelling purposes in the USA. The result apparently is that butter, in for example croissants, may be being replaced by artificially created fats, by mass food outlets including coffee shops.

The New York Times states that two ounces of ground beef would be over the trans fat limit, it raises the issue of natural trans fats in milk, and asks should they both legally be labelled as containing trans fats. I leave you to make your own mind up if you would prefer natural or synthetic fats.

11.29   Artificial Trans Fats–Until very recently the consensus was artificial trans fats presented no medical risks. A recent Canadian Report on artificial trans fats said *"Metabolic and epidemiologic studies consistently show that trans fats are more harmful than any other type of fat."*[vi] In 1981 a trial said "This study shows that the dietary trans fatty acids are differentially incorporated into the liver microsomal lipids and act as inhibitors for delta 9 and 6 desaturases."[vii]

---

v   Vaccenic Acid and cis–9,trans–11 CLA in the Rumen and Different Tissues of Pasture- and Concentrate-Fed Beef Cattle. Lipids. 2007 Oct 3 Shen X, Nuernberg K, Nuernberg G, Zhao R, Scollan N, Ender K, Dannenberger D.

vi   Transforming the Food Supply is the final report of the Trans Fat Task Force, co-chaired by Health Canada and the Heart and Stroke Foundation of Canada, which was submitted to the Minister of Health in June 2006.

vii Effect of dietary trans fatty acids on the delta 5, delta 6 and delta 9 desaturases of rat liver microsomes in vivo. Acta Biol Med Ger. 1981;40(12):1699–1705. Mahfouz M. PMID: 7345825.

The trial made the point the desaturase Six pathway is fundamental to the production of the chemical families of Omega Six [and the Threes would be interrupted too]. This was validated in a trial in 1982, "The biosynthesis of essential (n−6) fatty acids was depressed by the TRANS supplement in EFA−deficient as well as in non−EFA−deficient animals."[viii]

And in 1977 another trial noted "Trans fatty acids also influenced the fatty acid composition of testicular lipids, but much lower amounts of these acids accumulated in testes than in liver or serum."[ix]

It has taken 25 or so years despite early warnings of the potential impact of artificial trans fats, to begin to accept trans fats are an issue. How must these researchers have felt in the intervening years? Dr Enig reports trans fats have been associated with low birth weights, and more widely diabetes and coronary issues. A trial in 2003 suggested trans fats are incorporated in the mitochondria[x].

A trial dated January 2007 reported *"Women with a high intake of trans fatty acids instead of carbohydrates or unsaturated fats have an increased risk for ovulatory infertility"*.[xi] If artificial trans fats block conversion of the mother Omega 3 to DHA this would impact on fertility, and even Omega 6 conversion .

If this is correct, you have been long term participants in fertility trials on yourselves, in the search for artificial substitutes to make flaky pastry products 'just so', when natural alternatives like butter and coconut fat are available.

Is fertility worth risking for synthetic fat 'just so' flaky pastry?

11.30   Trans how much what foods−When you look at a chart of foods listing trans fats contents, the results are surprising. There is a very great deal more hydrogenated fat ['trans' fats] 'hidden' in food than you would imagine. If you enter "Fatty Acid Composition of Canadian Foods (Summer 2005)" into a search engine you will find a list.

11.31   Medium and short Chain Triglycerides−Some short/medium chain fats S/MCTs such as lauric acid (found in coconut) are reported as being very good fuel for burning (oxidation). As discussed above S/MCTs have a more direct route to the liver, and do not require bile salts for digestion.

Dr Enig reports they are an important part of infant formulas, as S/MCTs are part of natural breast milk [Lauric acid 5.8 per cent - Wikipedia].

---

viii Interrelationship between dietary trans Fatty acids and the 6− and 9−desaturases in the rat. Lipids. 1982 Jan;17(1):27−34. De Schrijver R, Privett OS. PMID: 7087680.

ix Studies of effects of trans fatty acids in the diet on lipid metabolism in essential fatty acid deficient rats. Am J Clin Nutr. 1977 Jul;30(7):1009−17. Privett OS, Phillips F, Shimasaki H, Nozawa T, Nickell EC. PMID: 879068.

x Dietary *Trans* Fatty Acids Alter the Compositions of Microsomes and Mitochondria and the Activities of Microsome D6−Fatty Acid Desaturase and Glucose−6−Phosphatase in Livers of Pregnant Rats J. Nutr. 133:2526−2531, August 2003 Elvira Larqué, Pedro-Antonio García-Ruiz , Francisca Perez-Llamas, Salvador Zamora and Angel Gil.

xi Trans Fatty Acid Intake Increases Risk for Ovulatory Infertility *Am J Clin Nutr.* 2007;85:231−237 Désirée Lie, MD, MSEd.

S/MCTs perform important functions in the body's defence strategy, and may assist in controlling some bacterial, microbial and viral agents, including it is reported HIV–1, Measles, Herpes, Influenza, Helicobacter pylori and others[xii].

"Monolaurin, a monoester formed from lauric acid, has profound antiviral and antibacterial activity". It is recognised that more research is required. But why are we so prejudiced against saturated fats in the face of such evidence?

What are the long term health effects of that prejudice?

11.32   Fats Oxidation Rates–Fats are oxidised at different rates in the body. Lauric acid 12 carbons long, found in coconut oil, palm kernel oil, [See page 287] and some in milks, human 5.8 per cent, goat 4.5, cows 2.2, is reported as being very efficiently oxidised. DHA is highly oxidised in the mitochondria. A trial suggested Omega 3s are better oxidised than the equivalent Omega 6, and there is a tendency to conserve the Omega 6 mother fat.

The most slowly oxidised were the mid chain 16 and 18 carbon long, saturated fats. The fastest oxidised by a long way was lauric acid, at 41 percent recovery in breath in 9 hours, followed by the mother Omega Three at about 25 percent. The mother Omega Six was about 20% oxidised, and the 16 and 18 carbon saturates came below that.[xiii] As usual it is complex, and oxidation rates will likely depend on what other foods are supplied etc.

Butter is a limited source of the very short chain fats, and good for variety. Replacing some animal fat, and palm fat, with natural unhydrogenated coconut fat, or palm kernel oil, may increase burn off of energy.

Replacing Omega Six with unhydrogenated animal, coconut, and palm kernel fat will provide benefits by different mechanisms. The variety of fats in butter, or dairy fats has a place too. Adequate supply of Omega Three is essential.

I must stress that variety is good, and it is accepted that excess saturates are undesirable in health terms. Generally in terms of fat, intake it is about appropriate proportions and variety. History suggests that optimal health fat intake is nearer war time ration quantities, than 2000 supersize portions.

11.33   Fats and Hunger Control–Several trials suggest that increased oxidation of fat in the liver is related to lower consumption and hunger. Short chain saturated fat intake is suggested to assist with hunger control. Short fats are more easily oxidised. Short fats have a more direct route to the liver. Short fats are more easily digested. Oxidation of fats, DHA, serotonin and dopamine, all interlink and are reported to reduce hunger [25.35].

---

xii   A review of Monolaurin and Lauric Acid Natural Virucidal and Bactericiadal agents. Shari Lieberman, Mary G Enig, and Harry G Preuss.

xiii Differential oxidation of individual dietary fatty acids in humans[1,2,3] Vol. 72, No. 4, 905–911, October 2000 James P DeLany, Marlene M Windhauser, Catherine M Champagne and George A Bray.

11.34   **COX and LOX enzymes and pathways**–The Omega 3 and 6 fats are converted into complex families of chemicals, by the insertion of one or more oxygen, by various enzymes [oxidation]. [See page 286 and Fig 1.19]

These enzymes include COX1, COX2, and the LOX families. These enzymes are applied to the raw materials of both the Omega 3 and 6 families. The exclusive Omega Three raw material is EPA. The exclusive Omega Six raw material is AA.

COX2 products have been mainly considered in this book, as COX2s were most often found in trials. The LOX pathways are also equally influential.

There are at least three LOX pathways each with it's own enzyme. Drugs, NSAIDs, block the LOX pathways alone, or both LOX and COX pathways.

11.35   **LOXs and Leukotrienes**–Leukotrienes are a product of the LOX enzymes pathways [P.286]. They like the COX products are central components of a chemical family "that affects essentially all organs and tissues in man".[xiv] There are Omega Six Leukotrienes, and Omega Three Leukotrienes.

The Omega Six LTA4, LTB4, LTC4, LTD4. LTE4 in general terms promote inflammatory reactions. Leukotrienes are involved in asthma, hay fever, allergic rhinitis, allergic reactions, cardiovascular issues, neuropsychiatric disorders, oedema, adrenocorticotropin release[xv] [precursor of cortisol the stress hormone], arthritis, gout, fertility, prostate cancer, breast cancer, vasoconstriction, broncoconstriction, chronic bronchitis, aneurysms, and vascular permeability. They also have a role in cystic fibrosis, inflammatory bowel disease, and psoriasis.

The leukotrienes link to the immune system through their interaction with the white blood cells the leukocytes. They were named leukotrienes because they were first found in white blood cells. [xvi]

Is excess Omega Six at least in part responsible for the growing numbers of allergies, and susceptibility to hospital bugs? I suspect it has a part to play. I don't pretend to understand the complexities. Everything inter links, and dietary trends such as avoidance of short chain saturates may also have a part to play.

I only seek to show you that the ultimate products of Omega 6, are very influential and complex chemicals, far wider than just the COX2 products.

LOX families also produce chemicals that control or influence critical pathways in the body. These pathways control western conditions such as asthma, and coronary heart disease.

An imbalance or excess of Omega Six has very fundamental impact on a huge range of critical body functions.

---

xiv   Leuchron Contract No QLG1-CT-2001-01521 The Leukotrienes Signalling Molecules in Chronic and Degenerative Diseases.

xv   Endocrinology, Vol 119, 1427-1431, Copyright © 1986 by Endocrine Society Role of arachidonic acid in the regulation of adrenocorticotropin release from rat anterior pituitary cell cultures AB Abou-Samra, KJ Catt and G Aguilera.

xvi   Brocklehurst, W (1960), "The release of histamine and formation of a slow-reacting substance (SRS-A) during anaphylactic shock", J Physiol 151: 416-35, PMID 13804592.

11.36 **Leukotrienes and Asthma**—Leukotrienes are the product of Omega 6. "Leukotrienes assist in asthma causing, or potentiating the following

➢ Airflow obstruction.

➢ Increased secretion of mucus.

➢ Mucosal accumulation.

➢ Bronchoconstriction.

➢ Infiltration of inflammatory cells in the airway wall" [xvii].

"As well as mediating inflammation, they induce asthma and other inflammatory disorders, thereby reducing the airflow to the alveoli." Leukotrienes are primarily responsible for bronchoconstriction.[xviii]

Leukotriene blocking NSAIDs are reported to prevent the inflammatory leukotriene chemical cascade so moderating the effects of asthma. LOX products may mediate the energy production pathways.[xix]

Arguably increasing the long chain Omega Three availability, and balancing the Omega Threes and Sixes, would also reduce the amount of LOX products, as well as blocking the pathways.

In addition DHA has been reported as an effective NSAID. There will always be a role for drug intervention, but should prevention not be the starting point?

11.37 **DHA and EPA moderate COX and LOX**—The body is controlled by a constant delicate balance of reactions, between the pathways, and dozens of chemicals in these pathways. Think of the supply of Omega Six as a flow of water coming out of a sprinkler nozzle.

The flow of water to the sprinkler is determined by how much the tap is turned on. In the body you determine the flow of Omega Six by how much you put in your mouth in your diet. Once the water is in the hose it has to go somewhere. The water in the hose cannot just disappear.

Omega Six put into the body is just the same. Omega Six cannot just disappear. Omega Six must be used to make chemicals, stored as fat, or burnt.

Stored fat is like a bulge in the pipe, it will appear at some point through the sprinkler nozzle. If you block or restrict one jet in the sprinkler nozzle more water must come out of the others.

If you convert less Omega Six to the long chain fats there is excess mother Omega Six to be oxidised in the arteries leading to arterial furring and damage.

---

xvii Wikipedia.

xviii *BMJ* 1999;319:90 (10 July) What are leukotrienes and how do they work in asthma? Abi Berger, *science editor*.

xix Novel Effect of Oxidised Low-Density Lipoprotein: Cellular ATP Depeletion via Downregulation of Glyceraldehyde-3-Phosphate Dehodrogenans. Circ Res 2006;99;191-200 Sergiy Sukhanov. Yusuke Higashi. Shaw-Yung Shai, Hiroyuki Itabe, Koichi Ono, Sampath Parthasarathy and Patrick Delaontaine.

MECHANISMS BY WHICH OMEGA THREE AND SIX INTAKE IMPACT ON BODY FUNCTION PARTICULARLY IN RELATION TO THE OMEGA THREE AND SIX FAMILIES OF CHEMICALS	
Fat	**Action**
Enzymes	COX1, COX2, and LOX are enzymes that make the chemical families from the Omega 3 and 6 fats.
	Desaturase 5 and 6 are the enzymes by which the mother Omega Three and Six fats are made into the longer fat children like DHA.
	There is a limited supply of all of these enzymes. Omega Three and Six are in competition.
	The body uses this competition, and limited supplies as part of its body regulation processes.
LA	Linoleic Acid LA is the mother fat of the Omega Six family. Excess LA blocks the body's ability to make long chain fats, and particularly those of the Omega Three family. Incomplete oxidation of Omega Six can result in cell damage.
DGLA	The child of Omega Six LA, and exclusive raw material for the COX1 pathway.
AA	The grand child of Omega Six LA, and exclusive raw material for the COX2 and LOX Omega Six pathway. It has preferential access before Omega Three to the COX2 conversion pathways.
ALA	Alpha Linolenic Acid ALA is the mother fat of the Omega Three family. The mother Omega Three is oxidised in preference to Omega Six. The body does not store Omega Three in quantity.
EPA	The grand child of the Omega Three ALA, and exclusive raw material of the Omega Three COX2 and LOX products.
DHA	The child of the Omega Three ALA. DHA has very important roles in the structure of membranes. The position and number of bonds gives it special chemical and structural properties [1.36].
EPA–Competition for COX2 enzyme	EPA competes with AA for the available COX2 enzyme production line which has a limited capacity.

Fat	Action
EPA – Competition for LOX enzymes	EPA competes with AA for the available LOX enzyme production lines which have a limited capacity. There are a number of LOX enzymes including 5, 12, and 15.
EPA – Raw material resolvins and protectins	The body makes resolvins and protectins from EPA. Resolvins and protectins close down inflammation, by working with immune agents, and inflammatory agents such as LTB4. The production of resolvins and protectins is blocked by certain COX inhibitors. [xx]
EPA – Less Inflammatory Products	The body makes a whole series of COX2 and LOX EPA products. Omega Three products are less aggressive than those of Omega Six, and connected more with repair.
DHA – Natural NSAID	DHA is a natural NSAID substitute, a COX and or LOX blocker – DHA is reported as being more effective than many drugs as a COX/LOX blocker. An advantage is it does not have the side effects attributed to various drugs. Drugs undoubtedly have a role but should prevention not be a starting point?
DHA – Blocks conversion of LA to AA	DHA appears to block the conversion of Omega 6 fats to AA the Omega 6 raw material of the inflammatory chemicals by switching down the conversion pathways.
DHA – Makes resolvins and alters T cell expression	The body also makes resolvins from DHA by a Lox enzyme. Aspirin triggers resolvins. [xxi] Resolvins switch down inflammation and related immune function. 22 long carbon chain chemicals are called docosanoids, and are an emerging subject.
DHA – Melatonin shuts down COX2	DHA increases levels of melatonin. Melatonin blocks COX 2 products, and shuts off release of Omega Six fats from stored fat tissue.
ALA – Competes for desaturase	Higher levels of the mother Omega Three compete with the mother Omega Six for the desaturase enzyme. A higher ALA to LA ratio leads to greater DHA production.

---

xx   Resolvins: Endogenous Omega–3 Fatty-Acid-Derived Mediators Nat Clin Pract Rheumatol. 2007; 3(10):570–579. ©2007.

Fat	Action
Saturated Fat− Improves Omega Three Six balance	Saturated fat replacing Omega 6 high products, improves the Omega 3:6 balance, and conversion so reducing inflammatory conditions. Short chain [C12] saturated fats improve metabolic rates.
Monosaturated Fat− Improves Omega Three Six balance	Monosaturated fat in the diet replacing Omega Six high products improves the Omega Three Six balance so reducing inflammatory conditions. Monosaturated fats are much better oxidised than Omega Six [but less well than medium short chain fats C12] so improving metabolic rates.
Gene expression	Omega 3s and 6s both modulate gene expression, and so impact on the proteins made, and the function of the immune system. DHA is reported to down grade inflammatory immune reactions.
Cell Membrane characteristics	Omega 3 alters the characteristics of the cell membrane making it more fluid. It influences calcium transport, and electrical conduction, is important to cell function, and key to heart function. Lipid raft function is sensitive to fat balance.
Fuel gauges	Fats act as hormone messengers and fuel gauges by interaction with substances called PPARs.
Mitochondrial function	DHA is a key element of cardiolipin, found in quantity in the inner membrane of the mitochondria. High levels of DHA are reported as impacting on membrane fluidity and function. DHA is more effectively oxidised then any other long chain fat.
Oxidation Rate	DHA is more effectively oxidised than any other long chain fat in the mitochondria. Oxidation is a key part of energy production. Highly reactive oxidation products are necessary to body processes such as thyroid function, and may be key to vision, immune function, cellular regulation etc.

xxi   Resolvin D1 and Its Aspirin−triggered 17R Epimer J. Biol. Chem., Vol. 282, Issue 13, 9323−9334, March 30, 2007 Yee-Ping Sun, Sungwhan F. Oh, Jasim Uddin, Rong Yang, Katherine Gotlinger, Eric Campbell, Sean P. Colgan, Nicos A. Petasis, and Charles N. Serhan.

12

LOW-LEVEL BODY INFLAMMATION

12   **Low-level body inflammation**–[Abbreviations listed at 1.1] . The body is all interconnected. If there is inflammation in one area the whole body is aware of it and impacted to some extent by it. Many functions of the body involve inflammatory oxidative processes.

Inflammatory chemicals are made in the fat cells and supporting tissue matrix. They are also made in all organs of the body including the brain. The fat cell matrix creates a background level of inflammatory chemicals. Your fat is a hugely influential chemical factory.

The fatter you are, the more production capacity you have. If you are overweight and have very high levels of Omega Six in your diet, and low Omega Three, it makes things even worse. The ovulation cycle, wound repair, obesity, cancers, and most 'western' diseases have been likened to, or linked with, inflammation.

It is a delicate balance between breaking down old tissue and creating the new. Whatever angle one searches from, one keeps coming across common threads that bind. Omega Six sits at the heart of these inflammatory processes. Omega Six is the master chemical from which the initiators and controllers are made.

No Omega Six = no inflammatory chemicals. Lots of Omega Six = lots of inflammatory chemicals. The body is designed to store Omega Six. The effect of excess Six is magnified by long-term fat storage levels. That is why excess Omega Six is fundamental.

Omega Three is absolutely essential to keep Omega Six in balance, and contain the inflammatory impact. In nature Omega Three would long term always exceed Omega Six, and so could be burnt as fuel.

We were never designed to run with long-term excess of Omega Six over Three. Omega 3 is not stored in any significant quantity. To counteract stored Omega 6, whilst Omega 6 fat stores are being reduced, it is essential to ensure adequate supplies of mother and long chain Omega 3s on a continuous basis.

12.1 Inflammation and obesity–

Obesity is considered by some to be a form of inflammation. There is a vicious circle. Long-term excess of Omega Six, combined with fat deposition, starts the process. Omega Six encourages storage and switches down the metabolism. Excess Omega Six is the catalyst for the production of inflammatory products. Excess inflammatory products lead to metabolic disorders, which include diabetes, impaired digestion, and vascular conditions. A self-fuelling inflammatory cycle is started. Metabolic syndrome develops, exacerbating the problems.

12.2 Digestion and inflammation–

If your digestion is not working well, you are not absorbing your food well. Digestion is fundamental to good health. The surface area of the small intestine is the size of a tennis court, which is a lot of membrane and messengers (made from fats in the membranes) to maintain. If your digestion is not working you may have inflammation, which activates the inflammatory factors that prevent digestion–a vicious cycle.

Elaine Gottschall's book *Breaking The Vicious Cycle* suggests limiting foods containing complex sugars for a while. It is a simple, short, thought provoking book on intestinal health. The gut has its own direct hotline to the immune controllers. Problems in the gut set up immune responses in the rest of the body.

Cells leak inflammatory agents into the blood stream. An inflammation call sets excess Omega Six into action. If Omega Three is short, there is no Omega Three to damp things down. A vicious cycle starts, which will not go away without Omega Three and reduced Omega Six. COX blocking drugs help, but do not deal with the problem.

Drugs clearly are wonderful and have a very useful function, but in 'western' conditions, removal of causes and prevention so far as possible, has to be the starting point.

12.3 Your medical advisor–

Please talk to your medical advisor before undertaking significant dietary change.

Tests for Omega Three and Six status do exist. Doctors that specialise in lipids also exist. It is clear that Omega 3 fatty acids have preventative and therapeutic benefits. More research is required to determine the mechanisms, and to develop age and Omega 3 specific recommendations.

Until there is a clear consensus it appears prudent to ensure intake of the mother Omega Three and include marine sources of Omega 3 fatty acids, via supplementation or fish consumption, throughout the life span. [101]

Bear in mind that fat testing based on blood products, has limitations in terms of its inability to determine your long-term status of stored fats, brain content etc. Testing of the blood will reflect recent changes in diet.

13

DIETARY RULES

13   **Key wider dietary rules**—[Abbreviations listed at 1.1] This is an alternate way to look at diet, and seek basic rules, rather than suggest ingredients or recipes. I end up confused by the variety of advice on diets, but am struck by some common elements. These common factors are clearly and usefully set out in a nutritional paper *"Origins and evolution of the Western diet: health implications for the 21st century"*. This paper suggests our current diet is in discord with the food choices our genes are used to, and looks at key factors.

13.1   **Sugar load**—*Avoid sugar, sugar substitutes, and refined processed foods.* I struggle to understand glycemic load, but on the ancestor diet/genes principle, beware refined food and sugars. Fruit is much sweeter than it was. Use fruit juices moderately. Fruit sugar is sugar, and stripped of fibre. Some dried fruits have high levels of sugars, including fructose.

    Fruit 'drinks', canned drinks, etc. are often high hidden sugar sources. Thirty-nine per cent of the U.S. diet was reported as being of high glycemic load. It was a mixture of sugars 18.6 per cent, and grains 20.4 per cent.

    Neolithic man had very limited access to grains and sugars, and no refined ones. [102] Lower calorie intake, helps long chain fat fabrication, EPA, DHA, and melatonin levels [27.3][103]. Undigested sugar is a big factor in digestive conditions such as IBS. [25, 25.41,42,43]. Fructose [25.20] and sugar [25.38] contributes heavily to obesity [25.6 and 25.39] and metabolic syndrome [25.21]. Obesity and metabolic syndrome closely link to many western illnesses.

13.2   **Fatty acid composition**—*Moderation in general terms. Consider cutting <u>right</u> down on high Omega 6 vegetable oils [p. 287].* Avoid artificial trans fats absolutely [11.29]. Avoid polyunsaturates in chip pans [11.4]. Cut down on fatty cuts of grain fed meat sources [11.25], **excess** butter, cheese etc. Eat some oily fish / fish oil, or use vegan [1.36] DHA, EPA supplements. Get some mother Omega 3 in flax seed or a high mother Omega 3 source [p.287, 30.31 and 26.5].

Virgin olive oil has known health benefits. [Processed olive oil may be high in Omega 6]. Coconut may assist in weight loss, and is an antibacterial [11.31].

Bear in mind many fats are unseen, in bakery products [11.21], processed foods etc. It is essential that you check labels.

There is controversy on saturated fats [11.25]. Clearly excess saturated fats are undesirable, but saturated fats are not 'lethal'. Saturates are essential to body function and membrane structure. Saturated fats are made in the body. Where saturated fats replace Omega 6 polyunsaturates, fat conversion improves.

Overall, extracted oils were not significantly available to our ancestors. Trans fats were not invented. Animal food sources had much lower fat content, and a better Omega 3:6 balance. So;

☞ Moderation within sensible limits.

☞ Balance the Omega Three and Six mother fats.

☞ Ensure a regular supply of Omega 3s as only a little is stored.

☞ Ensure a regular supply of long chain Omega 3s, DHA and EPA.

☞ Consider a sensible amount of coconut and butter.

☞ Limit fatty meats from grain fed animals.

13.3 **Macronutrient composition and density**—*Use whole foods as far as possible. Foods are a complex mix of nutrients, minerals, and vitamins. They are nature's pharmacy. Get as wide a variety as possible.* The body needs vitamins, minerals, and other chemicals, to make processes work. It has learned how to use the chemicals in food, in a giant balancing act. As hunter-gatherers, it is likely we had a much wider diet base than we do today.

Refining removes many nutrients, minerals, and vitamins, turning food into a pharmacy with bare shelves. Our domestication of plant food has resulted in falling nutritional density. We often tend to throw away the most nutritious bits, like the brown part of grains. A green powder with lots of different constituents can help widen the scope of your diet. Grass fed/wide grazing animals will have the best Omega Three–Six profile in milk and meat, and likely more nutrients.

13.4 **Acid-base balance**—*It is reported that in general, our bodies are too acid.* Our ancestors would have been, on balance, alkaline. This is because of our western diet. Long-term acid imbalance can have serious health risks. The professional says, "fish, meat, poultry, eggs, shellfish, cheese, milk, and cereal grains are net acid producing, whereas fresh fruit, vegetables, tubers, roots, and nuts are net base producing". Legumes yield near-zero mean acid values.

Salt is net acid producing because of the chloride ion. There are reported exceptions, such as acidifying vegetables, - corn, lentils, and winter squash, - and acidifying fruits – blueberries, cranberries, currants, plums, prunes, canned fruit, rhubarb etc. Opinions also vary between sources, for example olive oil is described as both acid and alkaline. So it is best to check on various web sites.

Generally, refined food, carbonated drinks, tobacco, beer, and artificial sweeteners are extremely acid forming. As a result, the experts say healthy adults consuming the standard U.S. diet sustain a chronic, low-grade pathogenic metabolic acidosis that worsens with age, as kidney function declines.

It is not about the acidity of the food, but the effect a food has on the acidity of the body. *Almost all pre-agricultural diets, were net base yielding because of the absence of cereals, and energy-dense, nutrient-poor, foods.* Foods introduced in the Neolithic and Industrial eras displaced base-yielding fruits and vegetables[104].

Urine test strips are inexpensive and easy to use. Acid and alkaline levels will change so don't panic based on one result. Several sites on the Web list the acid alkali forming status of foods. Balance, moderation, and variety are key.

13.5 Sodium-potassium ratio—*High salt intake (sodium) is outside the body's operational conditions in the manual. The body was designed to have much higher levels of potassium than sodium.*

The sodium-potassium balance is fundamental to cellular function, electrical function, the movement of raw materials into the cells, and waste product out. Cut down on your salt intake. Become an avid label reader.

The experts say, *"The inversion of potassium and sodium concentrations in hominid diets had no evolutionary precedent and now plays an integral role in eliciting and contributing to numerous diseases of civilisation".* ... Average sodium content (3271 mg/d) in the normal U.S. diet is much higher than the potassium level (2620 mg/d)[105].

This is due to salt in processed food, lower intake of fruit and vegetables, and displacement by whole grains and milk. Alcohol, coffee, sugar, and diuretics cause potassium loss.

13.6 Fibre content—*It's back to fruit and vegetables, pulses and whole foods.* The professionals say the fibre content of the normal U.S. diet of 15.1 g/d is much lower than the recommended value of 25–30g/d. In the U.S., refined sugars, vegetable oils, dairy products, and alcohol contain no fibre, and make up about 48 per cent of the energy intake. Eighty-five per cent of the grains consumed in the U.S. are fibre depleted.[106]"

13.7 Iodine—*Iodine is reported as a key nutrient,* and points to a shoreline origin. Deficiency in pregnancy may compromise the health of the foetus. The use of iodised salt is probably less prevalent. Seafood contains iodine[107]. Seaweed is high in iodine so a good source, but too much could provide excess[108][109].

Iodine supports thyroid function, deficiency can result in metabolic slow down, and weight gain. Conversion of iodine in the thyroid needs effective mitochondrial function. Effective mitochondrial function needs adequate DHA.

Required iodine intake is low and excess can have serious medical consequences. If you are concerned it is best to talk to a medical advisor.

13.8 **Dairy**–[See 9.4 11.25 11.17 13.9] *Fierce arguments rage over whether dairy products are good or bad in dietary terms.* Dairy products supply vitamins, minerals, an important range of fats, digestive flora, and were a healthy staple for many. Swiss mountain folk were a hardy race, and still are Vatican Guards.

Lactose intolerance [the inability to make lactase] is an accepted condition in some. However some northern Europeans continue to produce lactase into adulthood. Transformation into cheese reduces lactose. Hard cheese has the least lactose. The process of making yoghurt produces lactase, thus aiding digestion.

Dairy products can be high in added salts. Medication of cattle is an issue, and there are reports of cattle treatment hormones etc., in dairy products.

Dairy products are increasingly accused of being responsible for all sorts of allergies and disturbances, included as a possible trigger for diabetes 1. [See *The China Study*]. But what has changed? Many humans have a long history of high dairy intake. Is it some other factor related to dairy products that has changed?

Is increased susceptibility to dairy products due to, sensitisation of the immune system, the gearing up of the inflammatory system, immune stress, and poorer gut function, all caused by excess Omega 6 and lack 3? [29.29].

Grain feeding distorts the Omega 3:6 balance in the animals and their body fat. Grass fed animal dairy products have a much better Omega 3:6 profile.

13.9 **Fatty domestic meat**–[See 9.4 11.25 11.17 13.8] The farming industry does a wonderful job in feeding ever growing populations, and stocking our supermarkets year round. But if we are just eating more to try and find the nutrients we seek, and becoming sicker, is it not time for a review of our dietary aims, and farming objectives.

The fat profiles of intensively farmed, and wild, animals are very different. This comment is not against fat, it is about fat profiles, and what we feed our animals. Grain feeding has totally changed the fat profiles of animals. Lean meat content has dropped by 25 per cent, and storage fat increased by 21 per cent, with higher levels of saturation. In a wild animal, fat is about four per cent of the carcass. Farmed intensive animal fat is about 25 per cent [110] .

The impact in calorie terms is substantial. A gram of fat provides nine calories, and a gram of protein four calories. This effect is seen most shockingly in chickens. A wild partridge has 30 grams of fat per kilo (Figures from *The Driving Force*, Crawford and Marsh). A commercial chicken has over 200 grams. One has 300 calories, and the other 2,000 per kilogram. In commercial chicken, just meat and skin has about 1,300 calories per kg. Commercial chicken meat is also much higher in Omega 6 than 3, as are the eggs.

Whilst muscle has other nutrient content, minerals etc., fat is virtually devoid of additional nutrients. So, fatter grain reared animals are filling us with poorly balanced fats, high in calories, which are a storage vehicle for pollutants.

Fat is essential to human health. But they must be the right fats.

14

SIGNS OF IMBALANCE–TESTING AND SPECIALISTS

14.1 **Signs of fat imbalance**–[Abbreviations listed at 1.1] Signs of fat imbalance listed in *Smart Fats* by M. Schmidt include those below. Symptoms may be due to other conditions. Health concerns and significant changes of diet should always be discussed with your medical advisors. The list is in addition to the conditions listed in chapter 29.

☞ Dry or alligator skin.

☞ Dry unmanageable hair and dandruff.

☞ Excessive thirst and frequent urination.

☞ Brittle easily frayed or soft nails.

☞ Irritability.

☞ Hyperactivity.

☞ Attention deficit.

☞ 'Chicken skin' on back of arms.

☞ Dry eyes.

☞ Learning problems.

☞ Allergies.

☞ Poor wound healing.

☞ Lowered immunity.

☞ Frequent infections.

☞ Patches of pale skin on cheek.

☞ Fatigue.

☞ Weakness.

☞ Cracked skin on heels or finger tips.

Omega Three deficiency and excess of Omega Six is the more usual scenario. Omega Six deficiencies do happen [See 11.13]. Some people cannot, or are not very good at making either long chain Omega Three or Six, and so can be deficient in both. Testing a persons essential fatty acid [EFA] status may assume a much greater importance in the future,

Excess of Omega Three mother fat, and a deficiency of Omega Six is rare. I have not found much information on the results of long term mother Omega Three excess. I have seen suggestions including by Udo Erasmus in his book that thinner dryer skin may be a symptom of excess mother Omega Three.

So if on a diet high in mother Omega Three keep a look out for thinner skin round the susceptible parts like ankles. Changing body fats is a slow process. Most will have an excess of Omega Six in their body fat which may take some time to redress, but conversion ability is a key factor.

There is evidence that fat conversion ability diminishes with age. A lack of fat conversion ability would result in long chain fat imbalances and deficiencies of both long chain Omega Three and Six [See 11.13].

I am afraid there are not definitive answers as the necessary trials and observations have not been made. The only way to be more certain of fat status is to get tested - its on my list!

14.2   **Lipid specialists and fat testing**–Please bear in mind that testing of blood products is likely to give a limited view of the body's status, and will reflect short-term dietary fat change.

The body will take two and more years to rebalance fat reserves. Breast fat will show changes in months, but complete adipose fat tissue change can take five and more years.

Blood and plasma measurements will give different profiles to that of stored fat, although it will indirectly reflect long-term stores.

The fat stores of Omega Six will tend to work against dietary reductions of Omega Six[111]. Ensuring adequate Omega Threes can assist counterbalancing.

If on a 'low fat' intake diet, bear in mind you will be releasing historic Omega 6 consumption from fat reserves. Not much Omega 3 is stored at best. Many have diets that are low in Omega Three, so fat reserves will be even lower in Omega 3s. Body fat can contain 25% Omega 6 and well under 1% of Omega 3 in worst case scenarios.

☞ Low fat diets mean different things to different people.

☞ There is no definitive answer, but no matter what your interpretation of low fat, it may be prudent to supplement with the mother and long chain Omega Threes.

☞ Long chain Omega 3s may increase basal metabolism so helping with weight loss [23.52].

☞ Excess Omega 6 may lowering metabolism.[25.7].

15

FATS–WHAT, HOW, WHERE

15.1 **What is a fat?**–[Abbreviations listed at 1.1] A fat is a chemical made of carbon, hydrogen, and oxygen. The fats are wiggly, single-line, daisy chains. The daisies are the carbons, but they have four arms, instead of a stalk. They can use the arms to join to each other, or hold a hydrogen. If they use two hands to join up to one neighbouring carbon, it is called a double bond.

One end of the daisy chain is finished with 3 hydrogen. This end hates water. The other end is finished with oxygen and hydrogen. This end likes water.

The most common double bonds in nature are called Cis bonds. A double Cis bond makes the daisy chain curve. With six double bonds, the fat could be a circle, or a huge variety of chaotic crazy zigzag things [30.10, 30.4]. Shape making ability is important to chemical function, and structural cell membrane fluidity, including 'disorganised' membranes zones. [1.36].

Trans fats are not common in nature. Trans double bonds make straight chains [30.37]. Shapes are important as to how friendly a carbon daisy chain, can be with other chemicals. The positions of the double bonds, affects how well a fat can nestle up to, and join up with, other fats and chemicals.

Fats are stored by attaching them to a spine, that holds fats, which can be the same or different. Racks with two fats are used as bricks in the cell membranes.

The toast racks with two fats all line up, and form a membrane, like the skin of a bubble. The water hating bits all point inwards. Another parallel inner skin forms, and the water hating bits face the other skin. Watery substances are on the outside skins of the double skinned bubble, and water hating bits are protected in the middle between the double skins. It is simple and ingenious. [30.27b]

Storage fats toast racks, and structural membrane toast racks are different. Storage fats are held in threes, [30.38] and membrane fats in pairs. Storage fats are not used in cell membranes, so fats can be stored in different proportions to the mixes used in membranes. Different cell type membranes, need different fat mixes, to give them the required physical properties, like flexibility.

You see the natural behaviour of fats when you put a drop into water, and get a film of fat. That simple chemical reality effectively allows us to exist, and have a structure. Think about it next time you do the washing up. That greasy mix disappearing down the plug is our essence.

15.2   Body laboratories and fat factories–The human body can make all fats, except the mother Omega Three and Omega Six. Your cells are a series of incredibly complex laboratories and fat factories. They outshine any hi-tech process or lab facility.

The body's labs have huge flexibility, redundancy capacity, adaptability, secondary, and emergency options. The liver is the primary fat factory. All sorts of cells can manufacture fats, including brain cells.

Fat around your tummy [adipose], and elsewhere, is stored in cells called adipocytes [3.11]. Adipocytes are little factories too. They and surrounding support cells, use fats, and Omega Six stores, to make a whole range of important chemicals and hormones. The fat matrix has nerve cells and blood vessels.

The body needs a constant supply of hormones to function, as women know only too well. To have constant supply, there has to be a storage depot of raw materials. Raw material storage depots, are your fat cells, and their contents.

15.3   Fats we cannot make–The matriarchal essential fatty acids, EFAs, of the Omega Three and Six series, CANNOT be made in the body, by humans and the majority of animals. They are called Linolenic acid ALA 18:3 n3 (Omega Three) and Linoleic LA 18:2 n6 (Omega Six). LA and ALA have to be obtained from plants, or plant eaters, direct or indirect. The body cells however can elongate the mother fats into the longer chain children. For example ALA can be made into DHA and EPA (Omega Three), but Omega 3 and 6;

☞ *Cannot be used interchangeably by the body.*

☞ *Cannot be changed into each other.*

☞ *Have specific and distinct individual functions in the body.*

15.4   Fats we eat as fats–We get a huge range of fats in our foods. Fats are found in greens, seeds, nuts, meat and fish. Fats are found in all living things. Our body can make some fats, BUT Omega Three and Omega Six mother fats can only be got from food. The body can survive on very low fat intakes. We hear of a small number of fats. There are many more from the various families; they just do not figure highly in research.

15.5   Fats from carbohydrates–The body can and does make all fats, excluding Omega 3 and 6, from carbohydrates including sugars. The body can make Omega 7 and 9s [30.33, 30.34]. This raises questions as to how the body decides what fats to make and store. Fats made by the body from carbohydrates including sugars may be stored, used as energy, or used in cell membranes. Weight for weight, fats holds two times as much energy as carbohydrates.

15.6   **Other fats from fats**–We can do some nifty chemical engineering, and turn fats into longer or shorter chains, in the same family. BUT only if the conditions in the body are right. The longer the chain, the more complicated the process is, and the less that gets converted. There are a host of things that block the conversion pathways [11.13].

15.7   **In the liver**–The liver is the main chemical factory and warehouse for fat synthesis.

15.8   **In the cells**–Fats can be manufactured, extended, or broken down in individual cells of your body–tiny, amazing, sophisticated, factory complexes. Processing is done in sub cell units like mitochondria. The body is very organised. It manufactures in big factories like the liver centrally, or locally as needed.

Much of the immune response and repair, is organised and conducted at local cellular levels. This allows very unstable chemicals to be used that are too reactive, and unstable to transport around the body. It also enables initial responses to be virtually instantaneous. These chemicals are so powerful, for instance, that special ones are used in minute dosages to induce labour.

The system raw materials like Omega Three or Omega Six, are stored as the building blocks of the cell wall. They are taken out of the cell walls when needed to make immune and inflammatory chemicals. This saves delays and, for instance, the brain from sending a request to the adipose tissue, or liver, for immediately needed supplies. Cells use the fats they have and replace them after. The ratio of Omega Three and Omega Six fats, used as building bricks in the cell walls, reflects our diet. High Omega Six in diet = high levels of Omega Six in cell membranes.

When the body needs raw materials for immune or inflammation alerts, it knows what length of fat it is looking for, e.g. 20 or 22 carbons chain, but has no way of distinguishing a 20 long carbon Omega Six from a 20 carbon long Omega Three in the membrane. The body will simply take the fats on a random basis. The chemicals created will simply reflect cell membrane content, and so dietary intake. High Omega 6 dietary intake = high production of Omega 6 chemicals.

Your fat intake really does have a huge impact, at lots of fundamental levels, on the way the body operates. Omega 3 and 6 cannot directly or indirectly originate anywhere else but diet.

Imagine the fats are flowers grown for picking. You plant the seed (Diet). Seeds make flowers. (Membrane content). You randomly pick flowers (taking fat from membrane). The bouquet colours and design must reflect the flowers which reflect the seeds planted. (Chemical reactions reflect fat in diet)

Like a picking garden if the Omega 3:6 Six fat in diet (seeds planted) is imbalanced, the fat in your cell membrane (flowers grown) will be imbalanced. If the fats (flowers) in your cell membranes are imbalanced, your body's chemical reactions (bouquets) will be imbalanced. It is unavoidable and simple.

16

FATS-WHAT THEY ARE USED FOR
IN THE BODY

16.1   **Magic bricks**–[Abbreviations listed at 1.1] Fats are key structural building blocks. Fats are the bricks of cell membranes. An oil slick of your fats would cover 10 football pitches. [112]

You are very literally, what you have eaten. Skin is made of cell membranes, and they are in part what you ate. Skin is the largest body organ, about 16 per cent of a person's weight. It is a barrier and control gate, between the outside world, and the workings of our bodies. [113] Skin has a high requirement for fats, to maintain its integrity and function.

Fats are magic bricks. Wrong bricks, dodgy house. Wrong fats, wonky body functions. Fats are part of the magic wall of the cell membranes. Each fat type gives the membranes particular properties.

Fats team up in pairs linked by other chemicals. The more oil loving ends point inwards. The flirty water loving ends point out. The fat membranes lie next to each other, forming a double skin like a pair of concentric soap bubbles [30.27]. Parts of the membrane will be organised and regimented [30.24], and parts loose and chaotic [30.27b] [1.36]

Fats come and go from the membrane. The outer and inner skins are different. The type of fats in a cell membrane will define its character, flexibility, and function. For example nerve cabling has different physical properties than a brain cell.

A bit like people–the social characteristics of the group [organ] and individuals [cells] will define who is talked to, who is ignored, what is ordered, what is consumed, and who is invited to dinner.

Change the composition of the membranes and you change the properties of the cell. DHA has very particular properties [1.36], and is found in higher concentrations in mitochondrial membranes.

Mitochondria have specialist membranes. Without adequate Omega Three and Six, cells do not function 'properly'.

At times of shortage (famine/serious food shortage), the body tends to retain the DHA which forms part of the structure of the cell membrane. If there is a DHA shortage, there may not be enough DHA to properly make cell structures.

The use of fats for both structure, and as a source of raw materials for the manufacture of chemicals is an ingenious system. For example the mother Omega 3 is used first and foremost to protect the skin, and is easily oxidised. DHA has been shown to inhibit the growth of melanoma cells [114].

Imagine a house that kept you dry, but you could use the bricks, as food, protection, messengers, and the windows opened and closed automatically to let things in and out. Your cells do all this and more.

16.2   DHA in the membrane—Cell membranes are envelopes, little bubbles. They are waterproof walls that surrounds our cells, and us. DHA has a unique and irreplaceable role. DHA has a special shape. DHA is more energetic and chaotic [1.36]. DHA is used between lipid rafts [30.24]. Lipid rafts make highly organised sections, access loading bays, and production machines.

If your membranes do not open the doors at the right time, or have the right variety of doors, the right communication, and delivery systems, your body will not work. It is no different to any factory or supermarket.

DHA in membranes influences the passage of electric currents, like those that keep your heart going, it works with enzymes, and it is involved with neurotransmitters. If your membranes do not work properly, nothing does.

16.3   Storage—Fat cells are bubbles [3.10] acting as long and short-term fuel storage depots. Fat cells are petrol tanks. Fats cells stabilise fuel supply. Fats prevent wild fluctuations in hormones. Fats remove the need to eat all the time.

16.4   Destruction for energy—Fats contain a lot of energy, which is why we can run our cars on fats, and their cousins petrol and diesel.

Fats provide a major energy source for most tissues. The mitochondria of cells 'burn' fats to create energy. The heart can get 70 per cent of its energy needs from fat oxidation [115]. The brain uses about 20–25w, approximately 20 per cent of the body's energy consumption of about 100w [116] [2400kcal is equivalent to 116w]. The heart is the highest energy-consuming organ in the body. [117]

Mitochondria make energy, and process raw materials, in return for nutrients. They were originally symbiotes. DHA is the highest quality fuel, and present in significant quantity in the inner mitochondrial cell membrane. I guess adequate DHA in the membrane is essential to the efficient 'burning' of fat to produce energy. DHA is key to membrane fluidity and the correct electrical function.

By-products of the burning process are explosive compounds used in the body's defence and rubbish clearance. They include peroxides (same family as hair bleach) and aldehydes.

I guess that to get a clean and efficient 'burn' in the body's mini-boilers, the mitochondria, the fuel has to be in the right mix. Effective maintenance and combustion requires the right balance of DHA available in the cell. Mitochondria work with other cells like peroxisomes.

It is immensely complex, beyond me, and much is unknown, but it is clear that DHA has unique and fundamental roles in energy production, oxidation, and oxidation products. Peroxisomes break down fats and produce oxidants like peroxide. They also work with the mitochondria.

"Perilla and fish oils, compared to palm and safflower oils, approximately doubled and more than tripled, respectively, peroxisomal fatty acid oxidation rate. [118]"

Better control of mitochondrial oxidation may improve fitness, and reduce cardiovascular and metabolic disease, by making more essential proteins. [119.]

Omega Six is less well oxidised, and makes more damaging oxidation products, superoxides, which have been linked, for example, to clogging of the arteries. The wrong balance, and the mitochondrial powerhouses may clog up and fail. The weapons, immune and cleaning products, may not function to specification. Systems may fail without adequate DHA and EPA in your diet.

16.5   **Defence weapons**–The body uses the spare exhaust products of the cellular mitochondrial and peroxisomal processes, oxidants, as weapons and cleaning agents.

Subtle safety and security is required to keep weapons in control. If the weapons get out of control, they start destroying the good guys, as well as the bad guys. Part of that control system, is a supply of antioxidants. Part of the control system is factory maintenance, with the right fuels and production processes.

The antioxidants we eat help, but are a long way from the whole story. The combustion rates, processes and fuels used, are controlled by subtle interplay between factories, fuel fats, and antioxidants. The body creates some of the most powerful antioxidants, for example melatonin. Melatonin, is reported as being 20 times more powerful than vitamin C. Melatonin increases in pregnancy.

Substandard fuel and processes means less effective burning [oxidation], and poorer quality, or faulty weapons, which may mean damaged cells, or faulty DNA escape destruction.

Inappropriate cell destruction is a feature of autoimmune conditions. Failure to destroy damaged cells is a feature in cancers. The balances are very fine. DHA as a fuel is central to mitochondrial and peroxisomal function, which are central to body processes.

16.6   **Lubricants**–The body uses fats as part of the lubricants for joints, eyes, and bodily fluids. Fats are also used as antifreeze. The longer fats such as DHA are less prone to freezing. Fish in colder water have higher DHA levels, as do the feet of animals that spend a lot of time in snow.

16.7   Hormone messengers—Fats act as hormone and chemical messengers, to the fat storage, and burning processes. The hormones indicate what is available to burn, the levels of incoming energy from food, the muscle requirements, etc. The fats levels act in effect as a series of fuel gauges.

16.8   Gene expression—Genes are a really hot topic in the press. For a gene to have an effect, you have to own a copy, and it has to be switched on. All the genes you own are present in all your cells. But only a few are switched on dependant on the cell's function.

The more gene copies that are switched on, the greater the effect. Genes that are switched on are described as 'expressed'. Food can switch genes on and off. Different fats switch on different genes.

Omega Three and Omega Six can significantly alter expression of genes, and so the function of cells involved in fat storage and energy production. [120] Omega 3 and 6 change the expression of many genes including BRAC and HER2.

The effects of fats on gene regulation can be seen in hours. The effects are sustained as long as the fats are in the diet. [121] In a trial related to muscular structure in aged mice, significant differences were seen in gene expression between high Omega Three, and high Omega Six intake.

Of 588 genes surveyed, the high Omega Three group had 12 genes, including glucose regulators and tumour suppressors, that were expressed 100–340 per cent more than those of the high Omega Six group.

Twenty-eight genes including growth factors (ErbB–2 receptor), and immune regulators, were expressed 50–90 per cent less, in the Omega Three high group, than in the high Six group.

These results underline the importance of DHA, and the ratio of Omega Three and Omega Six in the diet [122]. Food changes the way cells work via genes.

16.9   Chemical pathway—"Western dietary patterns warm up inflammation, while prudent dietary patterns cool it down". [123]

The pathway is called the eicosanoid [20 carbon chain] pathway. It is a number of separate pyramids of chemicals, each made from an exclusive fat.

Mother Omega Three is the raw material for one (p.290). Mother Omega Six is the raw material for the other. Each of the pyramids is a separate, non-interchangeable, exclusive family. The families are complex and extensive as is evident from this diagram [Fig 1.19].

The two families have very different characteristics. They are fundamental to body function.

The quantity made of each family of chemicals, is dependent on the amount of the Omega 3 and 6 raw material present in the cell membranes. The Omega 3 and 6 content of the cell membrane reflects the fats stored, the level of fat conversion to long chain fats, the availability of the conversion enzymes, the long chain fats in the diet, and the current dietary intakes of mother fats.

Omega 6 is heavily stored in adipose tissue. Omega 3 is not. If there is more Omega 6 in the cell membranes, more Omega 6 chemical products will be made [p.286]. The amount of Omega 6 in our cells depends on how much we ate in our diet and how much is stored in our fat tissues.

This connects our body function to the environment. Our disconnect from the environment is relatively recent. Supermarkets, extensive farming, chemical structural modification of fats, mechanically extracted and heavily treated vegetable oils, and the extensive use of oils in preprepared foods including deep frying, are very new in our dietary history.

The body just takes the Omega 3 and 6 mother fats available in the proportion they are available, and processes them according to the instruction manual. If the Omega Three fats are not available, or in the wrong proportion, the whole process is thrown out of balance.

The chemicals made from Omega 3 long chain EPA, and Omega 6 AA, interact directly and indirectly in many processes, and are hugely influential in the function of;

☞ Immune, autoimmune and inflammatory systems.

☞ Hormones [including oestrogen and testosterone].

☞ Metabolic regulation.

☞ Fertility cycles and puberty.

☞ Brain function.

☞ Skin.

☞ Sleep and repair–the list goes on.

16.10 Melatonin, sleep, repair–[See chapter 21] Melatonin links our body chemically to light and darkness. Melatonin is another of those fundamental chemicals found in all living creatures, from algae to humans.

Melatonin is made in response to the dark by the pineal gland, and other organs, including the eye retina, lens, and skin. Some plants produce it.

Melatonin has an intimate cyclical relationship with DHA. Melatonin stimulates the production of DHA. DHA stimulates the production of melatonin, through facilitating serotonin production.

I suggest DHA shuts down the inflammatory Omega Six chemical production, which facilitates production of more DHA. So more DHA results in more melatonin. Increased melatonin results in increased DHA production.

DHA and melatonin by different mechanisms, shutdown the inflammatory Omega Six chemical production pathway. Melatonin and DHA work in a mutual self-reinforcing cycle.

The shutdown, sleep, damps down the Omega Six based inflammatory process, and Omega 6 fat release from adipose cells. Serotonin is necessary to make melatonin. Serotonin shortage in the brain is linked with DHA deficit, as are a host of brain functional issues. [124]

DHA deficit is linked to sleep disturbance, as are the Omega 6 inflammatory products, and immune markers. Sleep disturbance has been linked to asthma, [125] obesity, [126] and inflammatory conditions.

It is likely that the inflammatory products connected with obesity, cause sleep deficiency, and create a self fuelling cycle of less sleep and more inflammation.

It is clear metabolism changes at night, the impact is less clear. Higher PGE2 levels have been associated with being awake and activity. Increasing DHA in diet normalises melatonin levels in DHA deficient animals. [127] [128] Melatonin receptors are found in many organs including the immune system. The information flow is bidirectional. [129]

Increased melatonin damps down Omega Six inflammatory COX2 products of the eicosanoid pathways. [130] "Eicosanoid hormones are short-lived, local hormones affecting the producing and adjacent cells." They stimulate inflammation, regulate blood flow, "control ion transport across membranes, modulate synaptic transmission, and induce sleep... [131]"

In summary, melatonin triggers DHA production, which shuts down the Omega Six pathways. Melatonin also independently shuts down the inflammatory COX2 pathways. Increased DHA facilitates increased serotonin, which increases melatonin. Increased production of melatonin sets up a cycle with DHA, to damp down the inflammatory system.

Sleep is a slowing down, and alert step down. Melatonin acts as a powerful antioxidant to dampen activity. Lack of sleep increases the extent of inflammation in the body. If you want to sleep properly and give your repair paths a chance to work, cut down on Omega Six, and ensure adequate long chain Omega Three.

16.11   **Inflammation, obesity, sleep deprivation**—Sleep disturbance has been linked to asthma [132] and obesity. [133] It is likely that the inflammatory products connected with obesity, cause sleep deficiency. Obesity is linked to higher levels of circulating inflammatory agents. Obesity is also linked with lower levels of Omega Three.

Lack of DHA would restrict production of melatonin from serotonin. The combination of lower melatonin, and higher circulating inflammatory factors, would make it harder for the body to shut down.

On this basis, obesity may be a long-term cause of sleep deprivation. Interestingly, melatonin is reported as blocking the release of Omega Six from adipose tissue in sleep, and reducing metabolism of Omega Six. Sleep deprivation lowers leptin. [134]

Melatonin is a one use only antioxidant. Is night time oxidation, the mechanism that reduces melatonin levels, bringing the sleep cycle to a close, so allowing the Omega Six products back to work?

17

INTAKE RATIOS—HOW MUCH,
THE ENVIRONMENT, OTHER ANIMALS

17.1 **Omega 3:6 intake ratio**—[Abbreviations at 1.1] What is the ideal dietary intake of fats? It is a hotly argued subject. It is key to the discussions in this book. Neither we nor any other animal (excluding some worms) can make Omega Six and Omega Three mother fats.

Animals and we, can only get the mother Omega 3 and 6 from the food chain, greens plants, plankton, fish, etc. Land based greens, roots, and fruit flesh, on average contain equal amounts of Omega 3 and 6. So a 1:1 ratio of the mother Omega 3 ALA, and mother Omega 6 LA, is likely what we were designed for.

We also may have an underlying optimal need for additional long chain Omega 3 intake, above that available in our background survival plains diet, if we grew our brains with additional DHA from a shoreline marine diet.

Plains gatherers survived on relatively low energy diets. Swiss were healthy eating lots of mountain cheese. Polynesians fared well on fish and coconut. Eskimos did well on high marine fats. Yes they had other diseases of poverty, but not the western conditions we increasingly see in the ever younger people.

People on pre-industrial diets had much lower rates of western conditions, and according to *Nutrition and Physical Degeneration* by Weston Price, better jaw structures, less dental crowding, and very much lower level of decay.

All animals in a wild environment have a 1:1 Omega 3:6 ratio in the brain. Dolphins also have a 1:1 ratio in muscle tissue. They are a land mammal living in the sea. The ability of dolphins to metabolise excess long chain Omega 3s from the marine diet without harm, may suggest we should be able to as well.

Fish are high in Omega 3, so somehow dolphins are locating high Omega 6 sources in the sea, or more likely burning off most of the Omega 3 they acquire for heat and energy, and storing Omega 6s. Marine algae have much higher levels of Omega 3 than 6, which is why fish have higher Omega 3 than 6s.

On balance, the range of Omega Six to Omega Three mother fat in the human diet was possibly between 1:4 and 4:1 (a guesstimate). Exact answers are not available. Different schools of thought suggest different ratios as ideal. Like everything in life, each will confer slightly different advantages and disadvantages. So you have to do your reading and take your choice.

I aim to balance the mother fats, and take additional long chain Omega 3s in the form of fish oil/ oily fish. I ensure a supply of long chain Omega 3, to secure against conversion difficulties, the high levels of Omega 6 LA hidden in our diet, the importance of Omega 3 DHA to the brain, and to balance my historic fat reserves high in Omega 6. The mother Omega 3 ALA, and the long chain Omega 3s are metabolised differently, and balancing is primarily about the mother fats. An excess within reason of long chain Omega 3 will likely be burnt for heat and energy. If the conversion pathways are blocked supplementation is necessary.

17.2   DHA : EPA ratio—Fish oils vary in content, depending on which fish, and what parts of the fish body are used. EPA is higher in some, DHA higher in others. Some trials argue that EPA blocks the Omega Six pathways, and argue for higher levels of EPA. However DHA also acts as a COX blocker, and regulates Omega Six production as well. It is complicated and depends on, conversion rates, retro-conversion, consumption of conversion blockers, existing storage status, metabolism, and fats in the diet.

DHA is an essential structural element in the cell membrane, so an adequate supply of both DHA and EPA would seem to be the ideal. I am afraid it is something you will have to try and work out for yourselves.

I have found no trials which give a definite answer on this question, beyond that women's uptake of DHA drops of at about two grams of DHA a day, which itself would depend on the historic fat status, and intake of the women at the time. Recommendations for DHA vary between 200-300mg to 1 or two grams a day.

17.3   Less makes more—Lower fat intake levels improve conversion of Omega Three and Omega Six mother fats, to the long chain children. Interestingly, plant sterols also improve conversion. This would make sense in survival terms.

If you were a plains dweller, and there was no access to marine foods, you would have to rely on fats from greens, roots, seasonal fruit, insects etc.

Conversion to long chain fats would need to be as efficient as possible. Trials suggest this is the case. [135] To use other compounds in plants like sterols to assist with conversion, would be a good survival strategy.

When humans historically had access to excess EFA, it was primarily Omega 3, from the aquatic environment. Conversion rates to long chain fats could afford to fall. *Excess of Omega 6 or Omega 3 fat reduces conversion.*

17.4   Modern men do not convert well— Modern men are poor converters. Poor conversion has implications for social behaviour, including aggression and impulsiveness.

Lack of Omega Three and excess Omega Six may be a big factor in the behaviour changes we are seeing. If my analysis is correct, we are gathering a vast well of 'western' disease, and increased aggression for future years.

Conversion of EPA to DHA in the human body, is a complicated, and a difficult sensitive process. [136] A trial in young men, found very little mother Omega Three, was converted to DHA. Poor conversion in young men underlines the importance of supplementation. [137]

Survival in the wild in areas, with low access to long chain Omega 3, would require the ability to convert the mother fat. To what extent is poor conversion due to modern dietary elements? *Excess mother Omega 6 blocks conversion [11.13, p286, Fig 3.26]. Older men did convert but only .04 per cent.* [138]

Low dietary DHA or Omega 3 mother fat, and utilisation of DHA from the brain, eyes, and reproductive cell membranes, by rising alcohol intake has massive social and health implications.

In elderly males, there are rising levels of neurological degenerative disorders, dementia and Alzheimer's, which are not seen to the same extent in Japan.

We are seeing dramatic rises in liver disease in the young, and moderate drinkers. In young men and male children, we are also seeing rising neurological disorders, greater aggression, criminality, impulsiveness, lack of social cohesion, suicide, depression, ADHD into adulthood, all of which combine towards a less cohesive, more fragmented, less settled society.

17.5   **Women convert better than men**–A trial in women of reproductive age came up with the following result. (ALNA is an acronym for the Omega Three mother fat linolenic acid) "Estimated net fractional ALNA inter-conversion was EPA 21 per cent, DPA six per cent and DHA nine per cent." [139]

Levels of DHA in breast milk in the West suggest that both Omega Three intake and conversion are low. In a Canadian trial, almost all women were showing DHA levels in milk, that suggested intake below the national minimal recommendation [23.15]

Chinese women over a range of diets, exhibit much higher levels of DHA and AA. At low fat intake levels, Omega Three conversions may get preference, but low fat intake is relatively rare in the West. Higher levels of Omega Six, beyond the design parameters, may well also be disrupting conversion. [23.26]

Lack of raw materials will also contribute to low DHA levels. Greater conversion would suggest greater utilisation and need.

A combination of low mother Omega 3 intake, conversion blockage, and alcohol, is creating very low DHA levels in western women. This poses a significant future health risk to women, and their offspring, at very many levels.

17.6   Anti fat fanatics–A 'low fat diet', with no saturated fat intake, eating no fish and only high polyunsaturated vegetable oil, (grape seed, sunflower, safflower) is high in Omega 6 and very low in Omega 3, and so may be worse in Omega 3:6 terms than a 'take away diet'. Ironically a diet with burgers and butter, may be higher in Omega Three, than some low fat diets. Virgin olive oil is low in Omega 3, and contains about 10 per cent Omega 6.

Low fat diets in India[i] had high Omega 6:3 ratios, about 38:1, and linked to high levels of heart disease and diabetes. A reduction in the Omega Six–Three ratio to 9.1:1, reduced mortality by 40 percent.

This imbalance in low fat diets, may be why diet conscious women suffer from inflammatory conditions too. Low fat dieters could be creating a big imbalance of high Omega Six, high trans fats, and very low Omega Three.

17.7   Your pets –Cats are very poor at making the long chain Omega 3 and 6, neural fatty acids. They rely mainly on their prey, for long chain fats. (A good reason to ensure your pets get adequate EFA, why cats like fish, and why we are seeing diabetes in domestic cats!)

Producing long chain fats is resource expensive. So we trade things off for convenience. The example of felines, suggests that for those unable to make DHA and EPA, etc., supplementation is a valid option.

17.8   Brain ratio 1:1 –The Omega 3:6 brain ratio in many species is 1:1. Animals use different fats mixes in muscles and livers, but all species had the same 1:1 Omega 3:6 ratio of fats in their brains. [140] Departments of the brain are different sizes in different species depending on specialism, but overall fat balance remains the same. I have not managed to find figures on the lipid status of human brains. Brains in zoo animals show fats imbalances compared with wild animals

The importance of DHA to the developing brain is seen in the actions of the placenta, which will strip DHA even from a mothers brain, for the foetus. [141]

17.9   Lake, or shore dwellers–There is significant argument in *The Driving Force* that 'Aquatic Man' man evolved on the shoreline, or lake edge. Marine and shoreline food would provide adequate DHA for brain expansion.

They cite as evidence our love of water, ability to swim long distances to depths to forage, automatic heart rate drop reflex on immersion, need for iodine, fat under the skin in common with aquatic mammals not seen in savannah animals, inefficient water conservation techniques, and the innate ability of infants under six months to swim. The dolphin foetus has legs. [142] Dolphins have 3:6 a ratio of in muscle and liver stores, of 1:1. A cod has a 3:6 ratio of 40:1.

---

i   Effects of an Indo-Mediterranean Diet on the Omega-6/Omega-3 Ratio in Patients at High Risk of Coronary Artery Disease: The Indian Paradox *World Rev Nutr Diet. Basel, Karger, 2003, vol 92, pp 74–80* Pella D, Dubnov G, Singh RB, Sharma R, Berry EM, Manor O.

18

OMEGA SIX, THE ENVIRONMENTAL HUMAN MASTER-SWITCH

18.1   **Who is the boss, humans or nature?**—[Abbreviations at 1.1] Does nature respond to humans, or humans to nature? There is no question that we increasingly impact upon, and control, or have unthinking dominion over our environment. The degree of our impact and control, has vastly extended, as the human population expanded.

But we evolved to natures call, environmental conditions, and availability of food and resources. We did not historically 'terraform' the planet to suit our evolution or design.

The planet, nature, or God, 'people formed' us. The emergence of high levels of Omega Six arguably allowed the development by design or evolution of placental and sophisticated vascular systems.

We built a whole body system round Omega Six. When Omega Six was not freely available, systems shut down and went into economy mode. Lots of Omega Six meant the planet was blooming, and a lack meant famine. Our bodies adjusted to try and survive as best we could, according to the prevalent conditions.

We have now found a way to alter the availability of supply of Omega Six, nature's fundamental controller, very extensively in a very short time frame. Our body chemistry is unable to keep up.

18.2   **Emergence of placental land animals** —Without Omega Six, the female body cannot reproduce. Life originated in the seas where there is a predominance of Omega Three fats. Reproduction was primarily by egg laying.

At the end of the Cretaceous period new flowering high Omega Six sources, seed-bearing plants, enabled the development of placental mammals with the necessary vascular support systems. On board gestation allowed huge mobility to follow food sources, and so population expansion.

18.3   Environmental genetic master–Omega Six provides a direct genetic connection to our environment, its fertility, and seasons. Omega Three and Omega Six are essential to life and must be obtained from food directly (plants) and/or indirectly (animals).

A fertile land produces higher levels of seeds and nuts. We contain 'programmed' in-built responses to an environment that is bursting with food, or struggling to support us. Seeds and nuts are very high in Omega Six. Food changes gene expression.

It is a little like a rain sensor on car wipers. High Omega Six triggers fat storage. Stored fats are a source, of raw materials for the hormones, and of necessary chemicals for breeding. Stored fat gives hormone stability over a time frame of a year or more, in normal conditions.

In very lean times, the hormones are downgraded and the female reproductive cycle switches off as seen in anorexia and following deprivation. The body goes into economy mode.

A pregnancy with a negative outcome is a life-threatening risk to the mother, and may prejudice future fertility. In survival terms, a pregnancy is wasteful where the infant does not survive.

In summary Omega Six is intimately connected in the control of the reproductive pathways, fertility, [143] loss of periods in anorexia, [144] [145] early puberty, adhesion of fertilised eggs, general facilitation of stem cell type activity, cell splitting and migration, and so is a master food controller of body function.

18.4   Omega Six no 'off switch'– The body is hard wired with a prime directive to store Omega Six as fat when plentiful, because Omega Six is key to breeding.

Omega Threes are preferentially used as energy, and are a prime moderator of, and balance to the Omega 6 function. In nature, periods of plenty are seasonal and not indefinite. This has consequences for obesity.

I believe Omega Six directs the body to go into storage mode. There is no 'off [stop storing Omega Six] switch'. An 'off switch' was not necessary. There was never too much Omega Six.

High sources of Omega 6 –seeds, grains, and nuts–were scarce and seasonal. Today, in contrast, Omega 6 is permanently available in cheap, easy excess.

The results of permanent Omega 6 excess are a disaster, literally. Consequences of excess Omega Six include, obesity, metabolic syndrome, whole body low-level inflammation, oxidative stress leading to genetic corruption, and the acceleration or multiplication of a host of medical conditions.

The delicate dietary intake control mechanisms, through leptin, the storage of fats through insulin, and the supporting mechanisms are blocked in conflict, by the unstoppable prime directive to store Omega Six.

Whilst the body is supplied with excess Omega Six, it will continue to store it. Excess Omega Six is arguably a fundamental factor in rising obesity.

18.5   Warmth—If you live by the sea or lake, you have a constant source of Omega Three. If there was excess fat in the diet, it was likely to be Omega Three from marine sources, and so long chain Omega 3 DHA, and EPA, was more expendable for energy and warmth, than environmentally scarce Omega Six.

The ability to create body warmth is key, if you spend a lot of time in and around cold water. Omega Three was a plentiful available clean energy source for production of body heat, and higher basal metabolism. Omega Three encourages fat burning. Omega Three is not stored in significant quantity, almost no matter what the intake level.

This suggests that during our key evolutionary design time frame, Omega 3 food sources were relatively constant, and significant storage of Omega Three did not confer a survival advantage. This suggests we are 'aquatic' mammals.

18.6   Savannah living —A hunter-gatherer that does not live by the sea, or lake, will have less access to Omega Three. Wild herbivores are lean. Hunting is energy expensive. Prey may not be plentiful. Omega Three and Sixes are more or less balanced on the average in green plants and roots.

Hunger and low EFA fats intake, pushes up the conversion rates of the mother fats to the long chain fats. Plant sterols push up the Omega 3 and 6 conversion pathways. A lean forest dweller eating enough greens with odd bits of meat, insects, etc., should meet the minimum Three–Six requirements.

But these peoples did not have access to refined food, sugars, concentrated and frequent alcohol, which all conspire to inhibit manufacture of the long chain fats, or increase utilisation of EPA and DHA.

It is particularly important for vegetarians, who rely on the body's conversion for long chain fats, to be aware of the sources of Omega Three, Omega Six, and blocking factors. Vegetarians are reported as being Omega 3 deficient [1.36].

A vegetarian diet high in Omega 6 rich vegetable oils, combined with fat conversion blockers (High Omega 6 sources, sugar, etc.), could present significant health risks. Vegetarians often have high levels of Omega 6 in body fat.

18.7   Conflict between store and burn—Can the body store and burn at the same time? I have been unable to find answers, but this question may have significant implications.

18.8   Body knows best—Is the craving for fat, on a high Omega Six diet, caused by some unknown mechanism, leading the body to seek out Omega Threes that are associated with fatty foods?

Prior to industrial farming, land animals had a far greater amount of Omega Three, in adipose and muscular fat, than they do now. Some animals have been found to have ability to 'taste' and respond to Omega Six. Does such a mechanism exist in man for long chain Omega Three, and are we driven by it?

18.9   **Behaviour and breeding**– You have enough Omega Six stored in adipose tissue? You are ready to breed. If you have a high Omega 6 territory, it is a good strategy to protect that territory.

Protection of territory would confer advantage on aggression, size, and brawn over brain to an extent. In times of plenty, we could afford to be more selfish, more acquisitive, and less cooperative.

Are we breeding a more aggressive, less intelligent society. Is our more aggressive, less gentle, more self-interested society, an expression of lack of Omega Three and excess Six? I believe it is.

18.10   **Broken cycle**–The genetic connection to the environment through Omega 6, by gene expression is very sensitive to low levels of fat. *Nature never provided Omega Six by the shed load, AND with a year round permanent supply. We have thrown a massive spanner into nature's control mechanism.*

With mechanical extraction, vegetable, seed, and nut oils are freely available to excess on demand all year round. Stored fat profiles take 2-5 years to change. Excess Omega 6 is highly significant. The body never has an opportunity to rebalance.

18.11   **Master directive**–We obey our Omega 6 directives, and our drive to breed. We stuff ourselves stupid with Omega 6 until the body starts to 'break'.

We have no instruction set for this scenario. Double whammy, we have inadequate Omega 3 (because we have stopped eating and growing it). Omega 6 is the godfather of the heavies of the immune and reproductive system. Omega 3 is the gentle moderator of the immune and reproductive system.

When the immune system kicks off, there are simply too many heavies living on the street, leading to constant battles even amongst themselves. Heavies and moderators should be more or less in balance.

The content of your cell walls are the Omega Three and Sixes you have eaten. No body has told the body that the fuel had totally changed formulation. The body carries on as normal, taking fats units and processing them.

The body expects the Omega Three and Sixes will be more or less in balance. In evolutionary or design time scales, it has no experience of anything else. But man has created an unnatural distorted intake scenario. Rather than 1:1 or thereabouts, ratios are around 10:1 up to 30:1 and 50:1 in some instances.

A street with 90 Omega 6 heavies to each 10 Omega 3 moderators is likely to end up a problem. The worse the ratio, the more severe the problem, and shorter time to anarchy (illness). The western world is making itself and children, ill, aggressive, less intelligent, and likely to need expensive early medical services.

It is unavoidable. It is written in the body's chemistry. We may not be able to 'prove' it, but the writing is in day-glow, in big letters, and 'on the wall'.

BALANCE THE OMEGA THREE AND SIX MOTHER FATS

19

EXCESS OMEGA SIX, DOES IT EXPLAIN THIS RISE IN 'WESTERN' CONDITIONS?

19. Omega Six, and the rise in 'western' conditions?

Is excess Omega Six sufficiently fundamental in the biology of the body to be capable of providing rational explanations for the huge range of conditions and effects claimed?	Yes–By virtue of the multiple and fundamental direct and indirect roles Omega Six plays in the body including, hormones regulation, cellular building blocks, primary source of a vast range of highly influential chemicals in the eicosanoid pathway, energy storage and production, chemical messengers, fuel, peroxide and aldehyde precursors, T cell regulation, effects on lipid raft function, oxidation rates and reaction energy, cell membrane fluidity, calcium channel and electrical regulation, and ability to alter genetic expression.

Is it a factor that affects ALL people?	Yes—Omega Three and Six are essential fatty acids EFAs. The mother EFAs cannot be manufactured in human or animals. The EFAs are fundamental to the existence, the capacity to reproduce, and life itself. The availability of the EFAs are an externally controlled factor. The availability of the EFAs depends on the fecundity of the earth. We are all commonly bound by a need for a balanced supply of Omega Three and Six.
Is it a factor that is changing on a global scale?	Yes—Dietary intake of Omega Six has radically altered the world over, in the last 100 years. Vegetable and nut oils that were not seen 100 years ago are now staples. Usage continues to increase. The trend is very rapidly spreading to other populations including China. Most of these oils are high in Omega Six and low in Omega Three. Refined foods, and high sugar intake are undoubtedly significant contributing factors.
Is it an external agent, a primary metabolic factor?	Yes—Omega Six is an external agent. Omega Six is a primary metabolic agent. The body cannot make Omega Six. It is the originating raw material, no matter how far down the line you look. No Omega Six = no eicosanoid chemicals or related reaction. It is a direct and simple supply relationship (with the body's fat stores acting as a buffer).
Are there any historic population exceptions that would suggest that people historically lived healthily with very high levels of Omega Six and low Omega Three?	No—I am aware of no population that had access to high levels of Omega Six equivalent to, or near to, today's intake. Given the limited supply of Omega Six in nature, and competition for Omega Six, it is difficult to even conceive of such a scenario.

Genetic Change	Genetic changes of the extent that would be required to account for the enormous increase in 'western conditions' do not occur in the time frame of a hundred years. The expression of genes is altered significantly by food intake. Different Omega Three Six balances significantly alter body functions.
Do populations with a better Omega Three / Six fat profile have a lower incidence of 'western' conditions?	Yes (or didn't would be more accurate, show signs of these disease rises)–Eskimos, Japanese Island populations, Greek Islanders, poor South African fishermen living next door to their wealthy neighbours, all historically had lower reported incidence of 'western' conditions.
Is there another external factor that could obviously be so influential? E.g. Meat protein salt or sugar.	I have not found anything. Some suggest animal protein intake as a factor. There are some powerful arguments put forward. It is not an exclusive external agent. The constituent elements of protein can be made or found in other food. Populations like the Inuits rely in varying degree on high levels of animal/fish protein, and still have a lower incidence of western conditions. I do not think animal protein can be considered in the same category as Omega Three and Six as fundamental external agents. Dairy products were in use prior to this increase in 'western' conditions. Sugar consumption has risen rapidly but is not a unique external substance, being found in a number of forms in natural sources. Sugar is a fuel and does not have the same diverse influence in the body's chemistry. Salt is an external agent. Disturbance of the sodium-potassium ratio is reported as a factor in 'western' disease [146]. However, based on very limited searches, sodium's role whilst fundamental is much less extensive than that of the fats.
Pollution	The Japanese arguably suffer equally from 'western' pollution, but do not share the same rate of increase in 'western' conditions.

20

'WESTERN' DISEASE–WILL TO FUND PREVENTIVE RESEARCH?

20.1   Rising 'western disease', our legacy?–[Abbreviations at 1.1]
We in the West are becoming part of a more aggressive, more depressed, less intelligent era. Diseases of old age are increasingly being seen in the young. Is this our dietary legacy to the next generations?

Increasing rates of, childhood obesity, vascular disease in children of 10 and 12, ADHD, fertility issues, premature births, heart disease, asthma, autism, arthritis, cancers breast melanoma and prostate, osteoporosis, depression, suicide, brain-related disease, adult obesity, higher levels of aggression, self-interest, lower intelligence, is that our legacy?

For the fortunate western world, this is despite access to clean water, better food storage, more food choice, round the year availability, and greater medical knowledge. Some conditions like coronary attack are being held at bay by fabulous advances in surgical intervention and amazing drugs. Early detection may also be skewing increasing survival statistics.

But, it is unarguable that prevention, and of delay illness into true old age, is socially and economically a better option than the early onset of illness, and a lifetime of treatment, for both the individual and state .

Cardiovascular disease was so rare in hospitals at the turn of the 1900s, students are reported as rushing off to see a case, not wanting to miss it. Today they are more likely to be rushing to the next case.

20.2   Who will fund preventive research?–You have seen the list [2.3] of some of the conditions, that have been linked in trials to lack of Omega Three and excess of Omega Six. The trial conclusions are often 'promising, more trials required'. But who is going to fund the necessary prevention trials? Certainly not the drugs companies. There is no profit for drugs companies in improving so many conditions without drugs.

Is Government funding sufficient, and targeted adequately to prevention? It is reported that those on responsible government committees are often connected to companies, or research, in the drugs industry. If their life is immersed in the drugs industry, it is only natural for them to have a drug-centric outlook.

This is not to question motive or integrity. It is a simple fact that our environment, in the widest sense, affects the outlook of all of us. An aborigine looks at nature in a different way to an urban dweller.

Australians have recently begun to start looking at the economics, and wider implications, of prevention.

It will not be generally accepted excess of Omega Six and lack of Omega Three is a central factor in the long list of 'western' conditions, until it is the subject of trials. The Japanese and Chinese have greater focus on fats.

Prevention is just not 'sexy'. To give 'prevention' equal status to 'cure' requires a different outlook, reward, and financing structure. Prevention research, and positive results, have to be given the same razzmatazz, conferences, social reward and recognition as new treatments.

Governments need to devise strategies that direct sufficient research funds into determining cause and prevention. If not governments who else??

20.3 **Treatment or prevention, the cost to the nation** – If governments do not fund prevention, will it be funded at a sufficient level, and with sufficient determination, to achieve concrete indisputable results?

So many trials say, "Shows possible benefit, more research required", but the follow-up does not happen. We, the West, are turning ourselves into a sicker, less intelligent, more aggressive, population.

More illness results in greater, social healthcare, and unemployment costs. The West is reducing its ability to 'compete' in a global world, where some eastern nations are taking prevention very much more seriously.

For the avoidance of any doubt, I am in awe as to progress in medical knowledge and treatment. I am in no sense against progress. Without modern medicine, many of us would not be alive. But can we afford not to spend more on preventive research. Profit as a measure of success is driving funds into drugs research, with little consideration for the cause or long term prevention.

Single targeted treatments in 'western' conditions, however effective, are generally palliatives and not 'cures'. (This comment is applicable only to 'western degenerative' conditions, which are immensely complex and not 'external' conditions that may have less complex initiation pathways).

Side effects may not be visible, or associated with particular treatments, for years. Long-term drug outcomes, such as the homosexualisation of infants, are not the sort of concern that can feature in short term trials. Very long-term side effects are not easily spotted, and connected in trials to cause. Once a product is established, it is sadly human nature to resist any suggestions of defects.

The cost of conducting trials of products for every outcome, and for such long lengths of time, would be prohibitive. Once drugs are in use, there are strong commercial pressures, not to admit any deficiencies of the product.

It is my impression that once approval is reached, commercial pressure does not provide an imperative for ongoing long-term safety trials. The change in the status of trans fats is an example.

There were early potentially serious red flags. These warnings were ignored [11.29]. We were then sold the myth for many years, that trans fats were good for us. It is now accepted initial reservations were very valid. Trans fats are now accepted to be bad, but at what cost to the public over the last 40 years.

This is just the way it is, human nature, the market structure, and the human dynamic. The significant long-term risks of drugs intervention, in these fundamental pathways, must add to the argument for prevention as the primary objective.

20.4   Drugs intervention, COX blockers—Drugs are used to block the manufacture by the body via the COX and LOX enzymes of the Omega Six family of chemicals. They target the COX pathways. NSAIDs fall into this category.

NSAIDs are used in inflammatory related conditions, including pain. Intervention helps in the short-term, but poses unforeseen long term risks.

NSAIDs have a varied product dependent range of side effects, including indigestion, stomach bleeding, damage to the liver and kidneys, ringing in ears (tinnitus), fluid retention, high blood pressure, heart attack or stroke, [147] and impotence.

NSAIDs, in general terms, are intervening in the Omega 6 chemical family pathways, trying to undo downstream inflammatory effects of excess Omega 6.

The complexities of the systems that run the body are mind-boggling. The body is so complex, and so much is not understood, it is impossible to consider every possible long term consequence of treatments.

These drugs intervene in the most fundamental pathways in the body, including the reproductive pathways. The risks of long term unforeseen side effects are significant.

For example unforeseen long-term effects on fertility, and possible homosexualisation of infants based on animal trials, are very real concerns. Examination of humans for signs of homosexualisation consequent on COX blocking drug intake by the mothers, are in progress, it is reported.

A reduction in Omega Six, and increase in Omega Three, as part of a long-term dietary strategy, may have long term similar effects in reducing inflammation as NSAIDs, as well as of other benefits, with no significant side effects. DHA is reported to be a more effective NSAID than many NSAID drugs.

Is it not time at every level to look at prevention seriously, and then target funds at what cannot be prevented? Omega Six truly is the elephant in the room.

21

OXIDATION–GOOD AND BAD, ENERGY PRODUCTION, THE BODY'S ARSENAL

21.1 **What is oxidation?**–[Abbreviations at 1.1] Oxidation, can't live without it, can't live forever with it. Oxidation gives us energy and degrades us at the same time. The expression oxidation came from metals combining with oxygen and going rusty. Mr. Metal likes giving away electrons, very generous. Miss Oxygen likes collecting electrons. Mr. Metal and Miss Oxygen get married. The resulting couple is Mr. and Mrs. Oxide. As usual, it is more complicated. The term is used where a substance likes to give away electrons. It is mind bogglingly complicated once you scratch the surface. [148]

21.2 **What is an antioxidant?**–An antioxidant is a substance that likes to give away electrons more than its neighbour does. Not keen on Mr. Metal getting married to Miss Oxygen? Then introduce Mr. Antioxidant into the equation. Mr. Antioxidant, freer with his electrons, will see to Miss Oxygen's needs. Mr. Metal is kept away from Miss Oxygen.

21.3 **Oxidation good and bad**–By oxidation, the body, makes energy, processes chemicals, manufactures defence systems, weaponry, and cell rubbish disposal chemicals. Oxidation is key to life.

There are many oxidation based processes. An example of necessary oxidation is fats being 'burnt' in the mitochondrial energy furnaces. Another is the process by which Omega 3 and 6 fats are oxidised [Oxygen added into the fat structure] to make the Omega 3 and 6 chemical families.

Excess oxidation does immense damage. Inadequate oxidation compromises general function, cell destruction and rubbish treatment services. Insufficient nutritional resources means the body is unable to provide adequate repair and renewal due to, excess, under powered, or flawed oxidisation.

The garage cannot mend your car properly without the spares. The body is the same. Omega Three, and particularly DHA, is a very topmost fundamental nutritional resource, and can only be got ultimately through diet. DHA is much more readily oxidised by peroxisomes [16.4] and mitochondria than other fats. Spare oxidants ROS are used in the body's immune and defence systems

Cell death, is execution by very powerful oxidants, called ROS, reactive oxygen species. ROS can be useful or harmful. For example ROS are part of the process of electrical impulses that allow the eyes to function. ROS, in sunburn, results in skin inflammation. But ROS can cause DNA modification and damage.

Fats are a source of ROS when they are broken down for fuel. When they are produced in the wrong place and time, in systems that are not functioning optimally, damage may be the result. For example Omega Six produces high levels of damaging oxidants in regions of arterial dysfunction and furring.

If the oxidants you produce are not of the right type, or made in cell furnaces which are not adequately maintained, then your ROS may not have the energy to be able to kill damaged cells. It is accepted that cancer is in part a result of imbalance between cell growth and death[i]. Much is not known.

DHA produces more oxidants in the mitochondria and peroxisomes, than other fats, and importantly Omega Six LA . But Omega 6 can produce high levels of oxidants by chemical reaction in the cascades that make Omega 6 chemicals.

DHA is increased at night when melatonin levels are high. Melatonin is a very powerful anti oxidant, a weapons manager if you like. DHA, has been linked to higher death rates of cancer cells, in some trials.

This is only conjecture, but do special properties of DHA to produce high power oxidation, together with melatonin as an oxidation manager, combine operations at night, in sleep, to produce new cells and kill damaged ones.

Fats are key raw materials for cell membrane structure. You cannot viably kill old cells, if you do not have the raw materials to replace them. You do not change your old car, however much you would like, or the car needs replacing, if you do not have the money to buy a better one.

The body needs DHA to make new cells, and dispose of the old ones. No cash =no new car. No DHA = no new shiny top performance cells. No DHA = no top quality defence system. No DHA = Mitochondria without top quality structural membrane materials and fuel.

For example the thyroid and iodine metabolism is believed to involve strong oxidisation and free radicals. Decreased thyroid function lowers the metabolic rate[ii] and so may add to obesity factors.

If under maintained and resourced defence systems, weaponry, and rubbish disposal chemicals, get out of hand, they attack the body. Antioxidants keep the balance as weapons managers, but are unlikely to fix defective mitochondria.

---

i Environmental Stressors in Health and Disease Jurgen Fucs and Lester Packer.
ii Mitochondria, Hypothyroidism and Weight Loss, by Steven Wm. Fowkes, Ward Dean, M.D., and Thomas H. Nufert.

Excess antioxidants may be bad. Systems are complex and the balance delicate. Poor quality oxidation means, substandard defence and disposal. Oxidation of insufficient energy may impair consequent chemical processing. Oxidation of excess Omega 6 is linked to poor oxidation and arterial damage.

If damaged cells are not zapped, they can cause problems. The body was never designed for antioxidants to stop all oxidation. Antioxidants are the chemical process maintenance crews, and weapons managers. Oxidisation is a dilemma.

No oxidation = no energy, no defensive weaponry, no chemical reactions, and in simple terms no human life. But oxidation over time eventually burns out our boilers, and systems fail terminally.

21.4   **Antioxidants and serious malfunction**–Antioxidants will deal with small incidents. Antioxidants will not be able to sort out the underlying issues, and consequences, in case of system problems, the wrong fuels, damaged boilers, and consistent lack of maintenance. You need to fix the problem.

Excess Omega Six over Omega Three, and lack of long chain fats, is a system issue. The breakdown it causes, is outside the ability of the fire crews, no matter how many are available. The only solution is to bring the Omega Three : Six balance back within operating parameters.

21.5   **Oxidation, damage to genes**–The problems start when this amazing defence system gets out of control. [149] Oxidation required to zap intruders goes haywire. It starts attacking lots of things including genes.

Constant high-level oxidative attacks zap the gene defence outposts, telomeres. It appears repair systems, and anti oxidants, including melatonin, CoQ10, and oestrogen cannot get to work, and genes become damaged.

A telomere is a region of highly repetitive DNA, at the end of a linear chromosome, which functions as a disposable buffer. [150] Damage to the protective telomeres is caused by oxidative stress. Links have been suggested to cancer [151][152] and ageing. Oxidation of telomeres has also been linked to adipose fat, oxidative stress and inflammation.

Excess Omega Six has been linked with undesirable oxidation. Simplistically Omega Six is one of the poorer quality fat fuels. The mitochondrial fat, cardiolipin, appears to prefer Omega Three DHA, and the Omega Six LA. Omega Six LA is less easily oxidised in the mitochondria than DHA. But high Omega 6 levels in the membrane, would if triggered, result in oxidation via the chemical eicosanoid production cascades [1.19].

ROS, superoxides, are produced by the mitochondria. Superoxides, ROS reactive oxygen species, are "biologically quite toxic". Maybe Omega Six does not give a clean burn of sufficient energy level in the mitochondria, and produces undesirable eicosanoid by-products, leading to system breakdown.

DHA counter intuitively is reported as decreasing superoxide production.[iii]

---

iii   DHA-rich fish oil and regular moderate exercise: a combined intervention to improve cardiovascular, metabolic and inflammatory biomarkers in obesity. Alison M Hill School of Molecular and Biomedical Science University of Adelaide.

21.6   **Storage**—The body is no refrigerator. It is a warm place. Put fats in a warm place for a while, and there is oxidation. Fats go rancid. Antioxidants prevent this.

Antioxidants are maintenance crew not super-heroes. There comes a point where maintenance is not enough if the structure is falling into serious disrepair. When a building is in disrepair you need the construction gangs. Omega Threes and other fats in the right mix are construction workers.

21.7   **DHA cardiolipin and oxidation**—Fats are burnt in the mitochondrial cells by oxidation. The explosion of fuel in your car cylinder is controlled oxidationto create energy. Run your diesel on chip pan oil derivative, you are exploiting similar principles.

The body manages it with a very great deal more sophistication. DHA is essential to effective mitochondrial oxidation. Controlled production of oxidants can kill defective cells, and supplies free radicals to other processes.

Mitochondria are part of your very sophisticated inner world. Mitochondria are drawn as beans or sausages, but in living cells "they squirm, flex, elongate, and change shape almost continuously". They move in the cells "via dynein motors riding on microtubules, bulging the plasma membrane as they travel". [153]

Sounds like a description from a sci-fi film, but it's you and me! Properly controlled this is 'good' oxidation. Exercise increases oxidation. DHA increases "good" oxidation in the mitochondria. [154]

Cardiolipin high in DHA is found only in the inner mitochondrial membrane. It is a unique chemical with four fats in the rack. It is a big part of the mitochondrial membrane, 25 per cent in the heart. It is unusually sensitive to diet.

The amounts of Omega Three, Six, and Nine in cardiolipin depend on dietary intake. [155] The heart mitochondria function better with higher Omega Three in the cardiolipin. [156] Stress depletes cardiolipin.

Cardiolipin preferentially takes up DHA and LA by large amounts. (LA 33 per cent, DHA 44.5 per cent in the trial cited, with LA incorporation rates of up to 90 per cent reported). OA was taken up, but EPA and AA were not. DHA in the mitochondria produces five times more cellular oxidants than any other fatty acid. DHA also improves electron transport efficiency.

OA, LA, and AA diminished the mitochondrial potential by 11, 18, and 5 per cent respectively. DHA increased mitochondrial potential by 11 per cent. Mitochondrial oxidants produced by one measure showed figures of for OA, LA, AA, EPA, and DHA of 6, 35, 94, 40, and 429 per cent respectively. [157] [158]

I cannot argue the details but DHA clearly has a unique, and important role in the mitochondria and peroxisomes as an energy source, controller of electrical potential, and source of oxidants. Lack of DHA is likely to have serious functional consequences at many levels, and be reflected in poorer function of organs.

21.8   **Immune system, maintenance, and rubbish removal**–The immune system as one of its many strategies uses oxidation to zap intruders. It creates poisons and little highly unstable chemicals, which it uses to disable bacteria and destroy cellular rubbish. Destruction would include damaged cells that could be come part of a 'cancer'.

The oxidative control chemicals 'ROS' are so reactive, they can only be used in the immediate area of the cell in which they are made. They are short-lived and very unstable. We need quality controlled oxidation just like your car.

DHA is very effectively oxidised in the mitochondria, far more so than any other long chain fatty acid. DHA in the lab increases cell death rates in some cancers. Good quality high energy clean burn ROS superoxides are key to functions such as eyesight and thyroid function. Oxidation is a contradiction.

21.9   **Omega Three, an antioxidant**–DHA is oxidised in mitochondria. Oxidation creates energy as in your car, and by-products are important to growth factor responses, cell signalling and bactericidal functions. [160] [161] But trials suggest that Omega 3 reduces harmful oxidation. [159] Does DHA enable the production of protective antioxidants and act as an antioxidant? It appears DHA does both.

Omega 3 upgrades melatonin which is a powerful antioxidant. Omega 3s are increased by oestrogen which is an antioxidant. DHA may be sacrificially used.

The mother fats are far less protected from uncontrolled oxidation than their children DHA and EPA. High Omega Six may be a cause of chronic inflammation. The oxidation of linoleic acid Omega 6 LA is linked with vascular conditions. [162] [163] Yet oxidation of Omega 3 ALA is used and essential to skin protection systems.

Ultimately, it is all about very subtle balance and control. When the system goes out of control, there are very serious consequences for the body.

21.10 **Antioxidants**–There are very many antioxidants. Some we make. Some we cannot make. Some antioxidants are made in the body, and have multiple roles like melatonin and oestrogen. [164] [165]

Antioxidants can be found in plants, which need them for the same reasons as we do. Different antioxidants are found in different foods. Variety is good.

Some are minerals. Trial reports zinc as a strong antioxidant, and linked lack of zinc in chronic fatigue symptoms to oxidative stress. [166]

Water-soluble antioxidants include Vitamin C, glutathione, and lipoic acid. Water-soluble antioxidants act in the cells and plasma.

Fat-soluble antioxidants work in the cell membranes. They act synergistically and in complex ways, and it is necessary to have all co-workers present for things to be of use.

Foods are the first option as sources of antioxidants, because they are packaged with the things they need to work . Refining removes part of that package.

So get plenty of whole food rich in antioxidants, but antioxidants whilst helping are not the solution if you have a raging inferno. Like a forest fire, you need to cut off the fuel that is feeding the fire.

22

IMMUNE REGIMENTS

22 Immune regiments—The immune system is immensely complex. This section just tries to give a flavour based on my views through the mist. The point of this section, is that a link exists between Omega 3 and 6 intake, oxidation, and the immune function. Omega 3 and 6 are key to the immune system.

Many of the Omega Six COX2 chemical products are connected to the inflammation response, which is part of the immune response. The COX1 products are more connected to maintenance. COX1 is always present in cells at a constant level. COX2 only works on a call-out basis.

When the body senses a known invader, an unrecognised chemical, alien protein, bacteria, etc. it produces signalling compounds. Signalling compounds such as cytokines tell the body to make weapons to repel or neutralise invaders.

The weapons are oxidants, peroxides, and free radicals. They are produced initially as by-products of oxidation. Oxidation is in part both a cause and consequence of diseases, and stress. Oxidation is a subject on its own, as evidenced by a fairly technical book *"Environmental Stressors in Health and Disease"* [See section 12 of book] edited by Jurgen Fuchs, and Lester Packer.

There is always a certain level of leakage of oxidants from the burning of fats and carbohydrates for fuels. Presumably the signalling agents request or enable greater quantities of oxidants to be released. Some cytokine signalling agents like IL1 both fuel, and are encouraged by oxidants, so creating self fuelling cycles.

The oxidants and free radicals triggered by the signalling agents like IL1, act as the detonators, to release Omega 3 and 6 products into the chemical production line, and start the chain reactions that make the Omega 3 and 6 chemicals.

Omega 6 requires less energy to start a chain reaction than Omega 3 [*Fish, Omega-3 and Human Health* - W M Lands]. So if you have more Omega 6 available in store, you will prefer to make Omega 6 chemical cascades. Once Omega 6 cascades start, do the oxidants produced add fuel to the reaction chain, and so create a self-fuelling cycle?

DHA taken from the inner mitochondrial membrane for fuel, and DHA in peroxisomes produces more oxidation than Omega 6 LA. Also if there is more DHA in the membranes, there will be more Omega 3 chemical products.

Omega 6 LA burnt in the mitochondria produces less oxidation, but it is easier to trigger an Omega 6 cascade. If Omega 6 LA is being burnt, the raw materials are present to make Omega Six products. "Diets with high n-6:n-3 PUFA ratios may enhance the risk for both depression and inflammatory diseases"[i].

The body produces defence cells. These cells use the products of oxidation, with enzymes, for rubbish removal and cell destruction. They respond to signalling chemicals, and migrate to the site the messages are coming from.

The immune system response is also manipulated through gene expression, and activity in 'lipid rafts' [30.24] in the cell membranes. The relationship of Omega 3 and 6 to immune function is immensely complex.

Antioxidants do have a role in controlling and balancing Omega 6 produced oxidation. But the self fuelling Omega cascades, where Omega Six is in excess, may be beyond design specs. Consequently anti oxidants may be overwhelmed.

At a physical level Omega 6 increases inflammation. Inflammation causes degradation of the barrier between the body and the intestinal tract. This allows more bacteria and toxins to enter the 'body'.

Long chain Omega 3s reduce inflammation so protecting the 'inner' body from the hazards in the 'external' digestive system. Omega 3 assists the bacterial clearance systems, improving antigen response, and defence activities.

In animals infected with E.Coli the time to kill all the bacteria was almost halved in animals given Omega 3 rather than Omega 6. E.Coli bacteria measured in the lung were lower in animals fed Omega 3, than the control population, or those fed Omega 6. A multi centre study of 661 hospital patients, showed post operative / treatment reductions in infection levels. [E.g. sepsis].

Counter intuitively it seems that once the Omega 6 response is exaggerated, it is counter productive, and immune function is compromised. Omega 3 seems to reduce inflammation, without compromising immune function.

Excess Omega 6 increases inflammation and reduces immune function. Also "anti-inflammatory interventions ... depress host defence and place the patient at risk of immune compromise" *Omega 3 Fatty Acids in Clinical Nutrition* A R Heller, S N Stehr, T Koch. Excess Omega 6 and NSAID intervention are issues.

[It is my lay opinion a truly excellent, and highly thought provoking book. Some of the graphs and charts, on hospital stay and recovery times, for some conditions, have breathtaking implications. Even if only to spark debate, I believe it should be in every hospital library]. It concludes with the following:

---

i   Depressive symptoms, omega-6:omega-3 fatty acids, and inflammation in older adults. Psychosom Med. 2007 Apr;69(3):217-24 Kiecolt-Glaser JK, Belury MA, Porter K, Beversdorf DQ, Lemeshow S, Glaser R. Department of Psychiatry, Ohio State University College of Medicine, Columbus, OH 43210, USA.

"Supplementation with Omega-3 FA improves survival and accelerates recovery ... we found Omega 3-FA to be a valuable nutritional additive to improve outcome in patients with peritonitis, trauma, abdominal SIRS and sepsis, but also to reduce infections and complication rates in post-operative patients."]

The immune system talks to the prostaglandins through the cytokines, chemicals produced in inflammation. [ii] An imbalance in the Omega 3:6 ratio increases the pro-inflammatory immune markers, and predisposes us to an exaggerated response to stressors. [iii] Excess inflammatory response has been linked with rheumatoid arthritis, IBS, sepsis, asthma and others.

The immune system comes in two parts a burst of unthinking anger, and a more considered planned response, and reconstruction. For the body to achieve the most effective mix of shock and awe, and planned response and reconstruction, requires the right mix of resources. The Omega 3 and 6 families are a key part of the body's automatic chemical protection and defence resources.

If the body does not have the raw materials, or if the production and organisational processes are blocked, defence will be compromised. If there is excess Omega 6 and lack of Omega 3, the shock and awe is likely to be over aggressive, and the follow up and reconstruction delayed or insufficient, resulting in longer and less certain recovery.

An imbalance of Omega 3 and 6 is also likely to keep the body in a permanent state of excess alert, with a tendency to overreact, even if no real threat exists, with long term detrimental consequences.

22.1   **Fast reaction team**–Unthinking anger - The local cellular defence service, stores all the raw material they need locally. This includes fats. They react immediately, and autonomously, with short-term measures to local conditions and insults. They do not need to call central HQ, or the command structure.

The chemicals created are very unstable compounds, and do not travel safely. They act within the cells, and surrounding spaces between cells. They have very short lives. Many of these compounds are oxygen based. Some are like peroxide, some are chlorine based and more akin to bleach, some are nitrogen based. It is the instability of these compounds, which the body uses to destroy invaders, kill rogue cells, and remove damaged DNA. It is important these oxidation 'weapons' do not get out of control. Antioxidants marshal and manage the weapons systems.

---

ii   Central nervous system recognition of peripheral inflammation: a neural, hormonal collaboration. Hopkins SJ. Acta Biomed. 2007; 78 Suppl 1:231-47. Injury Research Group, Clinical Sciences Building, Hope Hospital, Salford, Greater Manchester, M6 8HD-UK.

iii   In humans, serum polyunsaturated fatty acid levels predict the response of proinflammatory cytokines to psychologic stress. Biol Psychiatry. 2000 May 15;47(10):910-20 Maes M, Christophe A, Bosmans E, Lin A, Neels H. Department of Psychiatry and Neuropsychology, University of Maastricht, The Netherlands.

Particular weapons systems require particular antioxidants. Antioxidants will not cope with systems breakdown. The type of defence force that turns out, will reflect the Omega Three-Six balance, and content of the cell stores and membranes. Poor quality defence which is out of control results in excess inflammation. This system is called the innate defensive mechanism.

22.2   **Long-term strategic defence**– A more considered response - The strategic defences, with long-term planning and intelligence teams, to recognise and destroy new threats, are organised on a body wide basis. This is called the learned system.

It is more efficient, effective, and targeted, than the fast reaction, local defence team, but takes longer to get organised. Defence strategies include up regulation of anti-inflammatory genes. [167] Special white blood cells come and engage in battle, engulfing their targets and releasing high power oxidants, and free radicals, to destroy their targets.

Excessive uncontrolled oxidants, and free radicals, cause tissue damage. The whole system is in a permanent delicate balance, between repelling invaders, repairing damaged tissue, and minimising short and long term collateral damage.

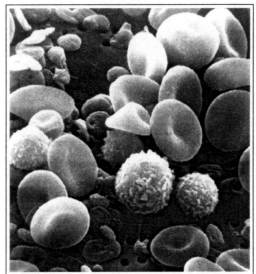

Thanks to Bruce Wetzel and Harry Schaefer (Photographers), National Cencer Institute and Wikipedia.

Fig. 22.2 A Scanning Election Microscope Image of Normal Circulating Human Blood

22.3   **Bone marrow**–The bone marrow is intimately connected with the immune system. Omega Three is reported as reducing bone loss, improving the cell levels in bone marrow, and so enhancing the immune function. [168] Omega Six increases fat storage in the marrow and lowers numbers of active cells, so reducing immune response.

22.4   **Autoimmune conditions**–In autoimmune diseases, you simply have too many emergency defence workers, programmed to defend and destroy. If there is no rubbish to tidy, or no threats to neutralise, and they are not switched off, they just becomes a job's worth. They attack healthy tissue for the sake of employment not knowing any better. Increased inflammatory immune status, connects to the Omega Six family, and shows evidence of being reduced by Omega Threes. [169 170 171 172 173]

23

PREGNANCY, POSTNATAL DEPRESSION, CHRONIC FATIGUE, DEPRESSION, PMT, FERTILITY ISSUES, OSTEOPOROSIS, PCOS, UTERINE AND BREAST CANCERS

23.1   **Fundamental to women's health**–[Abbreviations listed at 1.1. For PGE2 an Omega Six product; please see [30.35.]] I hope you will feel it worth investing the time, to try and gain a glimpse of why a balance Omega Three and Six mother fats, and an adequate supply of long chain Omega 3s, DHA and EPA, is fundamental to female health and fertility, brain maintenance, and everything.

Women have a very fundamental relationship with the Omega 3s [5.2], particularly EPA [30.14] and DHA [30.10]. Oestrogen increases production of DHA. Women make 10 times as much DHA as men. DHA defines women behaviourally, structurally, and hormonally. Omega Six, AA, [30.2] made from the mother Omega 6 LA, [5.1, 30.20] is the ultimate fertility controller.

Fats are essential to healthy babies. Fats control age at puberty. Fats feature in mental health, depression, and neurological degeneration. Women have more neurons in a smaller brain. DHA is essential to healthy neurons. Omega 3s moderate risks of cardiac disease. DHA controls basal metabolism. DHA is fundamental to the menstrual cycle and fertility. Omega 3 reduces the risk of osteoporosis, and breast cancer. Omega 3 can improve skin, hair, eyes, nails. . .

I believe the Omega Three and Six fats, are ultimately the controllers of the monthly hormone cycle. Even if it is not accepted that they are ultimately the controlling factor, it is undeniable that they have a very significant role in the monthly cycle, female fertility, and behavioural characteristics of women.

Hormones and steroids are made from cholesterol, in a set of interlinked production lines. [23.11 and Fig. 23.11b] If the production lines are out of balance, the hormones are out of balance. Fats, directly and indirectly, are the raw materials and controllers of 'sex' hormones, and steroid production.

Without adequate Omega 6 you cannot reproduce. Omega 6 is nature's way of controlling our fertility. Hormone and steroid production lines are controlled indirectly by enzymes made from Omega 6. Too much Omega 6, and a lack of 3, and the hormone production controllers (aromatase is one) are out of balance.

Very low Omega Six means low hormone levels. Too much Omega Six, and your hormones levels rise, and are thrown out of balance, with an increase in a host of fertility related conditions, including PCOS, and dysmenorrhoea.

I fear, that telling you to balance your Omega 3s and 6s, take some DHA and EPA, cut out the conversion blockers, and watch your fat intake, may not excite much more response than, "that is interesting". I try to bring an overview.

To see that this is fundamental to female health, you need a deeper understanding. You don't have to understand it all. I do not claim to see beyond outlines in the mist. The more I understand, the more I realise the less I know.

You only need to grasp the importance of Omega Three, and Omega Six, to reproduction, fertility, your health, and your child's health. The best scientists in the world, are still only beginning to explain the way the body works, in detail.

Each subject is a specialism. I am not in any sense an expert, but feel that when the evidence of others is lined up, the overall conclusion is overwhelming. This is a tiny peep into a wondrous world, where DHA and EPA are huge players.

***BUT** you cannot make DHA or EPA, without mother Omega 3 fat, the raw material, in your diet. If you do not eat the long chain fats DHA and EPA, and/or cannot make them efficiently from the mother fats, you will have a shortage of long chain fats.*

In this book I concentrate on DHA. The mother fat makes EPA. EPA makes DHA. [P286]. A shortfall of the Omega 3 raw material to make DHA, or a lack of direct intake of DHA in diet, has huge consequences for women, their babies, and children. Babies can be significantly affected for life.

Omega 3s are not stored in body fat in significant quantity, and are released for usage from the fat tissues before the Omega 6s, are used up first[i], for energy, and body chemical processes [25.8]. Omega 6s are heavily stored. [25.6, 25.7]

The body makes longer fats of the same family if the paths are not blocked. We can turn mother Omega 3 into DHA. Balance the Omega 3s and 6s, cut out conversion blockers, and ensure adequate supplies of long chain Omega 3 DHA.

---

i   Selective release of human adipocyte fatty acids according to molecular structure. Biochem J. 1997 June 15; 324(Pt 3): 911–915. T Raclot, D Langin, M Lafontan, and R Groscolas INSERM Unité 317, Institut Louis Bugnard, Faculté de médecine, Université Paul Sabatier, Hôpital Rangueil, 31054 Toulouse Cedex, France.

23.2 EPA and DHA deficit, the consequences—Most Western women's diet provides way too much Omega Six, very little Omega Three, and blocks their natural ability to make the long chain Omega Threes.

This is a health disaster. It is a giant time bomb. This imbalance creates a significant risk of a whole range of 'western' conditions in old age, including osteoporosis, and dementia.

Excess Omega 6, and lack of Omega 3, also upsets the hormone and steroid levels and balances. Omega 3 and 6 levels, indirectly control the hormone and steroid levels, through the Omega 6 chemical enzymes pathways [See 23.11].

Excess Omega Six, and inadequate Omega Three intake, carries a greater risk of infertility, PCOS, menstrual problems, diabetes, depression, alcohol-related conditions, atopic conditions, asthma, hirsuteness, uterine conditions, osteoporosis, papillomavirus, and various cancers, including breast cancer.

You are what your mother ate too. Your mother's diet, and hormonal status, may increase your risk of breast cancer and obesity. In pregnancy, there is heightened need for DHA. This is because the foetus rapaciously hoovers up DHA, for its brain growth. The foetus will take DHA from the mother's brain.

Some brains shrink in pregnancy. DHA deficit from pregnancy has serious long-term health impact, including PND [23.35], if the DHA is not replaced.

If the foetus cannot meet its nutritional needs, it too may suffer long-term consequences. We are what we eat, and what our mother ate and digested.

23.3 Fat sets women and men apart—Women have higher levels of DHA than men do. [174] Women through oestrogen make more DHA, from the mother Omega Three, than men.

LONG CHAIN OMEGA 3S DEFINE WOMEN. THROUGH OESTROGEN WOMEN MAKE 10 TIMES MORE DHA THAN MEN. IF YOU DO NOT EAT OMEGA 3S YOU HAVE NO 3S.

Men make between almost none, and one per cent of the mother Omega 3 fat, into DHA. Women can convert about 10 per cent [and maybe more] of the mother Omega 3 into DHA. DHA is linked to a range of female behavioural characteristics [See chapter 24 on the brain].

Low DHA has been linked to aggression, impulsiveness, criminal behaviour, violence, poorer spatial skills, temper tantrums, and lower 'intelligence'. [175] DHA, in general terms, links to attributes of women.

Women are gentler, more cooperative, less impulsive, and have better social skills, which may in part be due to the impact of DHA on brain function. [6.8]

Neurons have a high DHA need. Women's brains have a greater neuron density, and brain-bodyweight ratio. Is higher neuron density a result in part of higher DHA? Cognitive degenerative diseases link with neuron loss, and low DHA levels. Depression links with low DHA. Women have increased risk of cognitive degeneration after menopause, and depression brings a risk early menopause.

Women are at greater risk of Alzheimer's. Women with depression have greater DHA deficits in the brain, than men do, for no obvious dietary reasons. Is the greater loss of brain cells, neurons, with age in women, due to fall off in oestrogen leading to lower DHA levels after menopause?

Oestrogen boosts DHA levels. Women make this DHA for a reason. DHA is needed to regulate the fertility cycle, and build new tissue each month. Babies are DHA hoovers, in the hunt for the raw materials they need.

If women do not have an adequate supply of the mother Omega 3, ALA, and long chain children DHA, and EPA, the impact of a deficit is much greater in women than in men. Neural issues reflect the higher needs of women for DHA.

DHA may, by structural influences on the brain, through hormones, and chemicals such as serotonin, significantly shape the way women think.

23.4   **Fats control hormones**—Women due to oestrogen make much more DHA than men. The results of a DHA deficit for women are truly mind-boggling. Omega 6 is essential too, but a DHA deficit is the most common issue, due to western dietary factors. A DHA deficit may contribute to a wide range of menstrual and fertility issues. I suggest this is how DHA and AA may control the hormone cycle [See 23.11 for more detail].

Higher levels of oestrogen increase DHA and AA levels. [176] This was demonstrated by the effects of oestrogen, and testosterone, on transsexual men and women. [177] Oestrogens in oral contraceptives significantly increase DHA levels in men. [178] Testosterone significantly reduces DHA production in women.

With the different effects of testosterone, and oestrogen, on DHA production, we have the beginnings of the control of the menstrual cycle. DHA is fundamental to making babies, fertility, and maintaining a healthy monthly cycle.

Sex hormones, steroids, and the related chemicals, have both a daily, and monthly, cycle. In animals seasonal cycles of hormones and related chemicals have also been observed. Hormones and steroids, PGE2, melatonin, serotonin, cortisol and other influential chemicals, link through various mechanisms to AA and DHA, and all have a daily day/night cycle. Omega Six is an external agent.

The partner to DHA, in the monthly and daily cycle, is Omega Six AA. Pregnancy needs tissue destruction, creation, and inflammation, to make babies. Omega Six is a promoter of inflammation, tissue destruction and creation.

Chemicals of Omega 6 AA include PGE2, which works with aromatase and other enzymes, to control sex hormone production including oestrogen and testosterone [Fig 23.11b].

Constant background levels of hormones, are made in fat tissues, and sex organs. Sources of cycling hormones include cells of placenta, and cells in tissue relating to the preparation of the egg ready for fertilisation. During the monthly cycle new cells grow that produce hormones [Fig 23.11a].

In pregnancy, as the placenta grows in size, so it produces more cells that make sex hormones, so increasing hormone production. Rising oestrogen in pregnancy will lead to more DHA, and more Omega Six AA, being made.

The baby uses more DHA than AA. [Placental uptake uptakes of oleic, eicosapentaenoic [EPA], arachidonic [AA], and docosahexaenoic [DHA] acids were 15.36±4.1, 19.95±3.6, 28.56±8.1, and 62.25±9.5 nmol/mg of protein, respectively[ii]] I suggest that by consuming the DHA, the baby stops a rise in DHA. A rise in DHA would stop the rising production of Omega 6 AA chemicals, and so hormones.

The additional AA not consumed by the baby, will allow the growing placenta, to produce rising hormone levels until birth, when the baby's DHA consumption will suddenly stop. Omega Six AA will suddenly rise as it is no longer consumed by the baby, and result in an increase of PGE2, which initiates delivery.

After delivery, rising DHA levels will block Omega Six production, and sex hormone production. The production factory of the additional hormones needed to sustain pregnancy, the placenta, is no longer present, so hormone production falls dramatically.

Excess Omega Six levels, and lack of DHA disturb the production lines, and lead to hormonal imbalance, and the conditions as listed below. [23.11]

23.5   **Look after the liver**–DHA is made from the mother Omega 3 fat, by adding carbons and double bonds. DHA is also broken back down, and used to make shorter fats. The main fat conversion factory is the liver. [179] Individual cells all over the body, including the brain and heart, can and do make and breakdown fats, but the main factory is the liver.

A damaged liver is not able to make that essential DHA. Damage to the liver by alcohol is a multiple whammy for women.

☞ Excess alcohol blocks the conversion pathways, which make long chain fats. Poorer DHA synthesis leads to a host of problems.

☞ Alcohol damages the liver.

☞ Alcohol uses and releases precious DHA from the brain, which otherwise holds onto DHA.

☞ DHA deficit can impact very significantly on fertility, offspring, and the risk of a long list of 'western related' conditions as discussed.

An adequate supply of the mother Omega Three fat, may prevent low to moderate alcohol consumption, from causing damage by allowing the DHA used to be replaced. [1.30].

---

ii   Insulin and leptin do not affect fatty acid uptake and metabolism in human placental choriocarcinoma (BeWo) cells. Prostaglandins, Leukotrienes and Essential Fatty Acids, 2005 (Vol. 72) (No. 6) 403-408 Asim K. Duttaroy Aud Jørgensen Faculty of Medicine, University of Oslo, POB 1046 Blindern, 0316 Oslo, Norway.

23.6 **Omega Three and Omega Six in pregnancy**–This chapter highlights issues relating to women, pregnancy, infants in the womb, and young babies. If you don't understand it all, don't worry, I don't.

You just need to grasp that the Omega 3:6 fats balance, is fundamental to baby making, hormonal processes, chemical pathways and female health generally. Much is unknown and still to be learnt.

But overall, it is unavoidable that balancing the Omega Threes and Sixes, and for most supplementing the long chain Omega Threes, is an important step to good health. Long chain Omega Six is also fundamental.

Some, because of diet or genetic disposition, may not make enough AA or DHA, even if the raw materials are provided. Oily fish resolves the DHA supply.

Offal, eggs, and some marine products contain some AA. AA supplements are rare, and should be treated with extreme caution until more is known. Tests are available, and lipid specialists exist.

23.7 **Evolutionary fertility controller**–As explained in chapter 28, Omega Six is nature's way of controlling our fertility. The Omega Six family is connected to the development of the vascular system in land-based animals, and allowed the development of the placenta.

Pregnancy is the biggest expenditure of life force for a woman. Getting pregnant if the environment cannot support a child, is not a sensible species survival strategy. Unsuccessful pregnancy in the wild could equal death, for mother and infant. [180] This unique nutrient links us directly to the fertility of the environment, and stops us breeding, if there is insufficient food.

Omega 6 in nature is scarce, seasonal, and energy costly to collect. If the environment is fertile, and good for breeding, Omega 6 is available. Excess Omega Six is also connected with early puberty.

The body actively stores Omega Sixes in the fat. When stored levels of Omega Six are sufficient, to secure stable hormone levels, pregnancy can take place.

The family of chemicals including PGE2, derived from the Omega Six, AA, allows hormone and steroid production. Too much Omega Six intake from diet, at levels outside the body's design parameters, leads to severe problems. Insufficient fats, including Omega Six intake, results in the shutdown of the monthly cycle.

Omega Six arguably opens doors to stem cell activation. By eating diets unseen in history, we may be opening the door, and pathways, to design evolution. We have inadvertently and unknowingly, pushed the body beyond its operating parameters, by supplying excess Omega Six.

Some 'disease' [body malfunction], I suggest is one outcome of very rapid genetic evolutionary stress, through altered gene expression, in response to environmental change. It is easier to remove the catalyst of change, excess Omega Six, than suffer evolutionary, or design, pressure in the form of malfunction.

23.8   Babies, and almost everything–Women can and do make more DHA. So what you may say? The implications are enormous I say. Men can make one or two per cent DHA. Some men make almost no DHA.

Women make 10 per cent, and maybe more. Why, and what are the consequences? Probably the most obvious is that DHA is needed to make babies' brains, eyes, and other bits. No spare DHA = no babies.

In early pregnancy, neurons are made at 250,000 a minute. DHA is essential to neuron production. More DHA makes better brains, and bigger neurons. At birth, a baby's brain is approximately a third the size of the adults. The brain will more than double in size during the first year.

The brain is made up of 60 per cent fats, of which 25 per cent, and maybe more, is DHA. [181] (DHA figures quoted vary and are not easy to find). AA is an equally important building block, but for most lack of DHA is the primary issue.

The baby will take DHA from the mother's brain, and anywhere else, if the mother cannot/does not make/eat enough to supply the baby's need. Long chain fats are essential to babies, brains, eyes, sex organs, nervous systems, and bodies.

Formula fed babies are reported as having lower DHA than breast fed babies. Significant brain shrinkage, is seen in mothers in pregnancy, due to fat depletion. Babies are long chain fat hoovers. DHA deficit has been linked to depression, including PND. DHA deficiency may get worse each pregnancy if not replaced.

23.9   Long chain Omega Six deficit–Omega Sixes are equally important. For most, the deficit is likely to be Omega Threes, rather than Sixes. There is a lack of information, as to whether blockages in the long chain conversion pathways, lead to AA blockages as well as DHA, when Omega Six is supplied in excess. It is a factor that people should be aware of. However, much is not clear.

Trials suggest during pregnancy, conversion of the mother Omega Three and Six, to long chain fats increases. [182] Falling levels of the mother Omega Six fat LA, are reported in pregnancy. This would be consistent with increased oestrogens in pregnancy, prompting greater conversion of both Omega 3 and 6 mother fats to long chain fats, and usage of available LA Omega 6 body fats reserves.

It is essential to ensure adequate supply of Omega Three and Six mother fats, as raw materials for conversion to DHA and AA. Deficits are more usually in Omega 3s and DHA, but for some poor conversion could lead to AA shortage. This is a complex area, in which much more work is needed. We are all different, and you each must, with your advisors, look your circumstances.

23.10   Softer, more cooperative, less aggressive–Women's brains are more intelligent, in that they have more neurons in a smaller space. Women make much more available DHA, and their body is adapted to it. DHA is a fundamental, structural, and multipurpose factor in the human metabolism; it actually defines differences between men and women.

DHA, as well as being intimately linked with oestrogen, testosterone and progesterone, is key to the control of fertility, and the monthly cycle.

Lower levels of aggression have been linked to DHA. Higher intelligence has been linked to DHA. Maybe high DHA, explains why women have the same number of neurons, but in a smaller brain. Higher levels of DHA, in specific parts of the female brain, might explain character differences between the sexes. DHA promotes female traits. AA promotes male traits.

Also DHA makes cell membranes softer and more flexible. Your skin is made up of cells, so your skin will be softer. It is also likely to make fat stores softer. So, higher DHA in women could explain why women are 'softer' to the touch.

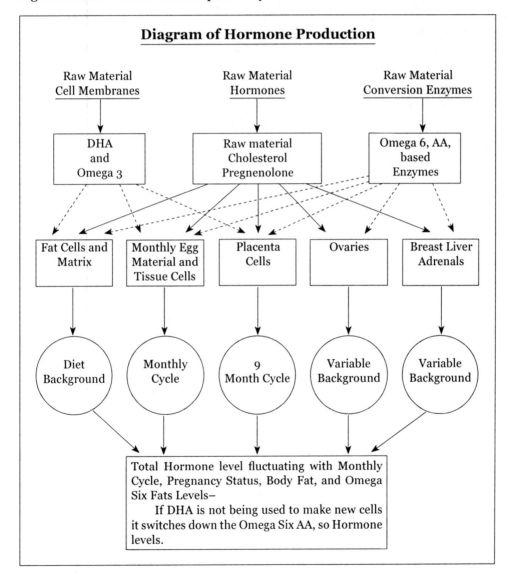

Fig. 23.II(a) Sources of Hormone Production

23.11   Fats fertility, and hormone–DHA and AA work in a subtle dance in the fertility cycle and pregnancy. DHA and AA, the children of the mother Omega 3 and 6 fats, and particularly Omega Six LA, connect us to nature. This is a view through the mist. There is much I do not know. I hope my joining of the dots proves to be an indication of the underlying mechanisms.

As discussed in the overview, and the chapters, on the brain and obesity, Omega Six is intimately involved in the promotion of inflammatory processes of the body. Ovulation has been likened to an inflammatory reaction. [183] Controlled inflammation is necessary to reproduction, body repair, and maintenance.

It is when inflammation gets out of control, that it is a problem. Omega Threes act as a balancing mechanism, dampening down, and modulating, inflammatory processes. In addition to playing a part in inflammation and immune function, the Omega 3:6 balance indirectly controls the hormone and steroid production.

Cholesterol, a fat, is made into pregnenolone, from which all hormones and steroids are made [23.11.b]. The amount of pregnenolone made, is controlled by messengers, including the sex hormones, so creating self controlling loops.

The mitochondria are closely involved in the process. Pregnenolone levels change in a day night cycle. The mitochondrial pregnenolone production controllers also have a day night cycle.

Sex hormones are manufactured in the sex organs themselves, the placenta, menstrual related tissue, and fat tissues, subject to availability of raw materials. Cholesterol makes the steroids and hormones, and Omega Six influences at least a number the hormone fabrication enzymes. [23.11.b]

There is also hormone activity in the breasts, liver and adrenal glands. I guess that maximum hormone production capacity of an individual cell is relatively fixed. Cells are little factories, that generally split into two factories, rather than becoming supersize factories, as it is more efficient [cell division].

Fat cells are an exception. Fat cells can expand many times. Larger fat cells make more hormones, and show higher gene expression, 20 times for some genes. Bigger fat cells make more Leptin for example[iii]. To provide hormones on a consistent basis, the body builds up stores of raw material in fat tissue.

Hormone producing sex organs, the testes and ovaries, are relatively fixed in size, so the maximum number of cells and production capacity of the organs, is likely relatively fixed.

---

iii   Separation of human adipocytes by size: hypertrophic fat cells display distinct gene expression The FASEB Journal. 2006;20:1540-1542 Margareta Jernås, Jenny Palming, Kajsa Sjöholm, Eva Jennische, Per-Arne Svensson, Britt G. Gabrielsson, Max Levin, Anders Sjögren, Mats Rudemo, Theodore C. Lystig, Björn Carlsson, Lena M. S. Carlsson and Malin Lönn Research Centre for Endocrinology and Metabolism, Division of Body Composition and Metabolism, Department of Internal Medicine, Institute of Anatomy and Cell Biology, and Cardiovascular Institute and Wallenberg Laboratory, Sahlgrenska Academy at Göteborg University, Göteborg, Sweden; and Department of Mathematical Statistics, Chalmers University of Technology, Göteborg, Sweden.

But, increased fat tissue and surrounding matrix, placental growth, monthly ovulation and uterine thickening, all result in increased cell numbers, or larger fat cells, with additional sex hormone production capacity. [Fig 23.11a]

Cells generally are factories with production capacity limits. Fat cells are an exception in that they can expand. Bigger cells in the fat matrix, means high background hormone levels.

Uterine and related menstrual tissue grows and declines on a monthly cyclical basis. More hormone producing cells in the uterine related tissue or placenta, = more hormone production capacity.

The hormone variable factors, that can be controlled by us, are fat tissue levels, and the type of fats stored particularly Omega 6. Stored Omega 3 [which is limited] and Omega 6 are a reflection of diet.

Omega 3 is metabolised before Omega 6. Omega 6 is heavily stored. Omega 3 is not heavily stored, so constant replenishment of Omega 3 through diet is important.

Rates of manufacture of hormones in the fat tissues appear to be sex independent.[74] So it is likely it is the content, number and size of mature fat cells, and the supporting matrix, that determines if the body can produce sufficient hormones to allow breeding. Mature fat cells also secrete other agents such as leptin, immune chemicals [IL6], and insulin related factors.

The monthly hormone / steroid / Omega 3/6 product cycles, are determined by the hormones/steroids, made by the new cells created during egg production and uterine thickening. In the monthly cycle uterine tissue growth, and in pregnancy the growing placenta and baby, act as control units, by consuming the DHA and some of the AA produced, to make new cells. New monthly tissue, and in pregnancy the placenta, produces more cells. More cells = more hormone manufacturing capacity, so increasing levels of hormones.

The ability of the cells to make hormones, is determined in turn by the availability of the necessary raw materials, pregnenolone to make the steroids and hormones, Omega 6 to make the conversion enzymes and new cells, and Omega 3 as a moderator of Omega 6, and providing Omega 3 material for new cells.

Oestrogen will rise cyclically with the growth in number of new hormone producing cells, in the monthly tissues, or the placenta in pregnancy. Oestrogen will increase production of DHA and AA, which is raw material for new cells.

This is a self fuelling hormone, and long chain fat, supply chain. More new hormone producing cells = more hormones = increased conversion of mother fats to DHA and AA = more raw materials for new cells = more cells = more hormones etc. Whilst DHA is preferentially used to make new cells, excess AA PGE2 production, will continue to keep hormones high and rising.

When DHA is not need to make any more cells, at the end of the monthly cycle following monthly shedding, or delivery of a baby, sharply rising DHA will shut off the Omega Six AA levels, and so hormone production, by restricting Omega Six activity.

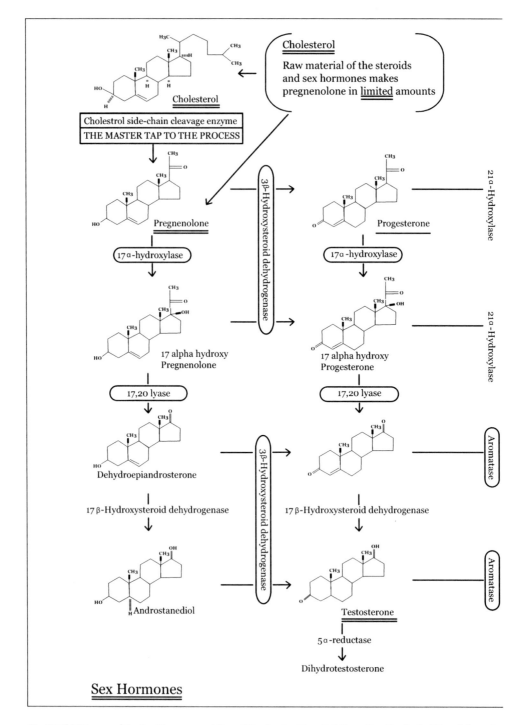

Fig. 23.11(b) Diagram of the Sex Hormane and Steroid Production Tree. It is like a Cats Cradle. It all Interlinks and is Interdependent.

Sex Hormones and Steroid Production Line Tree

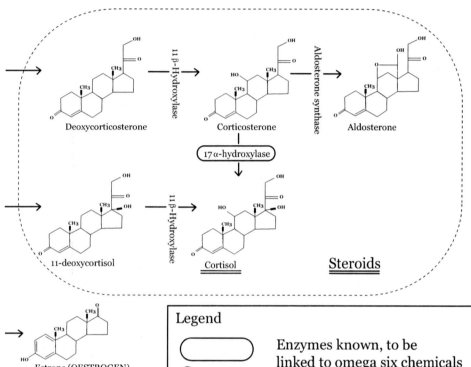

Deoxycorticosterone   11 β-Hydroxylase   Corticosterone   Aldosterone synthase   Aldosterone

17 α-hydroxylase

11-deoxycortisol   11 β-Hydroxylase   Cortisol   **Steroids**

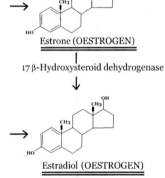

Estrone (OESTROGEN)

17 β-Hydroxysteroid dehydrogenase

Estradiol (OESTROGEN)

Legend

Enzymes known, to be linked to omega six chemicals through PGE 2.

The raw material for the process pregnenolone is limited.

Block any of the 17 paths (Taps) at any point and you change the output ratios. Reduce the raw material and you change all production.

Thanks to Wikipedia and Mikael Häggstrom Author of the original diagram which has been annotated.

The Omega Six derivative AA plays a key part in the ovulation process. PGE2 is a product of Omega Six. PGE2 stimulates aromatase, and other enzyme products, in the hormone pathways that convert androgens to oestrogens [184] and testosterone, and allows steroid production. [23.11.b]

Steroid production is linked to hormone production. [Oestrogens stimulate the production of DHA and AA. [185] [186] DHA reduces the production of the Omega Six derivatives of AA. DHA reduces testosterone. DHA increases progesterone and fertility. [187] Testosterone reduces DHA production. [188]] Progesterone increases melatonin. Melatonin helps shut down the Omega Six chemical pathways at night, increases DHA, and melatonin is a powerful antioxidant.

There are many interlinking threads and control mechanisms. Thus, the products of the Omega Three and Six long chain fats, are intimately involved in a delicate dance with the monthly cycle of hormones.

It is in a sense the availability of AA, that controls the fertility cycle, and implantation. AA is the product of Omega 6. Omega 6 is natures controller of the body, an external product that reflects environmental fecundity. In nature AA is scarce, and unlike long chain Omega 3 DHA, cannot be found in quantity in food. The essential ingredients of a control system for the monthly cycle are present.

Excess levels of Omega Six could well be interfering in the delicate monthly cycle. Excess Omega Six is raising levels of both testosterone and oestrogen above the norms, and leaving them high. These imbalances may be implicated in a failure to properly close down the monthly cycle, leaving the system on high alert.

Does a lack of DHA raw material, preclude rising DHA shutting down AA, and so hormone production, leaving hormones high at the monthly cycle end.

Does the body see lack of DHA, at the end of the fertility cycle, as being due to a fertilised developing egg, using the available DHA to grow new cells? The body does not know, the reality is you are not pregnant, but the DHA shortage is because you have not eaten the necessary Omega 3 raw material.

This confusion as to pregnancy status, could result in incomplete shedding, and partial closure of the fibrous sheath mechanisms, due to lack of clarity in hormone messaging. Imbalance may connect with a number of fertility disorders. Low DHA and high AA means hormone levels will not fall at the cycle end.

Given the intimate involvement of these fats, it is unsurprising if Omega 3:6 imbalances outside the body's design parameters, could lead to problems.

It is important that adipose fat production of sex hormones, is largely independent of the hormones made by the sex organs, an implanting egg, and placenta. [Fig 23.11a].

The fat matrix, makes background levels of hormones, based on the quantity of fat, and amount of Omega 6 the fat contains. High Omega 6 stores=high background hormone levels. The egg and related tissue in the monthly cycle, and the placenta in pregnancy, produce the additional periodic hormones.

Omega Six, AA, is a raw material for the enzymes, that enable and control hormone and steroid producing processes.

DHA shuts down AA hormone production. Lack of Omega Three DHA at the end of the cycle may mean the body thinks it is pregnant. As a result the body would be confused, and not have the DHA it needs, to shut down AA production, so leaving hormone production high, and so failing in the confusion as to pregnancy status, to properly shutdown the monthly cycle.

There is on the balance of probabilities, no provision in the instruction manual for Omega 3 DHA, to be unavailable when Omega Six levels are high, unless it is being absorbed by a developing baby. An adequate supply of Omega Six, but lack of Omega Three, is outside the body's evolution, design, experience, or operating parameters.

The above theory on DHA being the factor that shuts down the cycle, is one I have not seen elsewhere. If it is misplaced it is still clear that Omega 3 and 6 play a very big part in the fertility cycle.

23.12 Blocked conversion, declining DHA—Many factors in today's diet, stop women from making long chain Omega Threes, and possibly Sixes. These include age, diabetes, trans fats, sugars, mineral deficiencies, and high levels of Omega Six mother fat intake [11.13].

The combination of low Omega Three intake, poor conversion to long chain fats, and for some, pre-pregnancy alcohol depletion, presents potential for a serious range of conditions, for both mother and baby.

Intake levels of Omega Three are dropping in the West. If you do not eat Omega Three DHA, or the mother Omega Three, ALA, the raw material for DHA, you do not have the raw materials needed for baby making.

The body cannot manufacture the Omega Three mother fat [or Six] from scratch. The mother fat can only be obtained through diet.

23.13 Fats and hormones—Omega 6 is nature's fertility switch. Low Omega 6, seeds in berries and fruit, grain and nuts in the environment reduces our ability to breed. Lots of Omega 6 rich foods = eat, be merry, put on weight, "and do it like they do on the Discovery Channel"= Breed. A few fat facts:

☞ Fats are necessary as an energy store. For women in normal circumstances fats ensure constant energy supplies, for baby making, breast milk production, and hormones, over at least a year or so.

☞ Omega Six acts as a controller production lines for the hormones, and some, it not all, of the production enzymes of the steroids. [23.11.b]

☞ Fats are also chemical raw material stores. The body uses the fats directly, and indirectly, to make all sorts of chemicals, and hormones, including oestrogen, progesterone, testosterone, and steroids. The fats stores are raw material depots, and just like in a factory, ensure smooth production. Stop; start; is no good if you are trying to make a baby.

☞ Fats cells contain highly sophisticated mini factories, despite what fat looks like in the sink.

☞ The prime indirect controller, for most hormones and steroids is Omega Six. Pregnenolone, made from cholesterol a fat, is the raw material for sex hormones and steroids [23.11.b]. In adipose tissue, more fat plus Omega Six = bigger fat cells = a bigger factory with more raw materials. There is no Omega Six eating 'off switch' [See Ch. 25 on Obesity]. Nature never counted on you needing an 'OFF' switch for eating Omega Six and fructose. Nature never expected you to have access to so much Omega Six all year round.

☞ The variable production hormone factories, are the egg, connected tissue of the ovulation process, and placenta.

☞ The fat cells and surrounding matrix, provide a constant gender independent background level of hormones, proportional to the amount of fatty tissue, and its Omega Six content.

☞ Fat cells make 'inflammatory' compounds, that tear down and remake tissue. The same compounds are involved in making babies. A key raw material of some of these 'inflammatory' compounds is Omega Six.

☞ Babies' cell membranes, and so babies are made from fats. Brains require high levels of DHA and AA. AA appears to be made in preference to DHA. This may assist excess AA being available for hormones enzymes.

☞ In evolutionary terms you are fat because your world is full of fruits and seeds. If you are fat, you have a supply of raw materials to make hormones. Hormones are made in the sex organs (ovaries developing egg site, and placenta) as well as the fat matrix. The brain regulates and is regulated by the sex hormones. Small amounts of hormones are produced by other organs. Both the sex organs, and the fat cell matrix, use the same raw materials for hormones, which includes Omega Six. You make the hormones and steroids. The hormones tell you to breed. There is no 'off switch', to the ability of the fat cell matrix, to make a constant background level of hormones. The more Omega Six you have in fat cells, and the supporting cell matrix, the more hormone production capacity you have. The more Omega Six fat stores you have, the more testosterone and oestrogen manufacturing enzyme capacity you have. Excess fat tissue disturbs the hormone/steroid balance. Infertility and the risk of PCOS may link to the amount of excess fat you are carrying, your Omega Six levels, and your Omega 3:6 balance.

23.14 Deficit of DHA and EPA in pregnancy—Results in animal trials suggest that early DHA deficits in infants can in large part be reversed, but it takes time. Short-term changes happen quite quickly, but to fully rebalance the stored Omega 6s and Omega 3s, and structural cell membrane fat composition, will take time. [189] Compositional changes to the brain in animal trials take time.

There is some evidence that reversal of any DHA deficit, in pregnancy, in offspring may not be absolute in all respects. A regular adequate supply of Omega 3 is key, as it is not stored to any significant extent.

I have not seen specific trials on the recovery of mothers from a DHA deficit, resulting from pregnancy, but the implication seems to be that brain shrinkage can be reversed, with adequate supply of DHA post pregnancy.

23.15 DHA low in pregnant women–The recommended DHA intake level in Canada in 2005 was 300 mg a day, which is at the lower end of intake recommendations. Supplementation recommendations vary.

Only 10 per cent of women met the Canadian recommendation. Twenty per cent of the sample only had traces of DHA in their diets. The conclusion was that the low Omega Three intake, raised concerns, and implications for public health.

Breast milk across very diverse populations (Australia, Canada, Chile, China, Japan, Mexico, Philippines, the United Kingdom, and the United States) had only a small variation in AA by weight (.36 per cent to .49 per cent) although other trials in China and Africa showed rates from .8 per cent to 1.22 per cent [190].

DHA levels varied hugely (.17 per cent to .99 per cent; Canada and Japan) [191] to 2.78 per cent in Chinese marine dwellers. Generally DHA in breast milk is far lower in the West, than those on more traditional diets. [See 23.26, 11.28].

23.16 Trans fats in pregnant women–Trans fats in Canada averaged 7.2 per cent of the total fatty acids in breast milk. A 2002 report from a US National Academy of Sciences panel concluded with this recommendation: "The only safe intake of trans fat is zero."

Trans fats are incorporated in organs including the brain, which includes your baby's. Many artificial trans fats are new substances to the body, and the long-term implications are unknown. It is now being accepted artificial trans fats are a health risk. [11.29]

23.17 Fertility Male– Both Omega Three and Six are essential to healthy sperm production. Lack of DHA has been linked to infertility in men. A trial showed sub-fertile men had lower levels of DHA, and higher Omega Six, [n6] : Omega Three, [n3] ratios. [192] [193] Fats are a structural element in cell membranes. The balance between fats, governs the fluidity of cell membranes [30.27].

It is not hard to imagine that sperm with inflexible tails do not swim as well–a tadpole with a splint on its tail.

DHA sperm production in turkeys, was more than doubled by an Omega Three/vitamin E supplementation. [194]

The testes are reported to have higher levels of the "desaturase" enzymes that make the long chain fats, than the liver. DHA in ram's sperm has been reported to rise to 25 per cent of fats. [195]

There are a significant number of trials in male animals, chickens, horses, and turkeys that demonstrate clear improvement in sperm quality with improved Omega Three–Six balance.

In a trial on turkey, the sperm count was doubled by increased n3, and the susceptibility of the sperm to oxidation reduced. [196] In stallions fed DHA, sperm velocity improved, and had straighter trajectory. [197]

In cockerels, the highest levels of fertility were in those fed canola, and the worst those fed on sunflower. [198] Canola has about 10 per cent n3 and 22 per cent Omega Six.

Sunflower contains 65 per cent n6 and no significant n3. Sperm mass increased by 50 per cent and testis mass was 1.5 times higher in cockerels fed a high n3 as against n6 diet.

Where DHA was low, there was evidence of substitution for DHA by the nearest Omega Six fats 20:4 n6 AA and 22:4 n6.[199] Functional sperm needs a correct balance of n3, n6, and n9 fatty acid. [200]

So if you want to help those sperm become Olympic swimmers, ensure you have adequate levels of DHA in the diet. By another mechanism, fertility in men may be reduced by COX blockers.

NSAIDs including commonly used pain product are listed on the US National Library of Health Medicine as being a potential cause of impotence in men.

COX blockers could reduce the production of testosterone, and unbalance hormone production, by blocking the controlling PGE2 pathways.

More trials are needed on NSAIDs to determine if they are a factor in fertility.

23.18 **Testosterone** – Commonly used COX blockers such as Ibuprofen, and Indomethacin, block production of testosterone, which confirms the link between Omega Six and testosterone. [201]

Blocking of the long chain Omega fats pathways, and so hormone production could have serious fertility implications for both men and women [23.41].

Increased fat tissue levels result in sex independent higher hormone levels including testosterone and oestrogen. Does higher testosterone in obese women result in higher aggression, as they are likely to be more sensitive to testosterone, oestrogen being the default hormone, and conversely does higher oestrogen in obese men result in fertility issues as they would be more sensitive to oestrogen.

23.19 **Menstrual issues** – [See 24.1] Omega 6 controls the hormones and steroids, and so connects to the immune function, stress glands, and the brain. DHA, is needed for brain chemicals like serotonin and dopamine, which control mood, and link to the sex hormones. This is a vast simplification. But they all interlink, and DHA interacts with, and 'regulates' many of these agents. It is all immensely complex and the subject of great debate. The role of Omega 6 is evidenced by usage of NSAIDS for treatment of hormonally related conditions.

"For many years prostaglandins have been recognised as key molecules in reproductive biology by regulating ovulation, endometrial physiology and proliferation of endometrial glands and menstruation. [203]*"*

Prostaglandins are chemicals made from Omega Six and Omega Three. The Omega Six prostaglandins are intimately connected to the reproductive cycle. PGE2 is an Omega Six prostaglandin [p.286].

If your fats are out of balance, all sorts of factors in the body are upset, including steroids, hormones, [Fig 23.11.b] and chemical products of the fats pathways, which include prostaglandins. [Fig 1.19].

These imbalances could help explain PMT. PMT is also associated with PCOS [202] which itself is associated with excess Omega Six in the diet, and high androgens. Omega Six through PGE2, controls progesterone, testosterone, and oestrogen through enzyme pathways and aromatase [23.11b]. High levels of Omega 6 are associated with disruption of the fertility cycle [23.11]. Painful menstruation has been linked to higher oestrogen.

There is trial evidence that PGE2 impacts on oestrogen production in the granulosa cells in the ovaries as well[iv]. The major functions of granulosa cells include the production of hormones. This would give PGE2 a role in the major centres of oestrogen production.

Hormones are produced on a gender independent basis in the fat tissue of both men and women. Higher Omega Six and more and larger fat cells means higher hormone levels, irrespective of what is happening in the rest of the body.

Omega Six is highly stored in fat. More stored Omega Six means more capacity to make Omega Six chemicals. The production of Omega Six chemicals depends on the balance of Omega Three and Six in the cell membranes.

A combination of lack of Omega Threes, and excess Omega Six, could mean the cycle does not shut down properly. Improper shutdown would leave oestrogen and testosterone levels high, and disturb steroid production.[v] [23.11].

Many menstrual symptoms, depression, anger, lack of sleep, neural dysfunction, as well as fertility issues, [204] show links to fat imbalances. PMT and is associated with low serotonin. Low serotonin is associated with increased aggression. DHA is required to make serotonin. DHA increases dompamine [6.7, 6.8].

---

iv   Prostaglandin E2 increases cyp19 expression in rat granulosa cells: implication of GATA-4. Cai Z, Kwintkiewicz J, Young ME, **Stocco C**. Mol Cell Endocrinol. 2007 Jan 15;263(1–2):181–9. Epub 2006 Nov 13 Department of Obstetrics, Gynecology and Reproductive Science, Yale School of Medicine, New Haven, CT 06520, United States.

v   Increased 5alpha-reductase activity during the luteal phase of the normal menstrual cycle Endocrine Abstracts (2005) 9 P144 M Quinkler, BA Hughes & PM Stewart Division of Medical Sciences, Queen Elizabeth Hospital, University of Birmingham, UK; Dept of Clinical Endocrinology, Centre for Internal Medicine, Charite Campus Mitte, Berlin, Germany.

Higher oestrogen pushes up conversion of mother fats to DHA, but cannot make DHA levels increase, if there is no Omega 3 mother fat raw material, or if the conversion pathways are blocked [11.13].

DHA might also be used in the second half of the cycle, to increase oxidation and metabolism, to fuel the observed temperature increase [23.53]. DHA is required to build the additional cells to make the menstrual related tissues.

If DHA was already in short supply, usage as part of the fertility cycle would add to a serotonin shortage [6.8], and behavioural effects. Reproduction seems to have a priority call on resources.

Higher background levels of testosterone produced from the adipose fat cells, and the supporting matrix, would increase aggression, both directly, and by reducing the production of serotonin [6.8].

Imbalances in the hormone steroid pathway could also result in cortisol imbalances [23.11b]. Cortisol levels can be associated with moodiness. Balancing your Omega Threes and Sixes, and long chain Omega Threes may reduce the risk of PMT.

23.20 **Fertility and DHA**–There is significant evidence from trials on animals that improvement in the Omega Three : Six balance, and adequate DHA, will improve female fertility. [205]

Why this has not been checked in trials on humans is a puzzle to me. Anecdotal evidence suggests diet, and regularisation of Omega Three : Six intake, does improve fertility outcomes.

The essential fatty acids are so intimately bound in the reproductive cycle, it is not surprising if they are key to fertility. Chemicals made from Omega Three and Six, have key roles in reproductive tract conditions, including dysmenorrhea, endometriosis, menorrhagia, and cancer. [206]

Lack of Omega 3 intake, excess Omega 6, and the blocking of the conversion pathways, is driving the human system well outside its operating specifications.

The amount of Omega Three and Omega Six in your body depends on what you ate recently, and what you have stored in your fat reserves. Far more Omega Six is stored than Omega Three.

Omega Threes are used before Omega Sixes for housekeeping, they are more easily oxidised, and preferentially released from the fat stores. Omega Three is not stored in large quantity, and must be replenished on a constant basis. Omega Three and Omega Six are fundamental to the creation of offspring.

Omega 3, and 6, are both building blocks for cell membranes, and the precursors and controllers of development processes, cell division and migration.

Several trials in cattle and other animals, show that different Omega Three, and Omega Six content, changes the number and size of ovarian follicles, the ovulation rate, progesterone levels in the corpus luteum, and length of gestation. [207]

Trans fats have been linked with increased risk of ovulatory infertility. [208]

23.21 **Early puberty, PCOS, obesity, facial hair**–[See chapters 23.44 and 27.17, 17.18] The consequences of excess Omega 6, and fat imbalances, could include early puberty, PCOS, disturbances in the monthly cycle, greater predisposition to obesity, behavioural disturbances, aggression, greater disposition to 'western' conditions, including diabetes, and asthma.

Teenage girls on diets high in processed foods, polyunsaturated vegetable oils, and trans fats, are at risk of developing an imbalance of Omega 3s and 6s.

A certain level of body fat is necessary for the menstrual cycles to start. If the physical capacity of the cells of the ovaries [As distinct from ovulation process] to produces the sex hormones is relatively fixed by their number, then the variable hormone resource premenarche must be the fat tissue and supporting cell matrix. Increased levels of body fat containing higher Omega Six, would result in the trigger levels of hormones being reached at an earlier age.

Menarche in Norway in 1850 is recorded as about 17, dropping to 16 in the 1890s, and 13 in the 1950s, and is reported to have fallen slightly since then. Inuits are reported as having later menarche, which would be consistent with Omega 3 moderating Omega 6 product PGE2, and so oestrogen via aromatase.

A lack of Omega Threes, would mean that there were no raw materials, to down regulate Omega Six, and production of Omega Six derived chemicals, connected to the hormone pathways [23.11b]. Early puberty would result from higher oestrogen, consequent on high Omega Six availability, fat stores, and the lack of moderation by Omega Three DHA and EPA.

Very low fat diets carry their own risks as outlined elsewhere. Recovery from anorexia will be complicated, if the diet is imbalanced in Omega Six and Omega Three, and may explain cases, where weight recovery has not resolved the fertility problems. Low DHA can increase risks of future infertility. Increased AA, and lack of DHA, may lead to oestrogen and testosterone imbalance, and high testosterone levels in women.

Hormone and steroid imbalance has been linked to a number of conditions listed below, including PCOS [209], and levels of body and face hair. Early puberty has been linked to higher levels of Omega Six. Obesity would result in more stored Omega Six, which would result in greater hormone availability, contributing to earlier puberty.

Also evidence has shown that age of puberty can be influenced by maternal intake of fats. In rats, offspring of mothers fed a high fat high Omega 6 diet, followed by 'normal' laboratory food, had early puberty. Rats with restricted availability of AA Omega Six had delayed puberty. PGE2 was required to trigger puberty[vi].

---

vi   Essential fatty acid deficiency delays the onset of puberty in the female rat. Endocrinology. 1989 Sep;125(3):1650-9 Smith SS, Neuringer M, Ojeda SR. Department of Anatomy, Hahnemann University, Philadelphia, Pennsylvania 19102-1192.

Interestingly, the impact of a supply of higher levels of oestrogen (E2) was earlier puberty. [210] Oestrogen is controlled by PGE2. PGE2 is derived from AA, which can only be made from Omega Six.

Puberty is set in motion in part by prostaglandin PGE2. [211][212][213] PGE2 is also linked to the luteinising hormone that controls sexual development. [214] It has been shown that low levels of essential fatty acids delay puberty. [215]

The amount of PGE2 will, if consistent with other mechanisms, be based on the balance of Omega 3s and 6s in the cell membranes, which in turn is dependent on dietary intake and stored fats.

Excess Omega Six, and lack of Omega Three, combined with higher body fat, would be a credible explanation for early puberty, and rising levels of related conditions. High Omega Six, and low Omega Three, both separately contribute to early puberty, and combined, increase pressures towards early puberty.

Omega Six also is a link to the earth's fecundity and regulates fertility. Excess Omega Six is a message to the body that the environment is more fertile, so start breeding sooner (earlier puberty) to take advantage of current fecundity of the earth.

There is no automatic mechanism to tell the body, that this excess of Omega Six is due not to nature, but human intervention.

Omega Three will also work with melatonin to keep DHA high, lower PGE2 activity, and improve sleep. Higher melatonin, achieved through higher DHA levels, may also delay puberty through other mechanisms.

Omega 3 is likely to delay puberty by moderating the impact of Omega 6. A trial on 42 girls with dysmenorrhea, administered 1080mg EPA, 720mg DHA, and 1.5 mg vitamin E, daily, concluded "This study suggests that dietary supplementation with Omega-3 fatty acids has a beneficial effect on symptoms of dysmenorrhea in adolescents."[vii]

If Omega 3 is not available in the body through diet, it cannot moderate the impact of Omega 6.

23.22 **Diabetes 1 in the mother**—There are a number of trials and reports, suggesting the lack of long chain essential fats, may have a part to play in both types of diabetes. Omega Threes have been linked with reducing insulin resistance. [216]

Healthy babies born to mothers with diabetes type 1, have highly compromised levels of AA and DHA. [217] Uncorrected deficiencies could increase speech and reading problems. Lower IQ and test scores, and behaviour disorders, have been noted in some children born to Diabetes 1 mothers. [218]

---

vii   Supplementation with omega-3 polyunsaturated fatty acids in the management of dysmenorrhea in adolescents. American Journal of Obstetrics & Gynecology. 174(4):1335-1338, April 1996. Harel, Zeev MD; Biro, Frank M. MD; Kottenhahn, Renee K. MD; Rosenthal, Susan L. PhD.

A recent trial (September 2007) by J M Norris, on 1770 high risk children, followed between the ages of 1 and 6, suggested that high Omega Three intake reduces the risk of Diabetes Type 1 by 55 percent.[viii]

23.23 **Baby basics**—Babies are little people with a lot of growing and forming to do. The roles of Omega Three and Omega Six also apply to babies. Baby cell membranes like grown-ups are made largely of fats (body building blocks).

Babies need AA and DHA as key building blocks for their cells. DHA is particularly needed for eyes and growing brains. DHA is preferentially transferred to the baby. No AA and DHA, = no baby. Foetuses must get the necessary raw materials from their mother. Mothers need AA and DHA in correct proportions to control the process of pregnancy, sleep, and building the baby.

The baby brain grows from 100 gr. to 350 gr. in the last trimester. Omega Three can only be obtained through diet. Low DHA has been linked at varying levels to pre-eclampsia, atopic diseases, PND, lower cognitive skills in infants, lower visual acuity, pre-term low weight, possible greater risk of future breast cancer and obesity, and subtle changes of body type. Much of the research has been done in animals, and is considered a valuable source of information. [219]

23.24 **Baby's brain**—At birth, the brain weighs 350 grams, and at the end of the first year 1,000 grams. The brain grows nerve cells, insulates nerves with myelin, makes a vast network of branches, and forms synapses. The brain is wired for vision, feelings, movement and language. [220]

DHA is the principle fatty acid in the brain, comprising about 25% of the brain fats. Deficit of DHA is associated with problems in structural formation of the brain, deficits in serotonin and dopamine neurotransmission, cognitive issues, and in later life anxiety, aggression, hostility, increased risk for attention deficit hyperactivity disorder (ADHD), schizophrenia, and depression. [221 222]

Formula-fed babies historically have had worse DHA profiles than breast-fed babies. [223] [As noted elsewhere, DHA levels in western women are lower than their Eastern counterparts]. In summary, early life makes high demands for the structural long chain fats, AA, and DHA. DHA is often lacking.

Less research has been done on AA to determine how frequently AA status is compromised. Omega 3s are not stored at significant levels, so regular supply in the diet is essential.

23.25 **Obesity in babies**—(See Chapter on Obesity)

---

viii JAMA. 2007 Sep 26;298 (12):1420–8 17895458 Omega–3 polyunsaturated fatty acid intake and islet autoimmunity in children at increased risk for type 1 diabetes Jill M Norris, Xiang Yin, Molly M Lamb, Katherine Barriga, Jennifer Seifert, Michelle Hoffman, Heather D Orton, Anna E Barón, Michael Clare-Salzler, H Peter Chase, Nancy J Szabo, Henry Erlich, George S Eisenbarth, Marian Rewers.

23.26 Mother's milk –The DHA content of breast milk has decreased in the last few years. [224] Large portions of Omega Six, 60 per cent for breast milk, are drawn from tissue fat, and so breast milk is a reflection of past diet. [225] Remember, Omega Threes are not stored in quantity.

In China, DHA rates vary from .44 per cent rural to 2.78 per cent in a marine area. These are very large differences, and emphasise how low 'western' rates are, despite our access to food resources. AA the long chain Omega Six was fairly constant globally at between .36 per cent and .49 per cent [226], although trials in China and Africa showed rates from .8 per cent to 1.22 per cent. [227]

African women living in a lake shore environment but with access to liquid oils had DHA levels well above those in the West. [228] It has been noted that higher 'mother Omega Three', ALA, may not result in higher production of DHA. [229]

DHA in Canadian women in the third trimester were low. DHA in breast milk has decreased by 50 per cent in Canada and Australia in the past 15 years. [230]

In the USA the Omega Six mother fat, linoleic acid, in breast milk has increased from 5 per cent to 17 per cent between 1945 and 1995. In addition the ratio of AA: DHA is 1.8 times worse in the U.S. than Europe despite similar levels of Omega Three mother fat intake. Higher levels of Omega Six block the ability to convert mother fats to the long chain fats. In a recent breast milk meta-study, Japan showed a DHA figure of 1.1 per cent, some U.S. figures were under 0.2 per cent. [233]

Higher levels of Omega Six, as the result of some formula feeds, may lead to a predisposition to childhood obesity. [231] Omega Three rates in breast milk vary greatly. The West has generally far lower Omega Three content in breast milk than the East. [232]

23.27 DHA, EPA, AA, melatonin, infant milk formula–The mother Omega Threes and Sixes, also called essential fatty acids EFA, can only be got from diet. There are many questions [See 23.26, 23.27, 25.33, 11.31].

The long chain daughter Omega 3s and 6s, including DHA and AA, can be manufactured from the mother fats in the breast or liver, taken from body stores, as long as the pathways are not blocked, [234] or from what you just ate.

So mothers can influence breast milk through diet. If you use formula, look at the mother Omega Six and Three, EPA, DHA, and AA content.

Ideally, formula products will provide a balanced supply of Omega 3 and 6 mother fats, include the long chain fats, and short to medium saturated fats. Some formulas have a **very poor** balance of Omega 3s to Omega 6. [235]

Even those formulas that contain some long chain fats are unlikely to have the same range of fats as natural breast milk. Trials suggest that babies may not convert the mother Omega 3 and 6 to long chain fats well, and will have higher mother fats, and lower long chain fats, if fed on formulas without long chain fats.

Further, an Omega Three Six imbalance could expose a baby to the same risks of undesirable Omega Six oxidation as an adult.

Some formulas, even expensive organic ones, have a significant Omega Three : Six mother fat imbalance, and some have virtually no long chain fats EPA, DHA, AA, or necessary saturated fats, so check formulations, research, and speak to your medical advisors.

AND MELATONIN–*Trials suggest that babies at birth cannot produce melatonin, and the ability develops slowly over the first three months.*

Melatonin is produced in breast milk. A limited trial, shows that melatonin in breast milk follows the same nightly pattern as in the mother.[ix] This may synchronise the baby, to the mothers sleep rhythms.

This raises questions as to the possibility of sleep disturbance in newborns on formula feed. Are there any wider implications for babies, of the absence of melatonin in diet given its effects as a powerful antioxidant, and COX2 blocker.

Melatonin in adults has important functions in the body as an antioxidant [27.13], in addition to its roles in fat metabolism [27.11], sleep [27.18], inflammation [27.12], immune function [27.9] and regulation of brain hormones involved in mood [27.3].

From limited enquiries melatonin is not used as a supplement in any formula feeds. Melatonin is a very powerful agent, and supplementation of babies should NOT be considered, until research has been done to determine if it is safe, if indeed ever necessary, and most certainly not without specialist advise.

I report these observations to inform, and raise possible issues, and no more. Excess Omega 6, and lack of 3 may have similar impacts in infants, as in adults.

There are suggestions that sudden infant death syndrome SID may have links with melatonin deficiency. Melatonin is reported in being 50% lower in children that die of SID[x]. Excess damaging oxidation products are also noted in SID.[xi] Breast milk contains melatonin from the mother, formulas do not.

---

ix　Melatonin Rhythm in Human Milk Journal of Clinical Endocrinology and Metabolism 0021-972X/7703-0838$03.00 Helena Illernova, Milena Buresova, and Jiri Presl Institute of Physiology, Academy of Sciences, and Institute for Mother and Child's Care Prague.

x　Low melatonin production in infants with a life threatening event. Developmental Medicine & Child Neurology 2000, 42:491 Yakov Sivan MD Dana Childrens Hospital, Tel Aviv Medical Centre. Moshe Laudon PhD Neurim Pharmaceuticals Ltd Tel Aviv. Jacob Kuint MD, The Chaim Sheba Medical Centre, Tel Aviv. Nava Zisapel Faculty of Sciences, Tel Aviv University Tel Aviv Israel.

xi　Melatonin therapeutic use : Sudden Infant Death prevention and control Med-Hypotheses. 1997 Nov; 49(5): 425-7 Maurizi, C P.

23.28 Trans fats are transferred to babies—In a Canadian study, trans fatty acids [TFAs] averaged 7.2 per cent of the total fats in breast milk[236]. A trial in Prague gave a figure of four per cent TFAs.[237] In America, intake was between 2—5 grams of TFAs a day [11.29].[238]

Trans fats appear to be replacing Omega Threes and Sixes[239 240 241]. Artificial trans fats [11.29] are new to the body, so it is unclear exactly what other impact they have, in addition to reducing EFA intake. Trials have raised concerns.

Trans fats have no known additional nutritional benefit. So why take the risk? Once again, it appears to be the use of the law by consumers that has lead to change, and induced food companies to look at removing trans fats.

The fact that a company has agreed to settle in court for several million $US, says something about trans fats.[242]

It has been recognised that trans fats block the body's ability to make long chain fats. It is also now recognised that TFAs play a part in vascular illness. Steps are being taken to label or eliminate TFAs.

Omega Three is particularly vulnerable to being turned into trans fats in processing. Omega Three is considered undesirable in processed fats as it has a shorter shelf life. Omega Three and Six trans fats, are turned by the body into long chain trans fats, and have ended up in the brain.[243]

Some trans fatty acids are shaped differently, they don't fit to the nerve cell membranes as well as the normal Omega Three fats, so they *cause the nerve cells to communicate less efficiently, and the brain cannot function optimally.*[244]

23.29 Failure to make long chain fats—Many women appear not to be metabolising mother Omega 3 ALA, into the longer chain fats DHA and EPA.[245] This may be the result of a combination of mechanisms, partially blocking the pathways by which these longer chain fats are made.

Blockers include excess Omega Six intake,[246] trans fats,[247] alcohol for some, or alcohol in excess, mineral deficiencies, diabetes, possible inherited traits, and other factors. [11.13]

This is especially important in pregnancy. Fish oil has been suggested as a useful basis of supplementation for pregnant women. Consideration should be given to assessing AA levels as well.[248] If pathways are blocked, consideration as to why, and removal of dietary blockers would be a possible starting point.

The need of babies for DHA, increases toward the end of pregnancy.[249] Increasing oestrogen in pregnancy pushes up long chain fat conversion. Conversion to DHA is dependent on the mother Omega Three being available, and the pathways not being blocked. Trials show some women are not converting the mother Omega Three. If the mother Omega Three is not converted, supplementation is needed to supply DHA. Please discuss the matter of supplementation in pregnancy, with your medical advisors.

23.30 **Pre-pregnancy levels** – Pre-pregnancy levels of the Omega 3 family, are very important to fertility, and body condition, to meet pregnancy demands, particularly if dietary supply has been insufficient, or conversion is poor.

There is evidence that DHA, EPA and AA, are mobilised from the mother's cell membranes during pregnancy, to feed the foetus. There is also evidence of substitution of the long chain Omega 3s, by less suitable Omega 6s. [250]

For the mother this could have a number of consequences. Higher ratios of Omega Six to Omega Three in the cell membranes, could give rise to a greater predisposition, to all the conditions discussed in this book. This underlines the need to consider long chain Omega Three supplementation, pre-pregnancy, as well as during and after pregnancy.

Higher first pregnancy DHA levels, and falling levels with each pregnancy, might account for suggested advantages for the first-born. He or she would have had better DHA supply than subsequent siblings would.

23.31 **DHA depletion multiple pregnancies** – There is evidence in mice, that if Omega Three deficiencies are not corrected, that the maternal DHA deficiency gets a little worse each pregnancy, with implications for both mother and child. It would be interesting to compare fat profiles of siblings from subsequent pregnancies. Better supply of DHA, would be a logical possible explanation, for reported advantages in first-born children.

23.32 **Vegetarians and DHA** – Vegetarians generally have higher levels of the mother Omega 6. Some have higher levels of the mother Omega 3, depending on what oils they use. DHA is not found in vegetable oils.

There are risks that vegetarians may have low DHA levels, which may be reflected in breast milk. Trials suggest this is the case [251] [1.36]. High Omega Six fat intake from vegetable oils would block conversion pathways.

This is far from a statement against being vegetarian. I am sad that the availability of vegetarian long chain Omega Threes is limited. I simply point out particular fat intake risks for vegetarians.

23.33 **Conversion inability in infants** – A trial provides evidence that infants can convert the mother fats to the longer fats. [252] Other trials suggest fat conversion is not occurring, or is limited and insufficient to meet baby's needs. [253] There is no reason why pathways of children should not be blocked by the same factors as adults.

It may be the blocking seen in the parent, is reflected in the child, because of dietary and genetic similarities. Excess Omega Six, sugar, and trans fats would be likely risk areas. Trials show a need for DHA supplementation. [254]

It is not sufficient to supply the mother Omega Three, ALA, as babies may not have full ability to make the daughter fats, DHA, and EPA, although some ability has been demonstrated. [255] AA conversion many also be an issue for some.

23.34 **Pre-eclampsia** —Birth weights in the Faroe Islands are amongst the highest in the world. Post-term deliveries were 1.8 times more frequent than a comparable Danish population. The Faroe Islands diet is high in marine oils. [256]

"Expert Opinion on Investigation Drugs" said that fish oil supplementation looked promising as a treatment for pre-term babies, and more investigation should be undertaken. [257] Higher levels of Omega Six have been linked to pre-eclampsia. [258 259]

In sheep, higher levels of Omega Three have been shown to reduce estradiol, delay premature labour, and in two cases even reverse contractions to non-labour, when Omega Three was given by infusion. [260 261]

Pre-eclampsia has been linked to products of the Omega 6 eicosanoid pathway, through inflammatory factors, thromboxanes, oxidised fats, and decreased prostacyclin [262] leading to vasoconstriction and vascular inflammation. [263]

Increased PGE2 production, higher levels of AA, DPA, and all Omega Sixes, and lower EPA, have been linked with pre-term births. [264 265 266] PGE2 is administered to induce delivery and so is a relevant mechanism. PGE2 blockers are used to delay delivery.

Factors in pre-eclampsia may include a mix of excess Omega Six, inadequate Omega Three, and drain by the developing infant on the mother's DHA and EPA. Opinions are divided and more research has to be done.

23.35 **Postnatal depression**—A number of trials, suggest links between low levels of long chain Omega Threes, particularly DHA, and postnatal depression. [267 268] PND affects 10 to 20 per cent of women, and is as high as 50 per cent in some populations.

Pregnancy involves increased inflammatory and immune functions necessary to the creation of new life, and is enabled by Omega Six derivatives. Higher inflammatory and immune functions, are a factor in depression including PND.

Common mother hood events increase immune reaction and inflammation, including pain, sleep disturbance, stress and trauma.

"In the Adelaide Mothers' and Babies' Iron Trial, a 1% increase in plasma DHA was related to a 59% decrease in depressive symptoms postpartum".[xii xiii]

As explained balancing the Omega 3s and 6s will help control inflammation and immune response, improve sleep and reduce pain. Supplementation with Omega 3, and balancing of Omega 6, is suggested as being prudent. [269]

---

xii Rees A-M, Austin M-P, Parker G. Role of omega-3 fatty acids as a treatment for depression in the perinatal period. Aust N Z J Psychiatry. 2005;39:274–280.

xiii A new paradigm for depression in new mothers: the central role of inflammation and how breastfeeding and anti-inflammatory treatments protect maternal mental health Int Breastfeed J. 2007; 2: 6. Kathleen Kendall-Tackett Family Research Laboratory, 126 Horton Social Science Center, 20 College Road, University of New Hampshire, Durham, New Hampshire, 03824, USA.

Low DHA and EPA levels are reported in connection with depression, suicide, and a range of neurological conditions (See Chapter 24 on the Brain). Foetuses have been reported as taking DHA from any available source in the mother, including the brain. Brain shrinkage of three to five per cent has been observed in some in pregnancies. Shrinkage was larger in women with pre-eclampsia, and women with a pre-birth Omega Three deficiency. Mothers report forgetfulness and loss of menstruation.

Women have greater neuron density in the brain. Neurons need DHA to function. If not replenished, levels of DHA have been reported as dropping lower again after each pregnancy. DHA is reported as being replaced by the second rate Omega Six alternative DPA. [270] Ongoing DHA deficiency will have wider negative health implication, including greater risk of declining mental faculties in old age. Women are at a greater risk of neurological degenerative conditions in old age than men.

23.36 **Eyesight of infants**—It is recognised that an adequate supply of DHA is essential to the effective function of the eyes throughout life. The eye retina contains the highest concentrations of DHA of the whole body. DHA is essential to eye function. [271]

DHA deficiencies can impact on the vision of young and pre-term babies. [272] Breast fed babies had better visual acuity than formula fed infants.

Visual impact was most pronounced in pre-term babies. [273] Supply of the mother Omega Three alone will not solve the problem. [274] Evidence shows the effect of DHA deficit may become more pronounced each generation. [275]

23.37 **Babies' cognitive skills**—It is difficult to measure the cognitive skills of babies at an early age, but trials do suggest better cognitive function, visual acuity, visual recognition memory, and a means-end problem-solving results in babies who ingest higher levels of DHA. [276 277 278]

In animals, DHA deficit has lead to improper brain formation, serotonin and dopamine deficit, anxiety, aggression, and depression [279] [See chapter 24]. If the brain has insufficient DHA 22:6 n3, it will substitute with the nearest Omega Six 22:5n6 DPA. A trial on rats with an Omega Three deficient diet, showed significant decreases of DHA in the brain, 55–65 per cent, and significantly higher Omega Six DPA 22:5 n6 150–225%. [280]

There were also structural differences. Trials suggest that 22:5 n6 DPA functions less effectively in neurons and astrocytes. DHA supports greater neuron and neurite growth.

23.38 **Atopic conditions**—High Omega Six, and low Omega Three, are found in infants with atopic diseases, and the fat imbalance is reflected in their mother's breast milk. [281]

Another trial concluded that atopic conditions could be the result of disturbances in the fat metabolism in the mother's milk. [282]

Low levels of the mother Omega 3, and low total Omega 3, in mature milk from the mothers, may be associated with atopic sensitisation early in life, as well as disturbed relationships between the Omega 3 and 6 fatty acids. [283]

Levels of atopic diseases have been reported as increasing with poorer long chain fatty acid conversion. [284] Higher levels of Omega Sixes and AA lead to higher production of inflammatory products.

The body is put into a state of permanent low-level inflammation, and heightened immune alert by excess Omega Six intake, and Omega 6 body fat reserves. This could be exacerbated by lack of Omega 3, which would if present help shut down the immune inflammatory response. Atopic conditions are in essence inflammatory.

Fat imbalance may mean the body is more sensitive to insults, irritants and allergens, and overreacts. Atopic conditions are observed to run in families. Dietary habits common to the family might provide a partial explanation.

23.39 Allergies in children—Allergies in children have been linked with imbalances in the long chain polyunsaturated fats, (LCPUFA), and lower levels of Omega Threes, and higher Omega Sixes. [285]

23.40 DHA deficiency and foetal development—It is important not to get too hung up on this section. It emphasises the importance of the mother's diet, to the offspring at every level.

Trials are limited. These things are very difficult to measure. There is little point in worrying about the past. Trials do show, that deficits can be very significantly addressed, by subsequent appropriate supplementation. [286]

Potential effects due to DHA deficiency during gestation include, cognitive function, loss of visual acuity, time of puberty, risk of breast cancer, obesity, and bone structure alteration. [287]

There is evidence that whilst serious DHA deficiency is largely reversed, it is not possible to completely reverse the effects of it. [288] Trials in animals would suggest that levels of fullness of recovery would depend when DHA supply became adequate, during lactation or at weaning. [289]

Reversal is also dependent on the levels of Omega Six in the diet during supplementation. Consideration would need to be given to long chain Omega Three supplementation, and possibly assessment to determine if the Omega Six pathways were fully functional. Excess Omega Six will inhibit recovery. [290] It is possible in extreme circumstances that there may be long-term impact. [291]

23.41 Homosexualisation in the womb— *[See also 24.29]* In rats brain sexuality has been shown to be changed by certain drugs, which intervene in the fat pathways, and impact on hormone production.

These drugs are used in humans to delay or induce birth. It is accepted by specialists in the field of reproduction, that this is an area which requires further research. I have not found any reports of completed trials in humans.

It is important to differentiate between sexuality defined by the sexual structure of the brain, 'brain sex', and sexuality as defined by the sex organs, 'organ sex'. 'Organ sex' is defined by different mechanisms than 'brain sex'.

Sex organs are observed to continue to function, and drive behaviour [E.g. masturbation], even if the relevant area of the brain governing sexual behaviour activity, and desire, does not function.[xiv] Equally the brain may wish to engage in sexual activity, even if the organs or hormones are missing.

Chromosomes from the parent's sperm, and egg, together with hormones primarily define 'organ' sex. XX is a normal female, and XY is a normal male. There are other variants such as XYY super male, and XXX super female.

Brain sex is defined by hormones much later in gestation, towards, or during birth. We all start life as mentally female, and are by default 'brain' female. Testosterone levels at the end of pregnancy determine male 'brain sex', by turning the default female brain, male, creating a larger and different hypothalamic nucleus. It is observed in rats that testosterone levels will alter the size of the hypothalamic nucleus, and mental sexual orientation.

Autopsies on homosexual men who died of AIDS found that they had a small hypothalamic nucleus, which was the same size as those of women. Heterosexual males who died of AIDS, had a normal male sized hypothalamic nucleus.[xv]

It is suggested that the change in the structure of the hypothalamic nucleus is achieved with a burst of testosterone. Certain COX blockers, given in late pregnancy in rats, intervene in the hormone pathways, so reducing testosterone.

The offspring of rats have been reported as being made homosexual, by the administration to the mother, of certain COX blockers late in pregnancy. Male rats took on female mental and behavioural characteristics, including brain patterns.

[COX blockers restrict hormone manufacture and so testosterone production. The sexualisation seems to depend largely on testosterone and not oestrogen. Oestrogen levels are in any event high in pregnancy to the point of inducing lactation by male offspring at birth.]

These COX blockers included indomethacin. Indomethacin may be administered in humans to delay pre-term delivery, and is used in other conditions.

Even aspirin administration in rats had an observable if minor effect. An article suggest that expectant rat mothers administered aspirin may produce sons with unusually low libidos.[xvi]

---

xiv Essential Reproduction Martin H Johnson 6th Edn. Blackwell Publishing.
xv   Genesis of Sexual Orientation: From Plato to Dorner By Michel Odent Primal Health Research Center, London, England.
xvi Aspirin robs males of libido Caution urged for pregnant women as rats bear frigid sons. Helen R. Pilcher Published online 24 May 2004 | Nature | doi:10.1038/news040517-14.

Inversely administration of PGE2 (The substance blocked by the COX blocker, and used to induce delivery in humans) gave female rats male behaviour and male brains. Female rats wanted to mount and copulate with female rats in season.

This is highly complex and emerging science. There are not answers in humans, as trials have not been done. I am simply flagging up what could be a very serious issue. Rats and people are different. Trials are required, to see if certain drugs in pregnancy in humans, influence sexual orientation.

COX blockers, have been shown to block hormone production in humans, in trials on other medical conditions. COX blockers are used to treat fertility related conditions. The trials in rats on sexualisation, starkly warn of possible unforeseen long-term impacts, on the alteration of sexual orientation in pregnancy, by drugs such as pain relievers, and COX blockers.

We start life as effectively female.[292][293] The fact that changes in brain pattern to that of the opposite biological sex, were observed in rats, has very deep implications for our knowledge of homosexualisation, and our deeper understanding of the outlook and behaviour of people with cross sexualisation issues.

The potential for homosexualisation of a baby, by drugs that may intervene in the hormone pathways, like COX blockers and PGE2, and also conceivably pain killers [Morphine appears to impact on the COX2 pathways][xvii], during or prior to delivery have not been trialled in humans, so the answer simply is not known. Pressure on maternity wards is suggested to be resulting in higher levels of induced births so increasing exposure to these drugs.

Increasing levels of pre-term births are being seen. These factors could lead to greater use of drugs intervention. Is the issue of potential homosexualisation of human babies, as a result of drugs intervention in pregnancy, not an issue of such consequence, that it deserves examination and determination?

At the moment the effect in humans simply is not known.

[The same pathways are to a very very much lesser extent subtly impacted by diet. Excess Omega Six intake, combined with high fat stores, is leading to hormone imbalances. Higher Omega Six could result in higher PGE2, which would increase hormones levels, of both testosterone and oestrogen.

Effects at the end of pregnancy, could be magnified, by the high hormone manufacturing capacity of the mature placenta. It is reported that hormones do cross the placenta in both directions [Sulfated form]. Could slightly higher average testosterone levels, as a consequence of diet in theory, very subtly influence the sexual outlook, and brain formation, of infants in the womb?

Could excess Omega Six and consequent subtly higher testosterone, make women fractionally more male in outlook? Testosterone is the more influential hormone in sexual development and outlook, as our default setting is female.

---

xvii Celecoxib blocks morphine-induced tumor growth in mice ASCO report 26/12/2007.

23.42 Breast cancer risk—Trials in animals suggest that a mothers' diet can effect the future formation of the breasts of offspring, and the risk of breast cancer. [294] [295]

23.43 Obesity risk—High Omega Six intake in the mother may increase the risk of obesity in the child (see chapter on obesity).

23.44 Early puberty—[See also 23.21 27.17] Fat intake of the mother may impact on the future age of puberty. [296] There is evidence excess Omega 6 is linked to early puberty. Early puberty has profound social implications at many levels.

Age of menarche in Norway in 1850 was 17. Children do not have as long, to reach mental maturity, and for associated brain formation. What effect does the time available for the brain to reach maturity, have on mental function?

Could early puberty have subtle long-term implications, on brain formation, behaviour, or intellectual capacity of which we are as yet unaware? Brain formation slows down after puberty, and brains are reshaped in early adolescence.

This applies particularly in young males where, unlike in girls, there is no oestrogen increase with puberty, that would increase the conversion to DHA for continued brain growth [27.17]. [Adequate DHA in girls assumes Omega 3 mother fat is in the diet and conversion to long chain fats is not blocked.]

Permanent excess of Omega Six is nature's signal to humans to reproduce. There would be a survival advantage in breeding whilst environmental conditions were fertile, set against any disadvantage of shorter maturation time.

Reproduction is the biggest energy, and personal resource investment, a female will make in her lifetime. Omega Six availability is a major factor selected by design or evolution, to synchronise the body to the availability of food and the status of the environment as reflected by plants setting seed.

The best survival strategy is to breed when food availability is high. This link is observed in conditions such as anorexia, which can stop periods, and menstrual problems in those with low levels of Omegas in the diet.

Higher body weight, and higher intake of Omega Six, both would contribute to early puberty, by increasing hormone levels. PGE2 levels indirectly control oestrogen production. PGE2 is derived from AA, which can only be made from Omega Six. Puberty is set in motion in part by prostaglandin PGE2. [297] [23.21]

Obesity results in high levels of stored Omega Sixes. Omega Six stores in body fat as a percentage, have risen from mid single figures in the 60s and 70s, to 15-18% today. Adipose tissue contributes to the pool of sex hormones.

Puberty has been shown to be delayed by low levels of essential fatty acids.

In conclusion, a combination of stored Omega Sixes, and higher levels of Omega Six in diet, is increasing hormone production at an earlier age, and thus contributing to earlier puberty.

Lower DHA intake in diet may also result in lower melatonin, and higher PGE2, and less sleep [27.17]. Higher DHA, if available in the diet, would hold down Omega Six AA production, and so reduce hormone availability, and delay puberty.

This has wider social implications in children, and particularly males, where the increased DHA production necessary for brain fabrication, is reliant on the higher pre-puberty melatonin levels.

In girls after puberty, rising oestrogen increases available DHA levels. But in men there is no equivalent compensating mechanism.

Young men post puberty will require DHA for continuing brain growth [24.1]. They may, based on trials, convert little Omega 3 mother fat to DHA. This would be compounded by a lack of DHA in the diet. The situation would be even worse if Omega 3 mother intake was poor as well. Lack of DHA necessary for continued brain growth, combined with the effects of DHA deficit, including aggression and impulsiveness, may explain the teenage issues in young males.

23.45   Low growth in babies—Some suggest that AA may promote growth, in pre-term babies, and DHA restrict it. This is an obvious concern. A trial found that the impact of DHA on growth was not "biologically significant." [298]

A few studies conducted over the past decade suggest that formulas, supplemented with long-chain polyunsaturated Omega 3 fatty acids, may slow growth of pre-term infants.

Others suggest that a high intake of alpha-linolenic acid Omega Three mother fats ALA, the precursor of the long-chain polyunsaturated, or n3 fatty acids, also may limit growth. The majority of studies, however, have not shown an effect of n3 fatty acids as a precursor on growth.

At a common sense level, lots of high fish consuming populations have done well for a very long time, and arguably better in health terms than the average. [299]

23.46   PCOS 'The thief of womanhood'—Five to 10 per cent of women in the U.S. have PCOS. That is 10 million females. [300] There are suggestions that a significant cause of PCOS is too much male type androgen (testosterone), which disrupts the hormone cycle. PCOS is also linked to insulin resistance, metabolic syndrome, obesity, diabetes, hirsutism and cardiovascular disease. These conditions all link with Omega Three and Six imbalances.

Given the Omega Three and Six mother fats work in a delicate dance, and are indirectly the controllers of the sex hormones, it is surely prudent to provide them at the levels, and in the ratios, to which the body has over the millennia become accustomed.

It seems to me entirely reasonable, that unreasonable excess, will push the body into unknown territory. Excess Omega Six appears to relate to increased and persistent fibre production, and increased bleeding.

There is evidence from trials that AA, arachidonic acid, is involved intermediating testosterone in rats. [301] Trials suggest that dysmenorrhoea is connected with elevated prostaglandins of the AA pathway. [302] There is no question that the prostaglandin derivatives of AA, are involved in the regulation of the monthly cycle. [303]

I have seen a suggestion that one factor of PCOS, and related conditions, is the failure of the body to shut down the menstrual cycle, leaving the body unable to make up its mind whether to prepare for pregnancy or not.

The mechanism for incomplete shutdown would be as previously described [23.11]. NSAIDS are used in treatment options, which further suggests excess prostaglandins and hormone pathways are implicated. [304]

Whatever the mechanism, fat imbalance appear to be responsible at least in part for the rising levels of these conditions.

23.47 **Dysmenorrhea and Endometriosis**–Dysmenorrhea, monthly cramps and period pains are also linked to Omega Six. Prostaglandins are made from Omega Six [p 286]. Prostaglandins and AA both control the contractions of the uterus. Fats pathways imbalances may be the cause of abnormal concentrations of prostaglandins.

A trial on adolescents for two months showed marked improvements after administration of fish oil. [305] Fish oil contains DHA. DHA has been shown to act as a NSAID.

Doctors prescribe anti-prostaglandin drugs NSAID's [306] for these conditions. NSAIDS block downstream chemical prostaglandin products of the Omega Six pathways. Excess Omega Six combined with low Omega Three, may be what is leading to the prostaglandins being upgraded, through increased AA.

It has also been suggested that higher hormone levels might contribute to the problem. [307] Fats imbalances disturbs the hormone pathways [23.11]. Endometriosis has been linked to PGE2. PGE2 is a child of AA a long chain Omega Six [p 286]. PGE2 is a precursor of oestrogen through aromatase. AA increases testosterone production. As previously discussed high Omega 6 may result in higher levels of both oestrogens and testosterone [308] [309] [23.11].

If Omega 3s are not available in the diet, or the conversion pathways are blocked, DHA cannot be made in response to increased oestrogen. The Omega Three based close down of AA/PGE2/hormone production will not happen. These higher levels of hormones may result in disruption of the monthly cycle, and incomplete closedown as discussed in 23.11.

Endometriosis has also been linked to inflammation. [310] The Omega Threes act in a dance with the Omega Sixes, to damp down the Omega Six prostaglandins, and the consequent inflammation. If Omega Threes are not present, there is no mechanism to damp down inflammation.

23.48 **Osteoporosis**–[See 29.16 25.30] Osteoarthritis and inflammatory joint disease, afflict millions of people worldwide. A higher ratio of Omega Six to Omega Three, is found to link in both sexes with lower hipbone density.

Hormone therapy has been shown to increase oestrogen levels. Higher oestrogen levels increase DHA production. Higher ratios of Omega Three to Omega Six have been shown to increase bone density in the hip and spine.

Omega 3 supplementation, and a reduced Omega 3:6 ratio, reduces the level of prostaglandin production, increases calcium transport, calcium absorption, and decreases bone calcium loss. [311] [312] Fish oils, DHA, EPA and perilla oil depressed excretion of urinary calcium [314], and reduce PGE2.

PGE2 excess, the product of Omega Six, is linked to osteoporosis and arthritis, and is associated with bone loss. [313] Inflammatory cytokines linked to Omega Six inflammation, induce cartilage degradation [29.9]. Omega 3 reduces inflammatory cytokine production.

Osteoporosis has also been linked with excessive fat accumulation in the marrow. Melatonin [27.1] is reported as reducing fat creation in the marrow and the creation of new fat cells. [315]

23.49 Hirsutism–Hirsutism shares ground with acne, irregular periods, infertility, obesity and PCOS [316] [317], which all link to Omega Six excess (see 'western' conditions). Clearly, there are genetic elements, but male type hormones play a part too. [318] [319] The subject of hormones is immensely complex. The Omega Three and Six levels can influence sex hormones levels [23.11]. DHA and EPA are reported as mediating androgen actions. As above, AA has been shown to increase testosterone, and EPA / DHA moderate it. I have found no trials with DHA on hirsutism.

23.50 DHA blocks proliferation of human Papillomavirus–A trial suggested that DHA blocks the proliferation of the virus HPV16 and may kill it over longer time frames. When the DHA levels dropped, the virus started re growing. The trial concluded that women with precancerous lesions might benefit from increased dietary Omega–3 fatty acids. [320]

23.51 Selenium–A trial suggests that selenium is important to effective metabolism in the fat pathways. The trial was in animals but possibly a point to keep in mind. Selenium *deficiency*, in conjunction with a supply of fish oil, led to higher Omega Six to Omega Three ratios. [321]

23.52. Basal metabolic rate–Fats have different fuel values [25.5]. I have not found trials looking at human basal metabolic rate and type of fat intake.

A trial in animals suggested basal metabolic rate and body temperature has a part to play in obesity.[xviii] I saw a recent documentary on obesity where people claimed to have a low metabolic rate. Exercising rate metabolism was normal, but there was no discussion of resting / sleeping metabolic rates [BMR]. Basal metabolic rates [BMR] do change in nature, in response to environment, body process, and membrane fat content.

---

xviii Physiology of transgenic mice with brown fat ablation: obesity is due to lowered body temperature. Am J Physiol Regul Integr Comp Physiol 274: R287-R293, 1998 Susanne Klaus, Heike Münzberg, Christiane Trüloff, and Gerhard Heldmaier. The German Institute of Human Nutrition in Potsdam-Rehbrücke, 14558 Bergholz-Rehbrücke; and Department of Zoology, Philipps-University, 35043 Marburg, Germany.

BMR can be responsible for burning up to 70% of the total calories expended [*www.shapefit.com/basal-metabolic-rate.html*]. Membrane fat content is diet dependent to a large extent. BMR changes are seen during starvation, and food deprivation[xix], during the menstrual cycle[xx], and seasonally in some animals [Arctic Foxes[xxi]] and hibernators. Marmots and ground squirrels do not hibernate if given extra ALA [Greg Florant, Colorado University] .

It would make sense as a survival strategy to alter metabolic rate to reflect the current environmental conditions − like driving more cautiously if the fuel gauge is low, and the distance to the next open garage is uncertain.

DHA may have a part in increasing BMR. Oestrogen increases DHA. Neutering in female cats reduces the BMR.[xxii] Oral contraceptives in women significantly increases BMR.[xxiii] Metabolic disturbances occur after loss of ovarian function[xxiv].

DHA is associated with weight loss and appears to be more efficiently metabolised in the mitochondria. Melatonin may help maintain efficient mitochondrial function [See 27.3]. In sleep melatonin uprates DHA production. DHA deficit is linked with obesity and sleep loss. Lack of sleep has been associated with obesity.[xxv] Lack of sleep has been associated with increased hunger.[xxvi]

---

xix Adaptive reduction in basal metabolic rate in response to food deprivation in humans: a role for feedback signals from fat stores. Am J Clin Nutr 68 (3): 599. Dulloo AG, Jacquet J. Department of Physiology, Faculty of Medicine, University of Geneva, Switzerland.

xx   Menstrual cycle and basal metabolic rate in women. Am J Clin Nutr. 1982 Oct;36(4):611-6 Solomon SJ, Kurzer MS, Calloway DH.

xxi Seasonal trends in body mass, food intake and resting metabolic rate, and induction of metabolic depression in arctic foxes (Alopex lagopus) at Svalbard. Journal of Comparative Physiology 0174-1578 Norwegian Polar Institute, N-9296 TromsÃ¸, Norway.

xxii Effects of neutering on bodyweight, metabolic rate and glucose tolerance of domestic cats.
     M. J. Fettman, C. A. Stanton, L. L. Banks, D. W. Hamar, D. E. Johnson and R. L. Hegstad S. Johnston. Research in Veterinary Science; Vol. 62 Issue 2 Mar-Apr. 1997 p131-136. Department of Pathology and Department of Animal Sciences, Colorado State University, Fort Collins, CO 80523-1671, USA. Department of Clinical and Population Sciences, University of Minnesota, St Paul MN55108, USA.

xxiii The effect of oral contraceptive agents on the basal metabolic rate of young women. Diffey B. Piers L. S. Soares M. J. O'Deak. British Journal of Nutrition 1997, vol. 77, no6, pp. 853-862 The School of Nutrition and Public Health, and Deakin Institute of Human Nutrition Deakin University, 336 Glenferrie Road, Malvern VIC 3144, Australie.

xxiv Metabolic effects of the menopause and oestrogen replacement Baillière's Clinical Obstetrics and Gynaecology Vol. 10 Issue 3 Sept 1996 p449-467 John C. Stevenson.

xxv The association between obesity and short sleep duration: a population-based study. Singh M, Drake CL, Roehrs T, Hudgel DW, Roth T. J Clin Sleep Med. 2005 Oct. 15;1(4):357-63.
     Henry Ford Hospital Sleep Disorders and Research Center, Wayne State College of Medicine, Detroit, MI 49202, USA.

xxvi Sleep loss alters basal metabolic hormone secretion and modulates the dynamic counterregulatory response to hypoglycemia. J Clin Endocrinol Metab. 2007 Aug;92(8):3044-51 Schmid SM, Hallschmid M, Jauch-Chara K, Bandorf N, Born J, Schultes B. Department of Internal Medicine, University of Luebeck, Germany.

DHA determines metabolic rate at cellular function level[xxvii]. [See also Cardiolipin]. Insulin levels in humans increase at night[xxviii] which would provide a synergy with melatonin. Melatonin and insulin the both increase conversion of the mother fat to DHA [desaturase 5]. DHA increases metabolism.

Oestrogen levels rise through the fertility cycle. Increasing DHA may have a part in the temperature rises in the second half of the cycle. Oestrogen, melatonin, and insulin uprate DHA production from the mother fat, but cannot do so if the raw material is not available in diet. DHA may also uprate thyroid function.

Conversion pathways of the mother fat to the long chain fat may be blocked by age, diabetes, dietary factors such as sugar, and high Omega Six [11.13]. For the reasons given in the obesity chapter, and above, DHA may increase the resting metabolic rate, including during sleep, which may assist in weight control.

BMR is higher in more active animals. More active animals have greater amounts of DHA in their cell membranes[xxix xxx xxxi]. On this basis it would seem prudent to ensure an adequate supply of Omega Three DHA, and the mother fat in your diet.

23.53 Lower Incidence of Cardiac Events in Premenopausal Women – DHA is reported as offering some protection against cardiac events. Higher DHA in premenopausal women due to estrogen, would be a rational explanation for lower heart health issues in that group, compared with men and post menopausal women. A recent trial noted a significant relationship between Omega 3-6 profiles and risk for CHD in postmenopausal women, and said; "Healthy premenopausal women had a higher ratio of Omega-3/Omega-6 PUFA than postmenopausal women" [xxxii]

---

xxvii Docosahexaenoic acid (DHA) content of membranes determines molecular activity of the sodium pump: implications for disease states and metabolism. Biomedical and Life Sciences, Vol. 90, No, 11 Nov. 2003. Nigel Turner, Paul L. Else and A. J. Hulbert Metabolic Research Centre, and the Departments of Biomedical Sciences and Biological Sciences, University of Wollongong, 2522 Wollongong, NSW, Australia.

xxviii Diurnal pattern of plasma insulin concentration in the human. Diabetologia Vol.2 No. 1 June 1966 A. E. Lambert and J. J. Hoet Laboratoire de Recherches de la Clinique Médicale, Hôpital St. Pierre, Louvain, Belgium.

xxix Basal metabolic rate: history, composition, regulation, and usefulness. Physiological and Biochemical Zoology, 2004 (Vol. 77) (No. 6) 869-876 Hulbert, A. J., Else, P. L. 869-876.

xxx Life and Death: Metabolic Rate, Membrane Composition, and Life Span of Animals. A. J. Hulbert, Reinald Pamplona, Rochelle Buffenstein and W. A. Buttemer Physiol. Rev. 87: 1175-1213, 2007; doi:10.1152/physrev.00047.2006 Metabolic Research Centre, Institute for Conservation Biology, School of Biological Sciences, University of Wollongong, Wollongong, New South Wales, Australia; Department of Basic Medical Sciences, University of Lleida, Lleida, Spain; and Department of Biology, City College of the City University of New York, New York, New York.

xxxi Susan Allport. Queen of Fats.

xxxii Plasma free fatty acid level patterns according to cardiovascular risk status in postmenopausal - Clin Chim Acta. 2008 Feb 16 - Rhee Y, Paik MJ, Kim KR, Ko YG, Kang ES, Cha BS, Lee HC, Lim SK. - Dept of Internal Medicine & Endocrine Research Institute, College of Medicine, Yonsei University, Seoul, Republic of Korea.

24

THE BRAIN-DHA, EPA, OMEGA THREES AND ADHD, AGGRESSION, BIPOLAR DISORDER, DEPRESSION, DEMENTIA, DYSLEXIA, DYSPRAXIA, INTELLIGENCE, PMT, SUICIDE, SCHIZOPHRENIA, AND SOME PSYCHIATRIC CONDITIONS

24.1 **The brain, Doh!**–[Abbreviations at 1.1] Your brain is very fat. It is a fact to be proud of. Are they the right fats? Your brain is 60 per cent-plus fat.

Fifty per cent approximately of the brain is Omega 3 and 6 EFAs[i].

- ☞ Omega 6 AA, Arachidonic 15 per cent, and AD, Adrenic 10 per cent
- ☞ Omega 3 DHA, Docosahexaenoic 25 per cent - dry weight

These are the primary fats in the brain. EPA, DPA, and others are present in small amounts. Fifty per cent of retina membrane fats are DHA.[322] Fats are fundamental to brain function, the nervous system, and eyes. The brain has a particular need for DHA. Neurons are high in DHA, but AA is evenly distributed in grey [axions] and white matter [neurons]. So neurons rely on Omega 3 chemicals made from DHA. DHA makes better and bigger neurons, and brain connectors, neurites.

Women have greater brain neuron density. Women are twice as liable to suffer from depression. Women have a greater need of DHA, for brain maintenance and materials for the monthly cycle. Women are drained of DHA by babies.

---

i   TheDriving Force Michael Crawford and David Marsh p182 (Figures vary).

Women with significant depression are 3 times more likely to have earlier menopause[ii]. DHA is needed in the monthly cycle. [23.11].

Oestrogen in women makes more DHA, IF the Omega 3 raw materials are available AND the pathways are not blocked.

In animals DHA deficit leads to smaller brains. Lack of DHA links ADHD, suicide, depression, MS, Downs, Alzheimer's, and age-related degeneration.

DHA is a fat. All cell walls, including brain cells are made of fat. Fats make key chemicals. Fats are messengers. Fats are antioxidants. Fats work with steroids and sex hormones. Fats work with sleep. The brain needs DHA to work.

A lack of serotonin and higher testosterone is linked with irritability [6.8, 24.4]. DHA enables serotonin to be made. Depression occurs in the premenstrual period, when DHA is likely to be lower.

Dopamine and serotonin levels are increased by DHA. Noradrenaline a stress hormone is decreased by DHA. DHA is essential to neuron, neurite and astrocyte formation. Neurites are the cables and modems, that connect to the neurons. Astrocytes are huggy octopus like janitors. If you don't have enough DHA your brain cannot work at its most efficient. DHA is unique and irreplaceable.

Higher oestrogen leads to higher DHA, if the mother Omega 3 raw material is available and the pathways are not blocked.

If the Omega 3 raw material is NOT available, Oestrogen may extra boost long chain Omega 6 by increasing conversion.

There are clearly pathways, that connect sex and steroid hormones, to brain function. Many of the sex hormone and steroid production pathways are moderated by PGE2. AA is the raw material of PGE2. DHA moderates AA.

Pregnenolone [Fig 23.11b] is a product of cholesterol, the raw material of the hormones and steroids, and a neurosteroid involved in brain function. What controls pregnenolone is under investigation. PMT correlates with higher oestrogen [E2] and lower pregnenolone "a significantly higher level of E2 and a lower level of pregnenolone were observed in PMS patients ."[iii] High AA and low DHA would likely increase hormones and lower pregnenolone. If you do not eat Omega 3 or DHA, you will not have it. If the body cannot convert the mother Omega 3, linolenic acid, to the daughter DHA, and you do not have DHA in your diet, you have a potential long term problem.

24.2   **World peace, aggression, intelligence**–Lack of Omega Three, particularly DHA and EPA, combined with high levels of Omega Six, is linked with deterioration of brain and visual function. [323] [324]

---

ii   Depression and Its Influence on Reproductive Endocrine and Menstrual Cycle Markers Associated With Perimenopause Arch Gen Psychiatry. 2003;60:29-36. The Harvard Study of Moods and Cycles Bernard L. Harlow, PhD; Lauren A. Wise, MSc; Michael W. Otto, PhD; Claudio N. Soares, MD, PhD; Lee S. Cohen, MD.
iii   J Clin Endocrinol Metab. 1996 Mar ;81 (3):1076-82 8772579.

Changes function and behaviour observed include aggression, impulsiveness, criminal behaviour, violence, poorer spatial skills, temper tantrums and lower 'intelligence'[325]. Major depressive disorders link with higher Omega 3:6 ratios[326].

A very subtly more aggressive, [329] impulsive, selfish, less intelligent, less cooperative, high Omega 6 world, might have fundamental implications for global peace, cooperation over scarce resources, consumption, and our survival as a species.

24.3   **Omega 3:6 balance in nature** – Fats are the building blocks of cell membranes. These same fats are chemical messengers. Fats make hormones and steroids [23.11b]. Fats provide energy. Fats make chemicals. [1.19].

The fat content of the brain reflects long term diet. In wild animals, from dolphins to giraffes, the brain ratio of Omega Threes to Sixes is 1:1. In captive animals, brain Omega Three : Six fat ratios, are often a long way from 1:1. Brain trials show long term changes in diet have huge effect on brain fat ratios.

If very much more Omega 6 than 3 is stored in the cell membranes, the chemical reactions in the brain reflect that, just like a cake reflects it's ingredients.

Conditions linked to low Omega 3 and DHA, or improved by supplementation include, depression, suicide risk, [327] bipolar disorder, ADHD, dyspraxia, dyslexia, dementia, Alzheimer's, schizophrenia, [328] age-related mental degeneration, autism, and gliomas. The negative impact of excess Omega 6 is magnified by even moderate alcohol consumption, where Omega 3 intake was inadequate.

In extreme situations in animals, where DHA intake is very low, DHA brain content is under 10 per cent. DHA levels then rise above 30 per cent with even moderate supplementation. Lack of DHA is made up for with the second rate DPA n6. 'DPA n6' is an Omega Six 22:5 n6. DPA n6 has one less double bond than DHA, the shape is different, and it has one degree less flexibility. [See 30.10]

We have survived on very low fats, and high fats (Eskimos), and a wide range of diets and remained healthy, but until the last 30 years, never vast excess of Omega 6, adequate other fats, and very low Omega 3. Consumption of vegetable and trans fats, has risen considerably over the last 50 years.

In 1999 in the USA, according to the Department of Agriculture, combined consumption of fat products, excluding meat and dairy fat, totalled about 60 lbs. That 60 lbs. was made up of margarine 8 lbs., salad and cooking 29 lbs., baking and frying 23 lbs. excluding lard, butter, and tallow. Lard, butter, and tallow consumption was about 6 lbs.

Given the main vegetable oils consumed [Fig 3.26] are much higher in Omega 6 than 3 [Page 287], and lots contain almost no Omega 3, many of the population must have a severe imbalance in their Omega 3:6 intake. The body is not designed to work under these conditions. The Omega 3:6 balance is an issue for nations.

We are conducting a vast experiment on ourselves. If you changed a cake's ingredients by 60 per cent or much more, you would expect differences, if not a disaster. The principles are no different in the brain, except the brain is far subtler, more sensitive, and sophisticated, than a cake.

24.4   **Dopamine, serotonin, and melatonin**–[See 6.8 to 6.11]

Serotonin, melatonin, dompamine, and DHA, are intimately linked. All require DHA, directly or indirectly for their manufacture. DHA shortages may result in low dopamine, serotonin, and melatonin. The detail is fuzzy, but the ingredients are there for an explanation, that fat imbalances could result in a whole range of behavioural dysfunctions.

Fat also links to hormone and steroid production. Serotonin is a key factor in mood and behaviour control. Melatonin is key to sleep and body repair. Melatonin is dependent on serotonin. Serotonin levels are dependent on DHA.

Impaired serotonin function has been linked to long-term aggression, [330] violent behaviour, and sleep disorders in humans. Impaired serotonin function in animals has been linked to wounding and threat in monkeys, lack of impulse control, unprovoked and unrestrained violence, and aggression. [331]

Low serotonin function has also been linked to sexual behaviour, levels of sexual activity, and testosterone in free-living wild monkeys. [332]

Trials suggest, low levels of DHA, result in lower levels of dopamine. [333] Dopamine has many roles in the brain, including cognitive, motor activity, motivation and reward, sleep, mood, attention and learning function. Dopamine is particularly associated with pleasure and reward.

Disruption of dopamine, has been linked to psychosis and schizophrenia. Dopamine precursors are used in the treatment of Parkinson's. In conclusion, inadequate DHA, can significantly effect brain function, at very many levels via serotonin, dopamine, melatonin, the hormones and steroids, pregnenolone . . .

24.5   **Dopamine and addiction**–Opioid and cannabinoid products

in the brain modulate pleasure and liking. They can do this independently of dopamine. Alcoholics can have a mutation to the dopamine receptor gene. This mutation was also found in war veterans with post-traumatic stress disorder. Are mutations inherited, or due to stress, alcohol and factors such as diet?

Those with addictions have abnormal levels of dopamine and serotonin. Self-harm may be linked to abnormal low dopamine and serotonin levels. [334] Are addictions in part due to the body lacking the serotonin and dopamine to fill the receptors during withdrawal of the addictive agents from the brain, and also being present in sufficient quantity to undertake their other duties?

Low levels of DHA [and potentially high Omega Six] would result in low levels of dopamine and serotonin. Omega 3 deficiency reduces sensory function, and perception, [See 24.8]. Supplementation with DHA could increase sensory function, and so reduce the desire for alternative stimulation [1.36].

24.6   **ADHD**–(Attention Deficit Hyperactivity Disorder). [See 29.5] Fats deficits and imbalances, have been linked to ADHD. Resolution of fat imbalances has been claimed to have equal effect to drug remedies. Concerns have recently been raised as to the effects of some ADHD drugs in the longer term.

The FDA have recently required ADHD drugs to be labelled for side effects, including potential adverse cardiac, and psychiatric events.

A programme on memory on BBC Radio Four suggested it was estimated, that two children out of every class, were exhibiting learning disorders. The affected children were unable to understand multiple instructions, like get a green pencil, close the desk, bring your workbook, and go and sit on the carpet. Growing numbers are reported with ADHD.

This disorder was virtually unheard of 50 years ago. ADHD has significant consequences for the family and society. More males than female children show signs of ADHD, with a ratio of approximately 3:1. The ability of males to produce DHA [and AA] is lower than that of females, and is very low in some men [17.4].

In the young, the lack of sleep could exacerbate DHA deficits [27.3], and Omega Six inflammatory pressures. Puberty may worsen DHA deficits [27.17]. Alcohol intake, and dietary factors, would add to the problem.

There are consistent suggestions that lack of Omega 3, and excess Omega 6, leads to general degradation of brain performance, membrane differences, lower neuronal performance, poorer astrocyte formation, and inflammatory factors. Lack of DHA generally is linked to poorer neural function.

It is suggested that ADHD continues into adulthood. Estimates suggest that up to one half of all ADHD children, continue to exhibit symptoms into adult life. A higher proportion of women appear to be affected in later life. [335]

Omega 3 has been shown in a number of trials, to be of benefit. As ever, finding trials where the impact of both Omega 3 and 6, are examined together, is difficult. Omega Threes are relatively safe with few side effects, and offer a promise as complimentary treatment for ADHD. [336] If ADHD is in part due to blocked conversion pathways, then AA shortage for some may be an issue. Other trials suggest AA helps some too. Fish oil contains some AA.

Gene expression is altered by diet [See 7.15]. Gene expression examination in ADHD patients reveals abnormal fat pathway activity. Genes are switched on and off by foods. You have some control on the activity of your genes through your choice of fats and diet.

24.7   **Honey I shrunk the brain** – Alcohol, [337] and pregnancy both cause brain shrinkage. The foetus robs the mother's brains of DHA, if the mother does not have enough DHA in her diet, to supply the foetus.

Alcohol dissolves and uses DHA from the brain [1.30]. If the DHA is not replaced the brain will shrink. Excess alcohol also stops DHA being made. DHA is not stored in any great quantity in the body. The brain is the only available DHA source in times of shortage.

Baby comes first. Baby will strip DHA from the mother's brain to build its own [23.8]. If you don't even eat the mother fat, it is worse still. If you are pregnant, drinking, and have low Omega Three intake, it is maybe a triple whammy. Foetuses affected by alcohol have smaller brains.

24.8　**Pleasure, seeing, hearing, smelling**–Better brain function means feeling, seeing, hearing, tasting more vividly. Omega 3 deficiency decreases the perception of pleasure. Omega Three deficiency decreases brain function, as well as the function of the retina and inner ear. Sugar does not taste as sweet in those with Omega Three deficiency. [338]

Do women have stronger sensory perception than men do due to higher DHA? Does DHA explain women's appreciation of colour, and scent in flowers.

Women who improved their Omega Three intake were reported as having more satisfying conjugal relations. A man who had opted for castration, reported improved sensory experiences, colour perception, and vision.

24.9　**Most energy hungry organ in the body**–Brains are expensive to run. The brain is the most energy hungry organ in the body. It uses 20w a fifth of the body's energy of about 100w.

It weighs about 1.35 kilograms. A fin whale brain is about seven kilograms, and that raises a few questions! Different animals use different amounts of brain for different things. A human has 12 million smell receptor cells, a rabbit 100 million, and a bloodhound four billion.

A human brain is about 78 per cent water, 11 per cent fat and eight per cent protein. Women have smaller brains but greater neuron density. A baby in early pregnancy grows 250,000 neurons a minute.

An immature brain contains 50 trillion neurons, and 100 trillion connections. A mature brain has 100 billion neurons.

Our brains arguably deserve more consideration, than we give our cars, houses, and computers.

24.10　**60 per cent fat**–The brain, excluding water, is made of over 60 per cent fats. Some individual component parts are as high as 80 per cent fat. The roles of Omega Three and Omega Six have been set out in chapter 18.

Fats are used as magic bricks in cell structure. Individual shape and structure give each fat a different role. A builder's shovel and small gardening spade do different jobs, even if they both come from the same family. The interchangeability of fats is limited, and always second-best.

Each fat has a particular role in the structure and function of the brain. The brain structure has high levels of the Omega 6 long chain AA, adrenic acid, and Omega 3 DHA. Monosaturates and saturates have other uses, such as the nerve sheathing, which needs to be more rigid, like the plastic round electrical cables.

All fats are equally necessary, but the body can make all fats, except the mother Omega Three and Omega Six, which can only be got in food. In the brains of all wild animals, the Omega Threes and Sixes are in balance 1:1. DHA deficiency disturbs brain development, the composition and physiochemical properties of the neurones, and astrocytes. This results in brain dysfunction. [339]

24.11   **DPA a second rate substitute**–DHA is essential to brain function and structure. If you lack adequate DHA, your brain function is compromised. It is that simple.

The structure of brain cells is deformed if there is not enough DHA. Cells are less plastic. The body replaces DHA with the nearest structural equivalent, Omega Six 22:5 n6 docosapentaenoic acid, DPA. DPA n6 has less bonds in a different configuration and has a lesser shape making ability [30.10]. [340]

There is an Omega 3 DPA but if Omega 3 is short, it will not be available. DPA n6 is like using second grade fuel in your car. Your brain simply does not run as well. Trials have shown poorer electrical performance.

Astrocytes are octopus shaped cells of various types that hug neurons, and help them chat to each other. Some work in the brain, and some at the brain blood barrier. As well as chatting, they act as porters. [341][342] Astrocytes are poorly formed, and do not work properly, when a DHA deficit is filled by DPA. Neurons also do not function properly without adequate DHA. [343]

24.12   **Inflammation and stress**–Depression, stress, sleep disturbance, mental imbalance, hormone/steroid imbalance, neurological conditions, and inflammatory immune conditions, are all interlinked.

The latest medical thinking on depression, is that inflammation, is 'the' risk factor that underlies all others[iv].

Inflammation makers such as CRP are 50 per cent higher in people with depression. The brain, like the rest of the body, is very sensitive to inflammatory and oxidative stress. Low DHA in the brain uprates COX2 levels, increasing the rate of manufacture of the Omega 6 inflammatory family of chemicals [1.19].

Excess of Omega 6, and lack of Omega 3, is central to inflammation. Inflammation, increased immune response, stress, and hormone/steroid imbalances, create a self perpetuating, self feeding, circle. Excess Omega 6 provides an overflowing river of raw material.

There is no exit route, or way to leave the self reinforcing roundabout circuit, without Omega 3. Omega 3 will allow you to turn the steering wheel the other way and leave the roundabout.

---

iv   A new paradigm for depression in new mothers: the central role of inflammation and how breastfeeding and anti-inflammatory treatments protect maternal mental health. Int Breastfeed J. 2007 Mar 30;2:6. Kendall-Tackett K. Family Research Laboratory, 126 Horton Social Science Center, 20 College Road, University of New Hampshire, Durham, New Hampshire 03824, USA.

In the absence of Omega Three raw materials, increased conversion, just worsens the levels of inflammatory Omega Six products, creating a self-reinforcing worsening Omega Six cycle.

Higher levels of Omega Six has been observed in certain brain cancers.

Depression has been linked with inflammatory immune markers such as prostaglandins; cytokines, IL1ß, IL6, IL2 and TNF ...[344]

A trial with pneumococcal agents suggested that DHA and EPA assists in resisting inflammation in the brain. [345]

Excessive inflammation results in over-response to brain injury, restriction of blood supply, and high-levels of oxidants. Excess oxidants kill neurons.

Depression, mania, and stress link to high levels of AA, inflammation and increase immune reaction. The immune messengers, inflammatory cytokines, stimulate the pituitary, and adrenal glands, to produce stress hormones. The cytokines reduce L-tryptophan from which serotonin is made. Stress hormones can contribute to depression or mania.

If there is no Omega 3 to damp systems down, excess Omega 6 creates a self-fuelling self reinforcing cycle of inflammation, poor sleep, heightened immune factors, and hormone/steroid imbalance, leading to a susceptibility to stress which itself triggers inflammation, and poor sleep.

24.13 **400 miles of capillaries**–The brain has about 400 miles of capillaries. Capillaries remove toxins, supply nutrients, and act as a cooling system. Like your computer, no cooling system or wrong voltage = CPU function breakdown. Unlike your computer, a replacement CPU is not an option.

Omega Threes improve blood supply in a number of ways, including improved circulation. It is fundamental to keep the supply routes to the brain clear, and traffic flowing freely. In the developing foetus, the brain uses 70 per cent of the energy supplied by the mother, and 60 per cent of a child's energy in the first year of life.

Narrowing of blood vessels, and arterial disease, is now seen in young children, and is linked to an Omega Three:Six imbalance. [346] Excess of Omega Six, and particularly the mother fat LA, produce inflammatory superoxides, that are linked to blood clotting, and constriction of arteries.

24.14 **Production of DHA**–DHA and AA can be produced locally in the brain from the mother fats or related fats. [347] [348] [349] But trials in humans suggest conversion by the brain is low. [Could this be due to other factors in part, like high levels of stored Omega Six, and blocked conversion pathways, or does the brain simply have low conversion ability?]

The primary source of fat conversion is the liver. Short-term changes in blood fats, do not necessarily reflect the fat changes in the brain. Change in the composition of brain fats is possibly a long-term process that takes years to achieve in full. A very great deal is not known.

24.15 **DHA deficiency, reversibility**–Evidence varies as to the time taken to repair an EPA/DHA deficiency in the brain. It is unanswered, if all the effects of a serious EPA/DHA deficiency, is ever completely reversed. It is best to avoid depletion in the first place.

Much of the brain structure is formed in pregnancy. The brain continues to form into early adulthood. In rats and mice, nearly complete recovery of the neural system took several months rather than days. [350]

In human terms, time factors may be considerably longer. The organisation of neurons, it is reported largely takes place before birth, and largely remains for the subject's lifetime [351]. Much is not known.

It is not certain if recovery from DHA EPA deficit is absolute. [352]

24.16 **Core levels of DHA**–The body retains fiercely DHA, at or above minimum levels, at times of shortage. It is as if the body recognises, and is programmed as a safety mechanism, that a minimum level of DHA is essential to brain structure.

Alcohol depletes the brain of DHA, and may bypass this safety mechanism. Also a growing foetus may overrule this safety mechanism. It is important to ensure Omega 3 intake is adequate to protect DHA levels in the brain.

In trials in rats, "Compared with the adequate diet, 15 weeks of n3 PUFA deprivation reduced plasma DHA by 89 per cent and brain DHA by 37 per cent; these DHA did not change thereafter. [353]"

Omega Six DPA is the first choice substitute when DHA is short. Omega 9s, which can be made in the body, are used as substitutes of last resort. High levels of Omega Six DPA in the brain connect, with poorer neurological function.

24.17 **Inter-conversion DHA and EPA**–There is discussion as to whether supplementation with EPA, DHA, or both, is most effective in the treatment of mental conditions. We are all different, so we may have subtly different needs.

There are trials that suggest DHA is effective, and in others EPA is effective. In plasma, DHA is retro-converted to EPA, and broken down to make other fats. [354]

DHA and EPA fulfil different functions. Subject to usage for particular medical conditions, a source which supplies both, like oily fish, would seem to be a prudent course. Please discuss diet with your doctor.

24.18 **Fat and gene expression**–Changing the composition of fats in the diet, can regulate gene expression, in the brain, as well as other tissues [7.15].

EPA and DHA have different roles. EPA can alter the rate of uptake of AA from the cell membrane. [356] A change in diet from a ratio of 8.2:1 to 4.7:1 [Omega 6 LA to Omega 3 ALA] resulted in the significant change in expression of over 20 genes in the brain, including genes related to energy, lipid metabolism, and respiration. [355]

Omega 6:3 ratios in Europe are reported as being around 10:1 and higher. An ideal ratio might be between 1:1 and 1:3. Looking at gene expression based on these ratios in animals would be likely to produce much higher changes in gene expression.

24.19 **Cumulative fall in brain size over generations**—Brain size in newborn animals is dependent on available fat. Large litters with deficient nutrition, result in offspring with smaller brains.

Trials suggest that once a small brain is established, improved nutrition will not change it. Low EFA over three generations, produced a fall in the number of brain cells in generation three.

These effects have not been considered in humans, so far as I am aware, but maybe there is a warning as to decreasing brain size, for us here.

24.20 **Cognitive function**—Fats have wide ranging impacts on brain function.[357] Old mice fed a DHA rich diet, had significant improvement in brain function. Trials in animals suggest DHA may improve learning ability, visual function, and reverse decline in neural and visual function.[358]

24.21 **Diseases of wealth and poverty**—Campbell's *The China Study* noted the line between the incidence of 'western' diseases, and diseases of poverty is clear-cut. Tendencies to 'western' conditions run in common.[359]

24.22 **Infants, neural function, eyesight, and memory**—DHA deficiency in infants, leads to poorer visual acuity, loss in nervous system function, poorer, cognitive tests, visual recognition, memory means-end problem-solving, and generally loss of neural brain function.[360]

The risk of retinal damage in rats is related to the relative levels of DHA and DPA n6.[361] Deficits in Omega 3, and high levels of Omega 6, in pre-term infants, link to diminished photoreceptor function. Studies support Omega 3 for optimal maturation of visual and cortical function, in pre-term infants.[365v]

24.23 **Cognitive function and depression in children**—Trials suggest that EPA, and DHA, are significant factors in childhood depression, and warrant further consideration.

Other trials emphasise the importance of brain growth in the womb, and in early life, and the longer-term influences of DHA and AA shortages.[362]

A trial with 20 children, suggested Omega Three fatty acids might have therapeutic benefits in childhood depression.[363] Omega 3s and particularly DHA help improve cognitive function in children [See 23.24].

---

v   Essential n-3 fatty acids in pregnant women and early visual acuity maturation in term infants. - Am J Clin Nutr. 2008 Mar;87(3):548-57 - Innis SM, Friesen RW. - Nutrition Research Program, Child and Family Research Institute, Department of Paediatrics, University of British Columbia, Vancouver, BC, Canada V56Z 4H4.

24.24 **Neuron growth**–DHA makes bigger and better neurons, and other brain components. Much of the brain is formed before birth, and in early life. DHA in contrast with AA, DPA, and oleic acid, uniquely promotes growth in the hippocampus. [364]

24.25 **Impaired brain and retinal function**–DHA uniquely has six double bonds. The first bond is only three away from the end of the chain, as against six, for Omega Six. This gives DHA unique shape and electromechanical properties. [31.10]

DHA can get in close contact, and into the spaces, in which it needs to fit, to react much better than the nearest equivalent. Closer contact leads to a more potent reaction.

Impaired brain function, particularly as to thought processes, are associated with low levels of DHA. [366] Motor, and activity functions, seem less effected. [367] Lack of DHA has been associated with poorer neural performance, poorer formation of the astrocytes, general degrading of function, including poorer learning ability, and possible behavioural disturbance.

Degraded function in animals is seen in EEGs. [368] The sense of smell, memory, and spatial learning are also negatively affected. [369] Very low levels of Omega Threes, result in brain function abnormalities, and degradation of vision in animals. [371]

Photoreceptor membranes in the retina are dependent on both the number of double bonds and their position. [372] DPA has only five double bonds. Replacement of DHA with DPA results in degradation of neural function. [370]

24.26 **Aggression and irritability**–Excess of Omega Six over Omega Three, has been shown to increase aggression in animals. [373] Omega Three intake reduced irritability of patients suffering from bipolar disorder. [374]

Students taking 1.5 to 1.8 grams a day of DHA, versus a high Omega Six supplement, showed little change in stress and hostility during exams, but those on the Omega Six supplementation showed significantly increased levels of aggression. [375]

Similar effects have been reported on animals. EPA and DHA, has recently been demonstrated to reduce aggression, in substance abusers. [vi] [1.36].

24.27 **Antisocial behaviour, and impulse control**–Fats are increasingly shown to alter our behaviour. At an evolutionary level, this is unsurprising. Both wild animals, and we, are linked to our environment through availability of Omega 6. Omega Six is linked with aggression. [6.6]. When things are plentiful, we can afford to be more selfish, aggressive, and impulsive. When resources are short, we must co-operate to survive.

---

vi   Long-chain n-3 polyunsaturated fatty acids decrease feelings of anger in substance abusers. Psychiatry Res. 2007 Sep 25; Buydens-Branchey L, Branchey M. Research Service (151/BK), VA New York Harbor Healthcare System — Brooklyn Campus, 800 Poly Place, Brooklyn, NY, 11209, USA.

DHA conversely, links with agreeableness, self-restraint, impulse control, reduced aggression and neuroticism. [376] The implications for society are undeniably profound.

24.28 **Paedophilia**—Trials suggested that depletion of Omega Threes might cause alterations in serotonin usage, that might be connected with behaviour seen in paedophilia. The study looked at Omega Three, and Omega Six, levels in 27 paedophilic men, and 18 healthy volunteers.

In paedophilia, there was a significant depletion of DHA, and total Omega Threes. There was also an increase in Omega 6:3 ratio of AA : EPA. Based on the NEO Personality Inventory, depletion of DHA in paedophiles was reflected by impulsiveness, and lower agreeableness (trust, altruism, straightforwardness, compliance) and conscientiousness (self-discipline).

In addition, there was a lack of control of impulsiveness, and greater aggression. The trial suggested that DHA depletion observed in paedophiles, produced behavioural changes that are consistent with paedophile behaviour. [377]

Another trial noted low prolactin, and cortisol levels, in paedophiles.[vii] There is competition for raw materials between steroid and sex hormones. Low cortisol could be a sign of disruption of the cholesterol hormone/steroid pathways. Cholesterol conversion enzymes are mediated by Omega 6 PGE2 [23.11b].

24.29 **Homosexualisation in the womb?**—[See also 23.41] In rats, blocking the fats pathways with drugs in pregnancy can result in change in the mental sexual orientation of offspring, 'homosexualisation'. Sexuality as defined by the reproductive organs, and the brain are separately controlled.

Sexuality as determined by the sex organs, is largely defined by the chromosomes and consequent hormone production. Brain sexuality is determined by hormones at the end of pregnancy. There is a series of conditions called Congenital Adrenal Hyperplasia (CAH). CAH shows how blockages in the hormone pathways impact on sexuality. [Could COX blockers have any roles in CAH?- See following]

CAH is not the issue here, but is described because the conditions all are the result of failure, or blocking of the hormone/ steroid pathways, [23.11b] . The same pathways are involved in determination of the sexual identity of the brain.

---

vii Lower Baseline Plasma Cortisol and Prolactin together with Increased Body Temperature and Higher mCPP-Induced Cortisol Responses in Men with Pedophilia Neuropsychopharmacology (2001) 24 37-46.10.1038/sj.npp.1395585 Michael Maes MD, Ph.D, Dirk van West MD, Nathalie De Vos MD, Herman Westenberg Ph.D, Fran Van Hunsel MD, Dirk Hendriks Ph.D, Paul Cosyns MD and Simon Scharpé Ph.D Department of Psychiatry & Neuropsychology, University of Maastricht, Maastricht, The Netherlands. Clinical Research Center for Mental Health, Antwerp, Belgium. Department of Psychiatry, Vanderbilt University, Nashville, TN, U.S.A. Department of Psychiatry, University of Utrecht, Utrecht, The Netherlands. Department of Medical Biochemistry, University of Antwerp, Wilrijk, Belgium. Department of Psychiatry, University Hospital of Antwerp, Edegem, Belgium.

There are a number of forms of CAH. Effects are different, and range from monthly irregularity in women, to sexual mental and or physical identity issues. The most severe CAH is life threatening for infants. Hormone effects are so subtle, changes in behaviour and pheromone production are seen in healthy female mice, depending on their development position in the womb between males or females.

It is the same chemical tree, in which cholesterol is turned from pregnenolone into the steroids, and sex hormones [23.11.b]. Where pathways do not work in full, or part, there are two effects. The product of the pathway is not made. The raw material is redirected, leading to an imbalance somewhere else as well.

Drug intervention in the same mechanisms that cause CAH could lead to homosexualisation. The hormone enzymes are likely moderated by PGE2.[viiiix]

All brains are by default female. A burst of testosterone late in pregnancy, will instruct the body to change the critical section of the brain from female to male. Male and female brains are structurally different. The hypothalmus appears to control key aspects of mental sexual orientation and response to stimuli.

It is now being suggested humans like animals respond to pheromones. Pheromones are chemicals emitted by the human body which differ between the sexes. Production in women depends on the state of fertility. Research is looking at the role of pheromones in sexual behaviour.

Pheromone sensory organs have been found in the human nose. These sensors lead to the hypothalamus. (*Human Reproductive Biology, Richard E. Jones, Kristin H. Lopez*) Would a female type hypothalamus in a male, lead to the male responding to pheromones that a female would normally respond to?

It is possible to be male physically, and have female hypothalmus, and visa versa. A female hypothalmus appears to confer a female outlook. Autopsies on young AIDs victims, identified that homosexual men had smaller female type hypothalmuses, and heterosexual men had larger male type hypothalmuses.

On this basis the gender outlook is determined by brain type, and is not a matter of choice. A genetic male could have a male size brain, with a female controlling hypothalmus, so be a man with a brain that is sexually female.

It would be interesting to know what determines the higher brain neuron density in women. Do those with cross gender attributes have the ability to have both larger and more neuron dense brains?

---

viii Prostaglandin E2 is a positive regulator of adrenocorticotropin receptors, 3 beta-hydroxysteroid dehydrogenase, and 17 alpha- hydroxylase expression in bovine adrenocortical cells Endocrinology, Vol 129, 1333-1339 WE Rainey, D Naville, N Cline and JI Mason Cecil H. & Ida Green Center for Reproductive Biology Sciences, Department of Obstetrics and Gynecology, University of Texas Southwestern Medical Center, Dallas 75235-9051.

ix Sex, drugs and sports: Prostaglandins, epitestosterone and sexual development Medical Hypotheses Volume 69, Issue 4, 2007, Pages 829-835 Bryan K. Sanders College of Letters and Science (Alumnus), University of California, Berkeley, CA 94720, United States.

Gender differences have also been observed in other areas of the brain. Fats are fundamental to the hormone and steroid pathways [23.11b], and the production and levels of hormones. Prenatal exposure to certain drugs, COX blockers, like acetaminophen, and indomethacin, lead in a trial to irreversible change in sexual identity, homosexualisation, in rats.

It was reported in 2004, that a study was underway, to see if there is a similar sexual impact in humans. Doctors currently prescribe indomethacin, a COX blocker, to delay pre-term labour. Indomethacin and related drugs block PGE2.

PGE2 is a chemical made from Omega Six, which controls aromatase and other enzymes, which control the sex hormone and steroid levels [23.11.b]. Trials in rats suggest PGE2 has a part in the determination of sexuality of the brain during formation. Indomethacin, [A COX blocker] blocked PGE2, and so hormone production, in rats at a critical stage when brain sexuality was determined.

Male behaviour in rats was severely impaired. The brains of male rats were less 'male'. In contrast, female offspring given PGE2 exhibited more 'male' brains, and male behaviour, including a desire to copulate with fertile females. [378]

[High levels of Omega Six in diet, arguably also produce changes in the levels of PGE2. If PGE2 is leading to changes in sexualisation, high levels of Omega Six could by the same pathways potentially have a *very subtle* effect on sexualisation, including making women a tiny bit more male. These would be very much more subtle changes than by drugs interventions in the pathways.

Could constant high levels of Omega Six could on a very long term basis, through PGE2, create evolutionary pressure for change of sexual profile by altering hormone levels, and increasing testosterone levels in the same way as is seen in fertility conditions?

We are at essence female. Increased PGE2, increases oestrogen, and testosterone. Oestrogen, has limited influence at this stage, as we are already and by default brain female. Testosterone appears to influence brain sex status.

These observations beg many questions. Are high levels of Omega Six in humans, increasing testosterone levels throughout gestation, and childhood, (The brain continues to mature into puberty [379]), and so having *long-term very subtle but wide spread effects* on masculinisation of neural function, behaviour, and sexualisation in particularly women.]

COX blockers such as Ibuprofen, and Indomethacin, may block production of testosterone [380]. So potentially the mechanisms exist, to alter hormones with drugs at times of critical brain growth, sufficiently to change sexual orientation of the brain.

Homosexual men have in a small trial been shown to have female brains. Manipulation of the same family of pathways in CAH due to genetic effects can change brain gender identities. Brain sex change is observed in rats

Experts seem to agree the effect if any of drugs administered at the end of pregnancy on mental sexual gender in humans needs more research.

24.30 **Suicide risk** –[see 24.12] Trials show a link between lack of DHA and EPA, depression, stress, and suicide. A trial in China found that people with low EPA were eight times more likely to attempt to commit suicide.[381] In a 2 year study low DHA / Omega 3s predicted suicidal behaviour in depressed patients.[382]

24.31 **Psychiatric conditions**–Neural conditions such as schizophrenia, borderline personality disorder, bipolar and other psychiatric conditions presenting signs of irritability, may benefit from EPA or fish oil supplementation.[383]

Post natal depression is considered in section 23.35. A number of trials have shown benefits from EPA as an adjunct to medical treatment.[384] Deficits of DHA have been noted in depression[385] and schizophrenic patients.[386][387] Depression has been linked with immune dysfunction markers, seen in autoimmune disorders, and inflammatory markers.

Omega Three is a strong anti-inflammatory. Omega Six is a source of inflammatory products. Increasing Omega 3, and reducing Omega 6, is an anti-inflammatory strategy. Some anti-psychotic drugs have immunosuppressive properties, and so are active in the same pathways.

"Omega-3s show promise in the treatment of mood disorders according to a 2006 expert panel convened by the American Psychiatric Association. They do so, in part, by decreasing inflammation"[x]. "Diets with high n-6:n-3 PUFA ratios may enhance the risk for both depression and inflammatory diseases."[xi]

Depression has also been linked with pain and stressors, including sleep disturbance, hormonal changes, and steroid reactions, all of which fuel inflammation and immune response.

Reduction of inflammation, and inflammatory markers, reduces mania. Omega Six AA is the source chemical of inflammatory factors. Several of these chemicals have roles as chemical messengers, and are active agents in brain function neurodevelopment. AA may be a central pathway leading to the varied symptoms of schizophrenia.[388] Lower Omega Three levels were seen in schizophrenic patients, as well as disturbances in the Omega Nines.[389]

---

x   A new paradigm for depression in new mothers: the central role of inflammation and how breastfeeding and anti-inflammatory treatments protect maternal mental health Int Breastfeed J. 2007; 2: 6 Kathleen Kendall-Tackett Family Research Laboratory, 126 Horton Social Science Center, 20 College Road, University of New Hampshire, Durham, New Hampshire, 03824, USA.

xi   Depressive symptoms, omega-6:omega-3 fatty acids, and inflammation in older adults. Psychosom Med. 2007 Apr;69(3):217-24. Kiecolt-Glaser JK, Belury MA, Porter K, Beversdorf DQ, Lemeshow S, Glaser R. Department of Psychiatry, Ohio State University College of Medicine, OH 43210, USA.

"The preponderance of epidemiologic and tissue compositional studiessupportsaprotectiveeffectofomega-3EFAintake,particularly eicosapentaenoic acid (EPA) and docosahexaenoic acid (DHA), in mood disorders. Meta-analyses of randomized controlled trials demonstrate a statistically significant benefit in unipolar and bipolar depression."[xii]

24.32 Stress and students—Provision of EPA in animals reduces stress related behaviour.[390] DHA reduced stress and hostility in students under exam pressure to almost normal levels.[391]

DHA has been shown to reduce norepinephrine, a stress hormone, and increase serotonin production.

24.33 Violence and aggression—There have been a significant number of trials linking fats intake to aggression. Impulsive and violent offenders, had lower DHA, and higher Omega Six DPA, than non-impulsive offenders, and healthy controls.[392]

Generally, higher DHA and lower Omega Six, are linked to lower aggression and anti-social behaviour.

24.34 Brain tumours—Trials suggest that brain tumours have higher levels of Omega 6 and lower levels of Omega 3.[393] Higher levels of oleic acid were also noted.[394] In brain metastatic melanoma cells, AA stimulated PGE2, which stimulated the cancer cells, whereas DHA or EPA decreased PGE2 production.[395]

This has common elements to certain cancers, along with inflammatory factors, and the involvement of the fats pathways.

24.35 Wider nutrition—Essential minerals and vitamins that are reported to impact on brain function, include; the B vitamin group; vitamins E and K; and the antioxidant and energetic cofactors alpha-lipoic acid , ubiquinone CoQ10, and nicotinamide.

Acetyl L-carnitine, glycerophosphocholine, and phosphatidylserine were all reported as supporting mitochondrial function and improved brain function in double-blind trials. The Omega 3 long chain fatty acids EPA and DHA are key to neural function.[396]

What is the cause of the lack of long chain Omega Threes? Is the cause inadequate supply of the mother Omega Three fat, poor conversion, or lack of intake of the long chain fat? Trials show low conversion rates in men.

---

xii   Omega-3 fatty acids: evidence basis for treatment and future research in psychiatry. J Clin Psychiatry. 2006 Dec;67(12):1954-67 Freeman MP, Hibbeln JR, Wisner KL, Davis JM, Mischoulon D, Peet M, Keck PE Jr, Marangell LB, Richardson AJ, Lake J, Stoll AL. Women's Mental Health Program, Department of Psychiatry, University of Arizona College of Medicine, Tucson 85724-5002, USA.

Based on world vegetable oil consumption [3.26 p.287], it is all the above. Western dietary factors, sugar, high Omega 6, and excess alcohol, block conversion [11.13]. Western intakes of Omega 3 have fallen over the last 20 years.

24.36 **DHA – Anti-inflammatory** – The stimulation of inflammatory paths following neurotrauma, stroke, infection, and neurodegenerative disease (E.g. Alzheimers) results in an inflammatory response, which can include swelling and bruising.

AA in the brain is pro-inflammatory, and with over stimulation following trauma, oxidation products participate in cell damage, and cell death. [397]

DHA is the source of docosanoids, which are powerful counter-inflammatory mediators, [398] and generally mediate inflammation. [399]

Lipid messengers are essential to brain function at every level. Excess oxidation disrupts signalling and promotes neurodegenerative disease. [400]

24.37 **The need for professional medical consultation** – I emphasise the importance of medical consultation in making significant dietary changes. This is doubly so for those with existing conditions.

For the majority, reasonable DHA and EPA intake carries few risks, but there are those with abnormal metabolisms, at risk due to unusual lipid requirements.

Those taking blood thinners, or with related conditions, should be doubly sure to take medical advice.

The book does not profess that a change in diet is a cure. Evidence does suggest that balancing the Omega Three and Six mother fats, and ensuring adequate supply of the long chain fats, is a relatively painless way of reducing the average risk profile, to a range of 'western' conditions, with possible wider yet to be fully agreed benefits.

Those who may wish to consider, looking at their lipid intake and profile, should do so in consultation with their medical advisors.

25
OBESITY

25.1 Omega Three speeds up, and Omega Six slows down, the metabolism–[Abbreviations listed at 1.1] It is all in our design specs. Omega Six encourages weight gain, by setting the body to store, and reducing the metabolism. Omega Three, encourages the body to burn fats, increases the basal metabolism, and reduces fat storage. The table below compares the properties of Omega Three and Omega Six.

Omega Three	Omega Six
Omega Three speeds up the metabolism.	Omega Six slows down the metabolism.
Omega Three encourages smaller fat cells	Omega Six encourages more and bigger fat cells.
Omega Three is a trigger for the body to burn fat	Omega Six is a trigger for the body to store fat.
Omega Three is only stored in small amounts	Omega Six is stored in significant quantity.

25.2 Obesity–Shocking figures–Obesity is linked with heart and vascular conditions. Cost of a heart attack to the individual, and his family, – incalculable. Financial cost of ONE acute heart attack –$30,364 (2003),[401] with about one million heart attacks a year in the U.S.A. [402]

The global obesity epidemic has a major socioeconomic impact. Obesity and related inflammatory conditions, are a major drain on healthcare resources.

In the U.S., historic estimates suggest that one-third of adult women are clinically obese. In the U.K., by 2010, one in three adults will be obese. 27 per cent of girls, 11–15 years old, will be obese approaching child-bearing age. In the U.S.A., 65 per cent of adults aged over 20 are either overweight, or obese.

Metabolic syndrome, obesity, and type 2 diabetes, are occurring at epidemic rates in the U.S.A., and many parts of the world. [404] The estimated number of deaths ascribable to obesity was 280,184 per year. [403] From 1935 to 1996, type 2 diabetes often connected with obesity, climbed 765 per cent.

Global diabetes figures are predicted to rise 46 per cent, from 150 million cases in 2000, to 221 million in 2010.[405] More than 64 million Americans have heart disease, 11 million have type 2 diabetes, and 37 million have high cholesterol. Of postmenopausal women, 7.2 per cent have osteoporosis, and 39.6 per cent osteopenia. [406.] Excess Omega 6 is factor in these conditions and obesity.

25.3   **Omega Six and obesity**–Refined bottled high Omega Six vegetable oils are an invitation to increased risk of obesity, and disease and early death. They are cheap, and on a supermarket shelf near you. Vegetable oil is in many processed foods. You have been told Omega 6s are unreservedly good for you.

Omega 6 IS absolutely essential to health, but in EXCESS, or significantly out of balance with Omega 3, Omega 6 is long term, an invitation to an earlier risk of serious illness.

You have to eat Omega 6 and Omega 3 mother fats. The body cannot make them. The body can make all other fats. If you do not eat excess Omega Six, it cannot become a problem. The problem; we have a built in desire for Omega Six, and no 'off switch'.

Omega Six is the exclusive raw material for a family of very powerful chemicals [Fig. 1.19] that, control inflammation, interact with immune function, control fertility, significantly impact on metabolism, increase the risk of western diseases including obesity, and impact on many body functions.

An excess of Omega 6 inflammatory chemicals leads to permanent low level intruder alert, and low level inflammation status body wide. Obesity is considered by some to be an inflammatory condition along with many western conditions.

Simply, excess Omega 6, and lack of Omega 3, combined with excess fructose particularly, pushes the whole metabolism processes permanently off balance towards fat storage, lower resting metabolism and increased risk of obesity.

25.4   **Programmed to store**–We are programmed to store Omega Six because it is an essential raw material to breeding, and body function. In nature it is too rare and precious to waste simply on energy production.

We store Omega 6 in body fat. Omega 6 is 16–20 per cent of body fat in America, 24 per cent in Israel, 11 per cent in Europe, and historically much less. In the 1950s/70s it was in mid single figures. Body fat is a 5 year food diary.

Most now carry very large reserves of Omega 6. Your fat reserves regulate the Omega 6 levels in the cell membranes. Fat balances in the cell membrane determines body function. The important Omega 6 statistic is the *total* amount stored in the body, not just the percentage in a single fat cell.

25.5   **Metabolic issues**—Obesity, and metabolic problems, link in part to abnormal fatty acid metabolism. An imbalance in the Omega 3s and 6s, disturbs production in the main fat factory the liver, and body wide.

The Omega 6 mother fat promotes storage of fat, and lowers basal metabolism. Long chain Omega 3s increase basal metabolism [23.52]. In the fat tissue of the obese, Omega 6 is often high, and Omega 3 is low. [407] Obese adolescents have lower Omega 3, and higher Omega 6.

This is more marked in females. Women need DHA for the monthly cycle. Reproduction needs get priority usage. Oestrogen makes more DHA from the Omega 3 mother fat, BUT you can only make long chain Omega 3 if you have eaten mother Omega 3 first.

IF you have not eaten mother Omega 3, the body makes more inflammatory long chain Omega 6s instead. This fuels inflammatory chemicals, hormonal imbalance, and overproduction of immune chemicals. [408] Obesity is considered by some as an inflammatory condition.

Metabolic factors due to Omega 3 and 6 that directly or indirectly affect obesity through rest, sleep, and activity, considered elsewhere in this book include:

☞ The lower oxidative value of Omega 6.

☞ The higher oxidative value of DHA, and Omega 3s [21.7].

☞ The lower oxidation rate of mid chain saturated fats.

☞ The higher oxidation rate of short chain fats [11.32].

☞ Insufficient quantities of DHA in diet, or Omega 3 mother fat, which is the necessary and exclusive raw material for elongation to DHA.

☞ Blockage of fat conversion pathways from mother to long fats [11.13].

☞ Mitochondrial requirement for DHA, and the negative impact of excess Omega Six [21.3, 21.7].

☞ Higher melatonin may encourage greater number of mitochondria, which would allow a higher metabolic rate.

☞ Melatonin may protect mitochondria from oxidative damage, so maintaining mitochondrial function and metabolism. [27.13]

☞ The requirement of high quality DHA oxidation, for thyroid function. There is a nocturnal surge of thyroid hormone, consistent with higher metabolism, melatonin and DHA usage. Higher early night time basal metabolism included greater oxygen use in one trial. This would help to keep extremities warm in sleep, and reduce obesity [23.52].

☞ The lack of Omega 3, leading to the blocking of the leptin, and insulin, metabolic control functions [25.21].

☞ Fructose and insulin activating the SCD1 enzyme, which is related to the creation of fat from carbohydrate, potential metabolic blocks, and reduction in metabolism [25.21].

25.6   **Designed to store**–Sex again! Omega Six is nature's way of linking our fertility to the productivity of the environment. Omega Six controls production of sex hormones, steroids, and the inflammatory processes necessary to tissue creation. To breed you need Omega Six, and fat stores.

Hormones, and the chemicals for reproduction, are made directly, or indirectly, from fats. You can't have stop start hormones, and raw materials, if you are going to make a baby. Fat stores secure regular supplies of hormones, fats to build cell membranes, and energy to make babies.

This is the key. In nature Omega Six, and carbohydrate, (in the form of fruit sugars) come conveniently pre-packed in fruit. Like the bears, our ancestors would have got busy in the fruiting season.

Bears eat fruit and seeds, to save Omega Six, get fat from fructose, sugars, and carbohydrates, and breed. Nature is bountiful. Seasonality of seed and fruits in temperate latitudes, synchronises breeding to food and weather.

You do not make an entrance into the world with an instruction manual tightly grasped in hand. Your mother does not tell you the rules as you arrive. Your instruction manual is built in. It is automatic. Your whole body is simply programmed to do it. Omega Six and fats stores are key to breeding.

It is a survival strategy. Eat Omega Six and sugars, put on weight, and breed. BUT, with modern farming and industry, we have over-ruled nature. There is no way to reprogramme our body, to cope with new excess Omega 6 in vegetable oils, and the huge increase in fructose and sugars, in our diet.

It makes sense for Omega Six to be the master factor. In nature low background levels of Omega Six are found in green plants and roots. Green plants and roots are wide spread, but high level sources of Omega 6, seeds pips and nuts, are a scarce sought after [animals], largely seasonal, and an uncertain resource.

So, the body stores the Omega Six you pour into it. Omega 6 is here year round. It comes by the bottle. It is at a supermarket near you. It is cheap. You follow design instructions. See Omega 6, eat it, and store it as fat, to get into breeding condition.

Sugar and fructose come by the packet full, and canned with soft drinks. In nature if there is Omega 6 in seeds, there will be sugars, fructose, and carbohydrates in fruit and tubers. The body is designed to turn fructose into fat to store along with the Omega 6 from seeds and nuts [25.21].

THERE IS NO OMEGA 6 'OFF SWITCH'. It was almost impossible to get too much Omega 6. We did not have the stomach capacity to eat to many greens, and Omega 6 always came with Omega 3s in greens. Seeds nut and berries were seasonal, scarce, and there was competition for them from animals. No 'Off Switch' was needed.

Short saturated fats, and long chain Omega Threes would make us feel full, but we have stopped eating them. SO we have very plentiful supplies of Omega Six, and no off switch. We follow design instructions and get fat.

I suggest mechanisms for excess Omega 6 and fructose with a lack of Omega 3, as causes of obesity and metabolic syndrome, by hesitantly trying to join the dots of the work of others. [See 25.21 for more detail].

☞   When you eat sugars and fats in fruit and seeds, the body responds to glucose and Omega 6, AA, by increasing insulin. AA increases PGE2. PGE2 increases insulin. Insulin increases SCD1. SCD1 is a controlling part of the process by which the body makes **new** fat from carbohydrate.

☞   Fructose in fruit, also increases SCD1.

☞   Fructose increases leptin.

☞   Leptin tries to decrease SCD1, and so **new** fat production, but insulin tries to push up SCD1, as does fructose. Leptin has more influence with SCD1 than insulin, but it appears that fructose is the boss. So fructose effectively incapacitates leptin, and is reinforced in increasing SCD1 by insulin. *Fructose consumption keeps the body in make fat mode.*

☞   Leptin has no effect on the long chain polyunsaturates, and so no control over AA and PGE2. Long chain polyunsaturates may push down leptin, so reducing the ability of leptin to respond to stored fat levels, but AA and PGE2 is reported as pushing leptin up so creating a blocking loop.

☞   Insulin also pushes up the desaturase conversion rates, of the mother fats, to the long chain fats. The process is designed around more Omega Three than Omega Six being available, so normally leading to more DHA being made. DHA would increase metabolism and close down the creation of more AA. But instead, when the most plentiful mother fat is Omega Six, the effect of insulin increasing long chain fat conversion will be to push up AA and PGE2 exclusively.

☞   Increased AA and PGE2 keeps insulin high so creating a loop. *The body will continue to store fat until the supply of AA is turned off, OR there a supply of sufficient Omega Three, to block the supply of AA. Fructose compounds the effect of excess Omega Six.*

Omega Three will help balance the cycle by turning off the production of Omega 6, AA, and increasing metabolism. In absence of Omega 3, and ongoing supply of Omega 6, the storage cycle just continues. There is no 'off switch'. Fructose compounds the situation.

You must of your own free will cut your Omega 6 intake, balance it with Omega 3, and beware of excess fructose. There was never enough Omega 6, and fructose, in the 'natural' environment to need an 'off switch'.

Body processes were not designed for Omega Six excess, to be other than a short term event. Omega 3 supply in nature, exceeds [With marine sources], or is equal to [Vegetable sources], Omega Six for most of the year, except for short seasons when seeds pips and nuts are more plentiful.

We have broken our supply link with nature, and I am not complaining. Better nutrition has clear and undoubted advantages. We however need to understand our nutritional design parameters; what to select for our fuel tanks, at the supermarket.

If we had an effective off switch for eating Omega 6, we would be less likely to be obese, but we don't! [See 25.21].

25.7   Omega Six, makes you fat

☞ **Omega Six–Instructions to store fat**–Omega Six instructs the body to store fats [409]. Omega Six is saved and stored. In contrast Omega Three is used preferentially as fuel. High Omega Six reduces the ability of the body to make long chain Omega Three, which reinforces the store instruction.

☞ **Omega Six–Instructs to make bigger fat cells**–Omega Six and fructose, together via insulin and leptin, instruct the body to make bigger fat cells, and prepare dormant cells to receive fat.

☞ **Omega Six–Instructs to store fructose**–Omega 6 instructs the body to store the fructose eaten with the Omega 6, as fat. Fructose is found naturally in fruits, and berries. It is used heavily today as a sweetener. The body gives fructose a green light, to be made directly into fat. Fructose bypasses control processes glucose has to go through. Fructose does not need to be extracted as it does from sugar. Fructose is ready to make fat. The brain has a meter for glucose, but no meter for fructose.

☞ **Omega Six–In mothers may instruct more fat storage in babies**–Omega Six fed to mothers [rats] results in babies having more, and or bigger, fat cells [410]. [The comparison was to rats fed coconut].

☞ **Omega Six–Lowers metabolism**–The Omega Six oxidation rate does not increase with exercise rate [411]. [But oleic acid oxidation increased significantly] [This is potentially hugely significant, and would be consistent with the theory that the body conserves Omega Six for breeding, regarding it as a scarce resource].

25.8   **Omega Three, fat to burn**–Omega Three is the other half of our dynamic duo. Background levels of mother Omega 3 and 6 are found in green foods, roots and fruit flesh, in more or less equal amounts.

Omega Three and Omega Six are structurally and functionally different. They are not interchangeable. They cannot be made from each other. They perform different and unique roles.

It is believed that humanity were shore-based gatherers for a long time. The shore has food rich in Omega Three (Shell fish, worms, fish, etc.). So, shore based Omega 3, was generally available all year round in quantity and did not need cooking. Omega 6 in quantity was seasonal and scarce.

The body has a built in preference to burn Omega Threes, before Omega Sixes. [412] Omega Three is better fuel than Omega Six. The body releases Omega 3, in preference to Omega 6, from the fat stores.

The body stores only small amounts of Omega Three fat, 0.1–2 per cent approximately. By contrast, Omega Six storage rates are as high as 25 per cent.

If you needed energy to keep warm, the body is first instructed to burn short chain fats, then long chain Omega 3, then long chain monosaturates, followed by Omega Six and last mid chain saturates.

An ability to generate body heat would be important to aquatic fringe dwellers. Marine dwellers, dolphins, have a 1:1 Omega Three Six ratio, despite high fish intake, which is much higher in Omega 3 than 6.

The dolphin has an Omega 3:6 ratio of 1:1 in the liver store and muscle tissue [*The Driving Force* - Crawford and Marsh] which suggests dolphins are likely to be using the excess Omega 3 for energy and warmth.

Omega Three increases metabolism;

☞ **Omega 3–Pushes up metabolism**–Long chain Omega Three will encourage the body to burn, rather than store Omega Threes. [413] Omega Three pushes the body to burn, not store, **other** fats too. [414][415][416] Oxidation rates in rats are 50 per cent plus higher, on a high Omega Three diet. [417] DHA, fish oil, or a mix of DHA and EPA, is more effective than EPA alone, at triggering fat burning. In a recent trial, subjects lost weight without changing their diet, by adding fish oil, and exercise.

☞ **Omega 3–Increases metabolic rate**–DHA levels in heart cells linearly control the basal metabolic rates of the cells. Humming birds have more DHA than mice, which have more than lizards. DHA increases the metabolic rate, and available energy, etc. (Susan Allport–*The Queen of Fats* based on Australian research) [25.52].

☞ **Omega 3–Increases mitochondrial "burn"**–DHA is essential to mitochondrial function, cell membrane composition [more fluid 1.36], and as a high energy fuel. Fats are burnt in the mitochondria. The mitochondrial membrane constituent, cardiolipin, is high in DHA [3.14, 21.7]. Basal metabolism increases at night. DHA increases at night. DHA increases oxidation in the peroxisomes. DHA increases melatonin. Melatonin increases DHA. Melatonin protects mitochondria. If DHA is not available cardiolipin will contain high levels of Omega Six which is less effectively oxidised. Mitochondrial malfunction has been recognised as being contributory, if not causal in obesity related disorders. [418]

☞ **Omega 3–Fish oil increases metabolism**–A recent trial showed that young adults on an energy restricted diet, lost most weight, when fish oil was added to the diet. [419]

☞ **Omega 3–Thyroid function**–DHA may promote a higher resting and sleep metabolism, BMR, in part, through improved thyroid function. It is suggested, that thyroid function requires high level energetic oxidation, for the processing of iodine. The theory of Fowkes, Dean and Nufert, raises interesting questions about the potential wider influence of DHA. DHA is the most effectively oxidised of fats. Improved thyroid function may improve metabolism rates.[i] DHA provides high level oxidation, with possible night time increases. A trial in young rats, suggests that DHA uprates thyroid stimulating hormone, TSH, and adrenal corticotrophic hormone.[ii] TSH is central to thyroid function. Low THS is associated with lower metabolism, and thyroid dysfunction. TSH has been noted to be higher at night, which would be consistent with the role of melatonin in sleep, as a DHA promoter. Obese subjects have lower night time metabolic rates.[iii] Obesity is linked with poor sleep, and inflammation, which would be consistent with high AA, and low DHA, in the body [27.3]. Is this a self regulating loop? Does more DHA result in greater mitochondrial and peroxisomal oxidation, which creates greater thyroid activity and night time metabolism. Thyroid function is connected to metabolic rate.

☞ **Omega 3–Discourages storage**–Omega 3 discourages fat cells from growing, and inhibits new fat cells, preadipocytes from coming 'on stream'. [420 421 422 423 424 425 426 427]

☞ **Omega 3–Omega Three not heavily stored**–Little Omega Three is stored, including DHA. Omega Three is released from adipose tissue, in preference to Omega Six. The emergency Omega 3 DHA store is the brain. If you are short of Omega Three, and pregnant, your baby will raid the DHA from your brain [Postnatal depression 23.35]. Alcohol bypasses the body's mechanism to safeguard minimum levels of DHA in the brain if not available in the diet, to replace the lost DHA [3.28].

☞ **Omega 3–Reduces hunger**–Lack of energetic oxidation of fat in the liver, may relate to hunger. [428] More oxidation = less hunger. The fat oxidation rates in the liver may link to reduction of post meal hunger.

---

i   Mitochondria, Hypothyroidism and Weight Loss by Steven Wm. Fowkes, Ward Dean, M.D., and Thomas H. Nufert.

ii   Docosahexaenoic Acid Increases Thyroid-Stimulating Hormone Concentration in Male and Adrenal Corticotrophic Hormone Concentration in Female Weanling Rats. The Journal of Nutrition Vol. 128 No. 8 August 1998, pp. 1257-1261 Thomas Clandinin, Donna L. Claerhout, and Eric L. Lien Nutrition and Metabolism Research Group, Departments of Agricultural, Food and Nutritional Science and Medicine, University of Alberta, Edmonton, Alberta, Canada, T6G 2P5 and Wyeth Nutrition International, Radnor.

iii Sleeping metabolic rate in relation to body mass index and body composition International Journal of Obesity (2002) 26, 376-383. K Zhang, M Sun, P Werner, A J Kovera, J Albu, F X Pi-Sunyer and C N Boozer Obesity Research Center, St Luke's-Roosevelt Hospital Center, and Institute of Human Nutrition, Department of Medicine, Columbia University College of Physicians and Surgeons, New York, USA Mini-Sun, Fresno, California, USA.

A high percentage of the Omega Three intake is oxidised energetically. Omega 3 DHA is particularly oxidised in the mitochondria and peroxisomes. DHA is linked with higher dopamine and serotonin, which are linked with hunger reduction. Monosaturated fats such as olive oil are reported to increase oxidation. [429] SCTs [Short chain triglycerides] are also reported as increasing oxidation and appetite control. [430] Weight loss and hunger reduction is reported with coconut fat sources. SCTs, long Omega 9s and Omega 3s are all oxidised better than Omega 6. Mid length saturated fats are the least easily oxidised. My own perception is that fish oil and coconut reduces hunger.

☞ **Omega 3—Less fat accumulation**—Omega Three in diet results in less fat accumulation [431] **BUT** High levels of Omega Six intake prevent Omega Three, from reducing long chain Omega Six product AA. [432] [433] Omega Six AA levels are reduced, and Omega Three storage increased, if Omega Six is replaced with saturated fat.

25.9   Lose weight and keep your brain intact—

☞ **Cut Six**—Cut down on Omega Six sources. —(See general diet tips, etc.)

☞ **Regular Three**—*Get regular intake of all Omega Threes. Omega 3 is not stored in significant quantity, so needs regular and constant replenishment.*

☞ **Mother Three**—Get some mother Omega Three from vegetable sources.

☞ **Long chain Three**—Get some long chain Omega Three (fish, fish oil, or vegetarian equivalent).

☞ **Cut sugar**—*Cut out sugar, and particularly fructose, except in whole fruit.* (Not too much high sugar fruit, or sweet fruit juice intake).

☞ **Cut alcohol**—*Save your brain, eyes, and reproductive bits, from DHA depletion. Be alcohol aware. If you drink alcohol ensure you have an adequate supply of Omega Threes. Alcohol, in low to moderate quantities may improve fat conversion, which in the absence of Omega Three, may increase Omega Six conversion, so worsening the Omega Three Six AA EPA balance.* Alcohol will deplete the brain of DHA in the absence of raw materials to replenish it. Alcohol also contains carbohydrates.

☞ **Avoid trans fats**—Avoid trans fats.

☞ **Add a little SCT**—Short chain fats have a more direct route to the liver. are burnt preferentially, and trigger the burn of fats. Coconut also enhances anti-bacterial function. Butter adds variety of fats to a moderate fat consumption. [Page 287, 11.31, 11.32].

☞ **Check** all labels–Foods you might miss, that may be high in Omega 6 - Processed foods generally. - Factory farmed, grain fed, chicken and their eggs may be surprisingly high in Omega Six, which will need balancing. This is an issue particularly where a diet is highly reliant on chicken. The fat content of chicken, like ours, reflects their diet, whether raised in a field or warehouse. [We need better labelling. – Margarine is vegetable oil, so check which and how it is made [11.23].– Processed olive oil can be 50 per cent Omega Six–Nuts and seeds have health benefits for lots of reasons but in moderation, as they are generally high in Omega Six so need balancing – Be aware that soy is higher in Omega Six than Three. - Nutritiondata. com is a useful resource

☞ **Look at your wider diet**–Cutting down Omega Six, and balancing with Omega Three, will mean label checking. Aim for the usual healthy whole food options. Get as wide a variety as possible. Avoid processed foods using unspecified vegetable oil, until manufacturers catch up with labelling for Omega Threes, and Sixes. Organic fresh, etc. has to be best, but use what you can cope with, and afford. Include the usual diet recommendations, particularly lots of greens, coloured vegetables, some fruit, lots of variety, etc. Curiously, as your digestion and health improves, you will eat less.

25.10 **Raw materials for inflammation**–The quantity of inflammatory chemicals in the body, is dependent on the absolute quantity, and accessibility, of Omega Six AA in the cell membranes. Omega Six AA in membranes reflects fat deposits and current dietary intake.

Ratios of Omega Six fats, in fat cells, change with intake, and are within broad bands 5–25 per cent. The size of fat cells can change enormously. Looking at ratios in an individual cells, without looking at the total amount of Omega Six available in the body, is arguably flawed.

The amount of Omega Six immediately available, depends in part on cell membrane surface area, which will increase tremendously, although not linearly, with volume.

Bigger cells showed a tendency to secrete more pro-inflammatory factors and hormones. [434] The fat cells are mixed in a matrix of factory cells, which produce chemicals, and hormones, from fats.

Whilst the fat cells, and your waist line expand, your brain, heart, reproductive organs, and bones, do not. So in the obese, there is more Omega 6, and fat cell factory capacity, to service substantially the same sized key organs. Fat cells have been recorded as growing four or five times bigger.

The body stores Omega Six, and has more chemical production capacity, but there is no inbuilt body auto instruction or switch not to make more hormones, and inflammatory products, in the fat tissue matrix from Omega Six.

If there was an off switch to stop background hormone production by fat cells, the Omega 6 breeding control lever would not work.

Body fat with Omega 6 programs you to produce more hormones, steroids, inflammatory products, and immune agents, as certainly as night follows day.

The only way to break the chemical cycle is with regular long chain Omega 3 intake which will restock the cell membranes to some extent so giving a more immediate reduction of the impact of excess stored Omega 6.

25.11   **Wind and stomach problems**–This is a subject on its own. Digestion, the ability to absorb and process your food, is the start of good health. I summarise my own experience, based on what I have read, and found to work.

Tired of being between loose stools and constipation? Forgotten what a regular solid poo, at risk of being left in the pan, with positive splashdown, is like? Sort your digestion out. It will take time. I list useful references at the end. Sorting out digestion, is part of sorting out weight and health. Health begins with the digestion. Once digestion is normal difficult foods may again be tolerated.

If your digestion is not working, the most expensive food in the world is still largely wasted. You are depositing your scarce Omega 3's, health, and money, down the pan. Many digestive problems are due to a combination of whole body, low level inflammation, and high invader alert status.

To that, add, putrid undigested food leading to damaging bacteria. Add some excess mucus in the gut, which separates food from the digesting cells. Add generally degraded digestion. Add poor fat absorption, leading to loose, greasy stools. Poor fat absorption means lack of scarce Omega 3. Add undigested sugars and fructose, which contribute heavily to poor digestion, and wind.

You have a problem. The symptoms are often portrayed as food intolerance.

Food intolerance may be a part, but the first thing to sort out is excess, sugar, fructose, and Omega 6, and lack of Omega 3, leading to constant inflammation of the gut.

This site has a useful article on digestive problems. *www.westonaprice.org*. Section; *modern diseases* Article; *How to restore digestive health*. A book that explains sugars and digestion, simply and persuasively is Elaine Gottschall's *Breaking the Viscous Cycle, Intestinal Health Through Diet*.

25.12   **Outside design parameters**–The body's operating instructions, specify a seasonal scoff of fruit and seeds, or nuts, to get into breeding condition. An all year round permanent binge was not in the design specs. Trees do not grow bottled oil, or bags of sugar and fructose. The body has no plans for such excess.

The body does what it was designed to do. The body stores Omega 6 and fructose to get you to breeding weight and condition. You have to take the place of nature, and voluntarily cut on down fructose and excess mother Omega 6.

25.13   **Tipping the balance**—You can help reset the dials to burn rather than store. You can tip the scales permanently with the easy steps above.

But consume way too much energy (calories in fats and carbohydrates) and you will still be overloading the body, and put on weight. To see real difference you will have to eat better, and exercise too.

Once you have built up stores of Omega 6 in the body fat, the body will have high Omega 6 in the cell membranes. This will continue to turn down basal metabolism, even if your Omega 6 dietary intake is reduced.

Of course exercise and calorie reduction will help, but to tip the basal metabolism scales towards burn, you likely need to rebalance your Omega 3 and 6, and ensure a regular supply of long chain Omega 3.

This is not a short-term fix. Changing your fat composition, and improving digestion, is a lifestyle choice. Blood fat composition will start to change in hours to days. Breast fats take months to change. It will take two years, to see a significant difference in 'adipose' fat composition, and it will still be changing after five years. Brains may take longer still. Please discuss dietary change with a doctor.

This is not an absolutist solution. Fit it to your diet. Do it to the extent you feel happy. As with most things, there is a link between input and output. The better your 'diet', and the better you observe the 'rules', the better the outcome.

Some general truths on eating, are set out in the overview. I am still puzzling on this, but my own observation is that the inclusion of a moderate amount of saturated fat firms up fat deposits.

I ask the question and no more. Is our current love of polyunsaturates particularly excess Omega Six intake, and our obsession against saturates, leading to softening of fat deposits and distorting structure, and so a factor in sag, orange peel and related issues?? These are unanswered questions.

I reiterate I am not suggesting a return to large intakes of saturated fats, just not obsessive avoidance of saturated fats as part of a sensible dietary fat intake.

Just to reiterate, none of this can be divorced, from the general need for better diet, and exercise for optimal results. And finally some thoughts :

☞ **Saturated fats**—You will not lose weight if intake of saturated fats is high "Certainly, diets high in saturated fats have been shown to induce weight gain, insulin resistance, and hyperlipidemia in humans and animals." [435]

☞ **Low fat diets**—*Very low fat diets are not the answer, and have their own dangers. You need to balance the Omega 3s and 6s. More Omega Six than Three, and you are set to store,* [assuming your energy intake exceeds output]. There does not seem much point in having a very low fat intake, to replace fats, with refined carbohydrates. Balance in all things. Very low fat diets, with a high Omega 3:6 imbalance, places your health at risk. The same inflammatory factors are at work. Alcohol, will exacerbate the negative health impact, of a low fat, low Omega Three diet [1.30]. Low DHA, and a high Omega 6:3 imbalance, has long-term negative consequences, for a whole range of conditions. Low fat diets are popular. However, the decline in dietary fat consumption, has not corresponded to a decrease in obesity–in fact, the opposite trend has emerged. [436] How much fat, I do not know, but you need to balance your Omega Threes and Sixes. Dairy fats contain other useful nutrients and minerals.

☞ **Carbs**–Providing you manage the fats and exercise, there is not an absolute requirement to avoid unrefined carbs. Older men and women fed a high-carb diet containing 18 per cent fat, lost weight. Weight loss was increased with exercise. [437]

☞ **Alcohol and Omega Three**–Adequate Omega Three, may give you some protection from alcohol, at low to moderate doses. A combination of alcohol, and low Omega Three intake, and the body will be stripped of DHA, with disastrous health consequences. You will be at a much greater risk for the long list of conditions in the overview. Flax seed is a good source of the mother Omega Three. [438] If conversion pathways from the mother Omega Three to DHA are blocked, supplementation of EPA and DHA through diet is the only answer.

☞ **Balance - *THE AIM IS A BALANCE OF OMEGA SIX AND NOT AN ABSENCE. OMEGA 6 DEFICIT HAS ITS OWN PROBLEMS.***

25.14 Link to obesity–High Omega 6 and low 3 link positively to obesity. "The degree of obesity and central distribution of body fat were positively correlated with the total n6 PUFA content of adipose tissue (especially 18:2n6 content) and negatively correlated with the MUFA and n3 PUFA contents of adipose tissue." [439]

25.15 Little Omega Three stored–Levels of Omega Three storage in adipose tissue are low. [440] The amount of Omega Three stored in a Mediterranean study, was about one per cent, of which 0.27 per cent was DHA.

The amount of Omega Six stored was about 17 per cent, of which 0.44 per cent, was AA. Omega Nine stored, was 49 per cent. The amount of Omega Six and Nine stored, fairly closely reflected intake. [441]

Even when the intake levels of *long chain* Omega Three are high, and much higher than Omega Six, only a small proportion of Omega Three intake is stored. Omega Three is oxidised in preference to Omega Six.

25.16   **Omega Six aggressively stored**—Even if Omega Six intake is low, a significant amount of the Omega Six is stored. Intake lower in Omega Six than Three, still results in the storage of much more Omega 6 than 3.[442]

25.17   **Bigger fat cells**— Obesity results in an increase in fat cells size, and number. Fat cells can grow many times in size. The ability to make fat cells, is highest pre or around birth. Different levels, and types of fat intake in early life affect the number and size of fat cells. [443]

Your ability to store fat is shaped by your early diet. You have a mix of active and inactive fat cells. Omega Six, issues instructions to make bigger cells up to four or five times larger, [444] and to open up inactive cells, as required. Much is unknown, but there are several suggestions that early nutrition and status of the mother impacts on later risk of obesity.

Two factors in your mother's diet that make things far worse, are a lack of Omega Three and excess Omega Six. [See childhood obesity 25.31,32].

25.18   **Omega Six imperative**—We have broken our link to nature. Omega Six, fructose, and fat, are no longer scarce resources. Our bodies do not know that, and carry on as if Omega Six, and fat, were scarce resources. We are operating the body outside design parameters.

At a very simplistic level deep down in your instructions are buried some imperatives, which include:

☞ *Burn Omega Three for energy and body maintenance, in preference to Omega Six. (Except in famine).*

☞ *Store Omega Six (except in famine) together with the fructose it comes with as breeding reserves - and do not use it preferentially for fuel.*

☞ *To breed - Store as much Omega Six as you can whilst the going is good even if you are already have sufficient fat reserves.*

25.19   **Store to breed**—When the body is storing fats to allow breeding, it needs a range of fats, and not just Omega Six. You need a range of fats, and nutrients, to make babies, hunt, protect, and defend your territory—fats for energy—fats for hormone reserve—and fats as raw materials.

Men and women cannot live on Omega Six alone. Omega Six cannot be stored on it own, if it is to be of use. More stored Omega Six, must be accompanied by all the other fats the body needs. All the pressures are to fat storage.

We are programmed, to eat Omega 6, sucrose and fructose, and store it as fat. We do just that to bursting point. We have a 'taste' for it. It was just NEVER expected that Omega Six would be this plentiful. It was NEVER expected fructose and sugar would be this plentiful. Since plants started fruiting and seeding, there has never been this much Omega Six, and sugar.

25.20 A pre-packed whoopee bonanza – Fruits and berries are nature's pre-packed hunter gather, sex conditioner. Fruit and berry flesh high in sugars, are wrapped round a seed core, high in fats and Omega Six. Think berries with tiny seeds. Think bears.

Omega Six, fats, and lots of carbohydrate all come together in a neat bundle. Fructose is a sugar found in fruit. It is dealt with more technically below. Man met his normal energy need, so this was extra energy. This was really cool.

Over time, the body set up a process to put fructose, which was essentially spare energy, straight into storage. Neat thinking. Why create extra unnecessary fructose processing steps, if you are almost always going to store fructose as fat.

The body uses the fructose to make fats it would need for breeding. The body uses fructose to make the chemical storage fat-rack for Omega Six. The body does everything it can not to waste any Omega Six.

Omega Six and fructose, in nature come in one convenient ancestor fertility assisting package, with a hardwired instruction to store Omega Six, and make and store fat from fructose.

There is no limiter, no brake, no red traffic light, and no feedback mechanisms that I have seen. Trials suggest that higher fructose intake will contribute to obesity.[445][446] There is no STOP button to storing fructose, when combined with Omega Six. Modern diets oblige obesity, with cheap bottled Omega Six, and fructose and sugar everywhere.

There are always exceptions. Some people have genetic and other related conditions, as against dietary, or metabolic issues. This is in no way a criticism of a particular group. I see myself reading the label on a bar of chocolate, and reflecting on the sugar content, and my desire for that bar of chocolate.

For me sweet and fatty makes it difficult to leave an open packet unfinished. None of us are immune. Increasing Omega 3, and including some short chain fats and monosaturates, in our diet may dampen desire to eat fat and sugar for the reasons given.

Whilst our diet continues to contain excess Omega Six and sugar, and low Omega Threes , we will obey our Omega Six breeding instruction set. We do what we were designed to do. We stuff ourselves and get fat.

25.21 Metabolic X – The abnormalities in metabolic X, include, insensitivity to insulin and leptin, high levels of fat in the bloodstream, and obesity. I tentatively suggest possible contributory causes.

The bodies mechanisms all interlink. Stress and inflammation are also related factors. Obesity is considered an inflammatory related condition. Stress results from and causes immune activity and inflammation. For example noreadrenaline, a stress hormone, causes fats to be released into the blood stream.

Insulin resistance is largely due to modern westernised diets, and follows the rise in obesity[447]. This is vastly complex, interlinked, and the subject of much debate and research.

This section is a suggestion, and no more than that, as to factors that may be causal in metabolic syndrome. My head has spun trying to make sense of various reports I have read on this topic.

I suggest based on the observations of others, that lack of Omega Three, excess Omega Six and fructose, are likely at the core of metabolic X syndrome.

Omega Three, which pushes up the metabolism by increased oxidation, is lacking. Omega Threes are better and more readily oxidised than Omega Sixes. Omega 3s are released from fat stores before Omega 6s.

Insulin encourages the manufacture of DHA, by increasing conversion rates from the mother Omega 3 fat. DHA is easily oxidised in the peroxisomes, a good fuel, and an essential fat in the inner mitochondrial membrane. The mitochondria are the energy furnaces and chemical factories.

If there is no Omega Three raw material, and so no conversion and supply of DHA, then insulin cannot increase metabolism, by increasing DHA oxidation. The consequence is a blockade of the insulin mechanism, through a lack of DHA raw material, and excess Omega 6. Imbalance of Omega Three and Six has been suggested by others as a cause of diabetes.[iv]

Fructose has been suggested to be deeply implicated in obesity, by some researchers. Omega Six, instructs the body, to make bigger fat cells, and store fat. Glucose fructose sugars and Omega Six, are found in varying amounts in seeds and nuts in fruit and berries.

The body is programmed to save Omega Six, and fructose, to build up breeding reserves. In the modern diet, sugar and fructose come in bags, and Omega 6 in bottles, not just in fruits seeds nuts and berries. Sugar [fructose and glucose tied together], fructose [a sweetener], and Omega 6 in vegetable oils, are everywhere in processed foods.

The following are suggestions as to how body mechanisms combined with western diet may result in metabolic blockages. [See Diagram 25.21].

☞ **Glucose** - Higher glucose intake pushes up insulin levels.

☞ **Insulin** - Higher insulin forces the body to make and store fats.

☞ **Fructose** - Higher fructose forces the body to make and store fat[v]
*Fructose pushes up SCD1. Fructose and insulin in combination push up SCD1, creating a multiplier, doubling their individual effect, to make more **new** fat from carbohydrate.*

iv   Dietary fatty acids in the management of diabetes mellitus. Am J Clin Nutr. 1997 Oct;
      66 Berry EM. Department of Human Nutrition and Metabolism, Hebrew University-
      Hadassah Medical School, Jerusalem, Israel.

v   Insulin and dietary fructose induce stearoyl-CoA desaturase 1 gene expression of
      diabetic mice J. Biol. Chem., Vol. 269, Issue 44, 27773-27777, 11, 1994 KM Waters
      and JM Ntambi Department of Biochemistry, University of Wisconsin-Madison
      53706.

☞ **New fat**–BUT as usual it is more complicated. *Insulin increases the amount of fat converting enzymes. This includes BOTH the mechanisms to make long chain Omega 3 and 6 fats [Desaturase 5 and 6], and the SCD 1 mechanism for making **new** fats from carbohydrates* [Desaturase 1, SCD1 is an enzyme like desaturase 5 and 6, but which is suggested to somehow have a wider role in the creation of new fats from scratch, from carbohydrate. Blocking SCD1 in mice prevents obesity, but from what I have read exactly how is not clear, and my conclusion is a leap into the dark. The Mother Omega 3s and 6s CANNOT be made from scratch, and have to be obtained from diet, but can be converted using desaturase 5 and 6, into longer fats].

☞ **Insulin in a loop**–*Insulin is stuck in a self reinforcing Omega 6 loop.* Higher insulin pushes up conversion of the mother Omega 6 fats to the long chain fat, Omega 6 AA. Omega 6, indirectly pushes up insulin through its product AA. So insulin pushes up AA; AA pushes up insulin. Now insulin is stuck in a self reinforcing loop, with no way out. Glucose also pushes up insulin. The only way out of the insulin AA loop, is to supply Omega 3, and cut Omega 6, to balance Omega 6 and Omega 3, which through increased DHA will cut the AA supply.

☞ **Oxidation rate reduction**–Insulin and fructose increase SCD1, and so the manufacture of new fats. It is reported SCD1 may reduce oxidation rates and so metabolism. The mid chain saturated fats produced are the least easily oxidised, and the most effectively stored.

☞ **Leptin fructose insulin battle**–Leptin is a hormone which regulates fat levels, and metabolism. Leptin is made by fat cells. Leptin production increases as stored fat increases. Leptin tries to increase the body metabolism, to stop the body storing fat. Leptin, and SCD1 are increased by a high fat, fructose, and sucrose diet [448.] There is a conflict between fructose leptin and SCD1 [See Diagram 25.21].

☞ **Fructose wins?**–Fructose may override leptin's attempts to increase metabolism, and reduce fat storage. Leptin is involved in a conflict with itself insulin[vi] and fructose over SCD1. Fructose increases SCD1. Fructose increases Leptin. Increasing leptin normally decreases SCD1. Insulin increases SCD1. It looks as if fructose has the upper hand, and the body has an overriding instruction to store fructose, which would be consistent with fructose's association with Omega 6 and breeding.

☞ **Fructose raises uric acid**–Fructose has been reported as raising uric acid, which appears to contribute to metabolic syndrome [beyond me].[vii]

---

vi   Leptin suppresses stearoyl-CoA desaturase 1 by mechanisms independent of insulin and sterol regulatory element-binding protein-1c. Diabetes. 2006 Jul;55(7):2032-41 Biddinger SB, Miyazaki M, Boucher J, Ntambi JM, Kahn CR Research Division, Joslin Diabetes Center, One Joslin Pl., Boston, MA 02215, USA.

vii A causal role for uric acid in fructose-induced metabolic syndrome Am J Physiol Renal Physiol 290: F625-F631, 2006.Takahiko Nakagawa, Hanbo Hu, Sergey Zharikov,

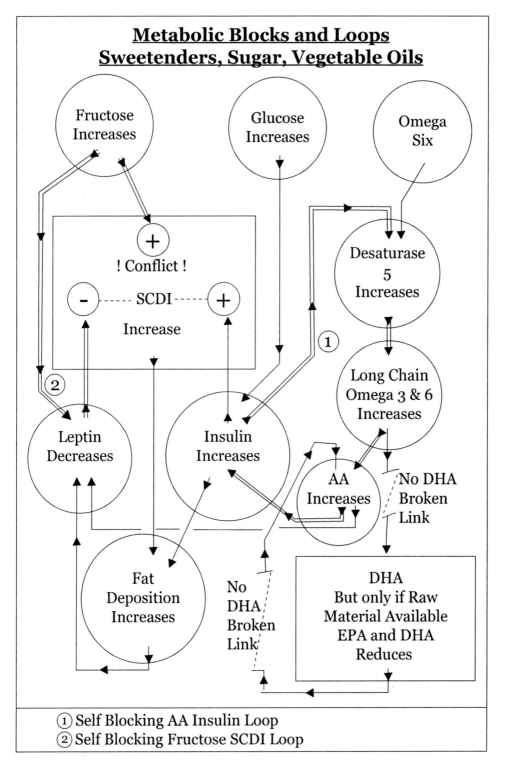

Fig. 25.21 Possible Mechanisms Contributing to Metabolic Blocks and Obesity

☞ **Impact of DHA and EPA**–*Increasing DHA would turn up the metabolism, and turn down fat producing AA pathways, so reducing the storage of new fat made from carbohydrate excess.* A trial suggests fish oil and exercise, will induce weight loss, even maintaining existing diets. A trial suggested, replacement of a proportion of Omega 6 intake, with Omega 3, prevented sugar induced insulin resistance in rats. The trial concluded "Thus, inclusion of fish in the diets or use of fish oil supplements may be beneficial for alleviation and prevention of insulin resistance and for reducing the risk of associated chronic diseases". [viii] If there is no Omega 3 in the diet, the consequence of increasing fat conversion rates, is that manufacture of the Omega Six long chain fats is even further increased. Omega 6 long chain fats include AA. AA increases storage by increasing insulin, and insulin increases SCD1...

☞ **Leptin no influence on Omega Six**–*Leptin appears to have little influence on the manufacture of long chain Omega 3 and 6 fats,* so leptin can try and turn down **new** fat manufacture, but not the storage of Omega 6, or the production of long chain fats including AA in the absence of DHA. Increasing AA through insulin increases SCD1 so blunts and opposes leptin decreasing SCD1. AA may also increase leptin. Leptin may be the master in this process, but it is clear there is a basis for conflict. *Thus letpin can regulate fat deposition by switching down SCD1, and so production of new fats, but whilst Omega 6 is high it is in competition with insulin over SCD1. Does leptin have any mechanism to stop increasing Omega 6 AA and PGE2 levels.* Leptin does not significantly influence storage of polyunsaturated fats, and may even be reduced by them. Increased PGE2 and AA increases Leptin so creating a cycle of increasing Leptin, as AA rises. In the absence of Omega Three leptin is in a blocking loop. AA promotes insulin[ix] and leptin production. Leptin is

---

Katherine R. Tuttle, Robert A. Short, Olena Glushakova, Xiaosen Ouyang, Daniel I. Feig, Edward R. Block, Jaime Herrera-Acosta,, Jawaharlal M. Patel, and Richard J. Johnson Division of Nephrology, Hypertension, and Transplantation, University of Florida, Gainesville, Florida; Department of Research, The Heart Institute of Spokane, and Biostatistics, Washington State University, Spokane, Washington; Division of Nephrology-Medicine, Baylor College of Medicine, Houston, Texas; and Departamento de Nefrologia, Instituto Nacional de Cardiologia Ignacio Chavez, Tlalpan, Mexico.

viii   Dietary (n-3) Long Chain Polyunsaturated Fatty Acids Prevent Sucrose-Induced Insulin Resistance in Rats1 2005 American Society for Nutrition J. Nutr. 135:2634-2638, November 2005 Ghafoorunissa2, Ahamed Ibrahim, Laxmi Rajkumar and Vani Acharya National Institute of Nutrition, Indian Council of Medical Research, Hyderabad-500 007 A.P. India.

ix   Exogenous arachidonic acid promotes insulin release from intact or permeabilized rat islets by dual mechanisms. Putative activation of Ca2+ mobilization and protein kinase C Diabetes, Vol 37, Issue 11 1453-1469 SA MetzDepartment of Medicine, University of Colorado Health Sciences, Denver 80262.

trying to stop fat storage, Insulin is trying to increase it. *They are both in a battle over storage of mid chain new fats. But the battle is controlled by Omega Six and fructose.*

☞ **No Omega Three and hunger**–If Omega Threes are available, the production of DHA will increase. DHA will turn down the AA inflammatory pathways and hormones levels. DHA will increase metabolism by increasing mitochondrial oxidation, thyroid function etc. The body status will change from store to burn. Increased oxidation in the liver will result in signals to the body it is less hungry. Higher DHA will increase dompamine and serotonin further reducing hunger. Omega Three will, if available, push leptin down. Leptin will also to push insulin levels down. Excess fructose and glucose would still likely push the body to storage and conflict, but be working against Omega 3 trying to increase metabolism, rather than with Omega 6 trying to increase storage

☞ **Key Omega 3, 6 and fructose**–To reduce obesity it is likely necessary to balance the Omega 3s and 6s, ensure a supply of long chain Omega 3s and reduce fructose , which would include indirect sources like sugar.

There is an important metabolic conflict between Omega Three and Six. Marmots fed Omega Three mother fat do not go into hibernation. Marmots fed Omega Six, go into hibernation on time, even if food is available.

More DHA equates in more general terms to more active animals. [449] Toads have less DHA than mice. Mice have less DHA than humming birds. So, high levels of Omega Six are turning down our metabolism, at the very time we need to turn it up, to get rid of that excess fat.

But only Omega Three can turn off Omega 6 storage routines, and turn up the basal metabolism. [23.52] We have inadequate intake of Omega Three, reduced short chain fat intake, and blocked pathways. Omega Threes have been shown to have an anti-diabetic effect. [450]

The hunter-gatherer body never saw high levels of fruit (or packets of sugar either) on a permanent basis, so store all you can get, was an instruction that conferred an evolutionary advantage. [451]

The switches between Omega Six based storage, and DHA based burning, cannot happen, if conversion to DHA is blocked due to lack of raw material. Omega Six AA, and insulin create a self fuelling cycle.

In summary there is a conflict between leptin, insulin, and fructose. Glucose pushes insulin up, which pushes SCD1 up. Insulin increases AA, which increases leptin and insulin. More stored fat pushes leptin up, which tries to push SCD1 down. Leptin does not have any significant influence on the storage of polyunsaturates, and fat cells may even be stopped from producing leptin by long chain fats. [See 25.37].

Insulin and fructose just keep on instructing the body to make fat directly, and by insulin increasing AA levels. Insulin leptin and fructose are locked in a cycle, that can only be broken, by reducing fructose and Omega Six, and increasing Omega Three. A lack of high level oxidation in the absence of DHA, may mean that the satiety signals are not effectively generated.

It is dreadfully complicated, my understanding is very limited, the subject is huge and immensely complex. My suggestions as to blocking mechanisms may be embarrassingly badly flawed, but the underlying reality, I believe is that we simply do not run properly, on permanent excess of Omega 6, high supplies of sugar and fructose, and lack of Omega 3. The body is not designed to cope with this scenario.

Was mother Omega 6 ever designed as a significant fuel for the body? Omega 6 is low in marine sources. Is the primary use of scarce Omega 6 as a raw material for the chemical and hormone pathways, and to facilitate breeding? Excess Omega 6 in chemical processes results in high levels of harmful superoxides which damage tissue. Is Omega 6 a second rate fuel for energy?

High level Omega 6, and fructose, were only ever available in nature on a seasonal short term basis. They were both scarce and precious. The body was designed to work where Omega 6 and 3 intake were in balance, or there was excess Omega 3, and fructose was limited. Omega Six by the bottle, and fructose by the bag, were not in the body design specs.

25.22 **Inflammation, and immune response** – Omega Six from adipose fat stores, facilitates hormones and inflammatory products. Large amounts of Omega Six are stored in fat. The tissue matrix surrounding the fat cells also releases inflammatory agents. [455]

Obesity is an inflammatory condition. Obesity equates to sub-clinical inflammation of adipose tissue, and chronic activation of the innate immune system. [452] [453]

Prolonged low-level immune inflammation, induces the formation of adipocytes, and may be responsible for weight gain seen in those with immune conditions. These reactions are increased by Omega Six, and reduced by Omega Threes (fish oil)[x]. Low-level inflammatory conditions therefore may contribute to weight gain.

It really is a multiple self-fuelling whammy. Many of the factors of inflammation are common to cardiovascular disease, (IL1, IL6, [454] TNF, CRP, etc.) obesity, and other conditions [7.13]. An imbalance between Omega 6 and Omega 3, links with metabolic syndrome.

---

x   Adipose tissue and the immune system Department of Biological Sciences, The Open University, Milton Keynes Prostaglandins, Leukotrienes and Essential Fatty Acids Volume 73, Issue 1, July 2005, Pages 17–30.

Obese people potentially have much larger stores of the Omega Six chemical, arachidonic acid [AA] in total terms (sum of amount in every cell). [456] Excess Omega 6 promotes a low level permanent inflammatory state in the body, by production of high levels of inflammatory Omega 6 chemicals—the eicosanoids.

Low levels of Omega Three are stored, and EPA is used first. [457] The mother Omega Three, ALA, has shown beneficial results in reducing inflammatory markers in several trials. [458] When the body is in an inflammatory state, it pushes fats into the blood stream as part of the defence reaction. [459]

Stress aggravates the inflammatory process [460] and results in higher levels of fats including linoleic acid in the circulation system, and higher deposits in the arteries. Oxidation of linoleic acid produces higher levels of damaging superoxides, leading to arterial damage.

Omega Three can moderate the low-level inflammation caused by Omega Six, if Omega Three, is present in the diet, and conversion pathways are not blocked. Children who had pneumonia, recovered from the inflammatory effects more quickly, when DHA was administered. [461]

Fish oil has been shown to reduce the inflammatory Omega Six eicosanoid products. [462] DHA in animals shows an anti-inflammatory effect. Various trials looking at other conditions, suggest that DHA or EPA do reduce inflammatory markers in humans. [463] [464] A study in elderly Japanese with high fish intake, suggested CRP levels, an inflammatory marker, were reduced. [465]

In a community, study of 1,123 persons, total Omega Threes "were independently associated with lower levels of pro-inflammatory markers (IL6, IL1ra, TNF, Creactive protein) and higher levels of anti-inflammatory markers (soluble IL6r, IL10, TGFß)". [466]

A similar result was found looking at fish consumption in men. [467] Similar results have been recorded in a trial looking at depression. [468] The optimal solution is to ensure adequate Omega 3, reduce Omega 6, and to balance the 3 and 6 mother fats, with long chain Omega 3 intake supplements if needed.

Why is there a lack of effect in short-term trials? My guessplanation is the short-term effects, of what are often small doses, are overridden by, preferential oxidation and usage of Omega 3s, and the high adipose stores of Omega 6.

There is a need for stability of hormones, and inflammatory agents, in pregnancy. Fat stores provide this stability.

Blood and membrane levels of Omega Threes, seem much more sensitive to short-term manipulation. [469] [470] [471] The short-term manipulation of Omega Six in the blood fat, is always subject to the longer-term influence, of the fats in storage, which stabilise the system, and so resist short term change.

Visible results in humans will generally require long term studies, using Omega Three types and doses that recognise the preexisting high levels of stored Omega Six, the blockage of fat conversion pathways, alcohol intake washout, the different roles of the fats, and that take account of Omega Six levels in the body.

25.23 **Inflammation and fat quantity**–The amount of inflammatory agents in the body, must reflect the total quantity of the raw material, Omega Six, accessible through cell membranes, which is a reflection of the total body quantity.

As hunter-gatherers, we would have gone through an annual fat cycle. We would have been on average fairly lean. Today, we store what are huge amounts of fats in historic terms. Links between variation in fat content in individual cells, and disease, is only part of the story.

Two people may have the same fat profile, say 20 per cent Omega Six, but different levels of obesity. The more obese person, will contain much more stored Omega Six, and bigger fat cells, than the lean person will. In consequence, one would expect, and we see, different health outcomes.

Omegas Threes as a proportion are not heavily stored. Low storage of the mother Omega Three is consistent with it being used, and released from fat stores by the body, in preference to Omega Six.

Figures are difficult to find. The mother Omega Six, 18:2 n6, in a breast milk trial in China, remained between 18 and 20 per cent of total fats, marine pastoral or urban diet. [472]

In a Mediterranean trial on the obese, linoleic acid the mother Omega Six was about 15 per cent. [473] In The Nurses Trial, linoleic body fat content, was about 18 per cent, and AA .7 per cent. [474]

In Israel, linoleic acid body fat content was 25.6 per cent. [475] AA appears globally to be stored at around between .4 to 1 per cent. [476] Omega 3 storage is generally below that of Omega 6 AA, and in a significant amount of Westerners very low.

The direct impact of AA is dependent on the Omega Six AA in and accessible through cell membranes. If an inflammatory call goes out in response to immune threat or tissue injury, the call goes through the blood stream to all cell membranes.

All relevant membranes that get the message will respond. The output of inflammatory chemicals by fatty tissue cell membranes, will reflect the total manufacturing capacity, a function of cell size, and Omega raw 6 material in the fat cells and supporting matrix.

More and bigger cells are present in obesity. More and bigger cells provide more manufacturing capacity, and greater stores of raw material. Secretion rates of chemical agents by fat cells links to the size of the fat cell. [477]

Fat really is responsible for excess inflammation. The impact of fat on the production of immune and inflammatory chemicals by the fat cells and surrounding matrix, was confirmed by surgical removal of internal animal fat. A consequence of fat removal was that inflammatory markers dropped significantly, and insulin was normalised. [478]

25.24 **Low fat and Omega Three**—Omega 3 and 6 levels in the diet, can be imbalanced even if fat intake is low. Cell membrane Omega 3:6 balance will be distorted with the consequent results.

Historic stored fats are a significant factor. A change to a low fat diet, may simply result in release of the past reserves of Omega 6 from fat storage. Without adequate Omega 3 intake to balance the release of Omega 6 from stored fat, the result will be increased inflammatory pressures. Women are at particular risk.

To change your metabolism, and fat storage instruction, it is necessary to balance the Omega 3s and 6s. A low fat, very low Omega 3 diet, is for many a damaging option releasing stored Omega 6, and causing a deficit of Omega 3.

An Omega 3 deficit will lead to greater susceptibility to alcohol damage, hormonal issues, and other conditions discussed. Lack of the Omega 3 mother fat, and long chain fats will each have their own effects. They are all necessary.

25.25 **Inflammation, wider impact**—Inflammatory factors have been linked with a number of conditions including depression, [479] problems with sleep [increased PGE2 and IL6 is seen in depressed and sleep disorder patients], [480] a host of 'western' conditions, and have a role in cancers.

25.26 **Fat has personality**—Fat stored in different places has different characteristics [481]. Fat deposits are more, or less, active depending on the storage site. They have different roles, and impacts. Fat is not just fat. Fat allows you to function without eating. It is your long and short-term petrol store. Like a car, you are not going far without a petrol tank. Fats store energy very efficiently. Fat stores are used to smooth, nutrient and hormones flows to assist in breeding, hormone and steroid availability, and energy release and storage.

25.27 **Fat on the inside**—Visceral fat is the harder storage fat (10 per cent average, 25 per cent in the very obese), found deep in the body protecting the organs, insulating, and shock absorbing. The fat you see around kidneys at the butchers is visceral fat. [Fig. 3.12] Omega 3 may suppress visceral fat tissues. [483]

"If it really is what's on the inside that counts, then a lot of thin people might be in trouble....", internal fat, unseen and unfelt, may be as dangerous as external fat. [482]

A trial cited above connects visceral fats to the inflammatory agents. Some with fat imbalances might look relatively lean, but have high visceral fats, which could result in conditions such as fatty liver. [Fig.3.12]

25.28 **Fat on the outside**—Subcutaneous fat is the stuff you can grab hold of on the outside, hips, tums, bums, arms, etc. This keeps you warm, provides some cushioning, and acts as a storage depot. It too has a blood supply, and nerves. It, with the surrounding cellular matrix, is a source of hormones, adipokines.

25.29 **Intramuscular fat**—Intra muscular fat, is the fat in muscle tissue. Intra muscular fat is the marbling you sometimes see in beef. Muscles use it for energy. If the body runs out of fat storage space, it forces fat to be stored in muscle. You see it in beef but not venison.

25.30 **Fat in bones osteoporosis**—"Recent findings show that high adipocyte count in bone marrow is directly related to bone loss, as fat cells replace osteoblasts (or bone-forming cells)."[484] [See 23.48].

25.31 **Diabesity**[485]—[See 25.26] Some suggest diabetes 2 should be renamed diabesity, because of the close link with obesity. A trial in India, looking at urban and rural populations, and diabetes 2, found a remarkable straight-line graphical relationship, with Omega 6 consumption. In another trial, women with diabetes, had higher Omega 6 levels, than normal women, and conversion of fats was altered.[486][487][488] Insulin up-regulates desaturase 5 and 6[489].

25.32 **Children—Heart disease,**[490] **obesity, diabetes,**[491] **asthma**— These conditions are now seen in children, and arguably the scene is being set in the womb. Inflammatory imbalance, in the mother due to diet, at the time of birth, may impact on the health of the infant.[492] A large number of reports and trials, are alarmed by this trend. Children reflect the trial findings in babies, that higher Omega Six is correlated with obesity, and insulin issues.[493]

25.33 **Obesity in babies**—Low DHA and Omega 3, high Omega 6 and fructose intake by mothers and infants, may explain rising obesity levels in the young.[494]

    The balance of Omega 3 and 6, also determines the number and size of fat cells. Early influences potentially have long-term impact. Animal trials suggest the balance of fats in early feeding may impact on diseases including obesity and breast cancer in later life.[495][496][497] Increasing obesity in children, is following a trend of increasing Omega Six, and falling DHA in the diet.[498]

    Trials suggest, obesity in mothers, can be passed onto their children[499] through metabolic trends, based on the child having a similar nutrient supply to the mother. Fructose and excess Omega 6 link to obesity. [See 25.6]

    Sugar is half fructose. www.netmums.com has useful information.

Baby food like fromage frais from major trusted manufacturers contains fructose. An apple and blue berry baby food was approximately 15% sugar.

Infant formulas may contain high mother Omega 6 LA, and no or little mother Omega 3 ALA, or long chain EPA or DHA [See 23.27], and lack medium short chain saturates.

The ingredients listed below have <u>limited mother Omega 3</u>, <u>no long chain Omega 3</u>, and <u>little short medium chain saturates</u>.

For example an infant formula (breast milk substitute) contained skimmed milk, ... Vegetable oils - palm oil, rape oil, sunflower oil ... [See p 287] [11.31] [AA may well also be necessary if babies cannot convert the mother fats]

Most vegetable oils are high in Omega Six, again please see the chart at end of terminology section chapter 30 p 287. Palm oil and palm kernel oil have very different profiles.

Nutritiondata.com is a useful free site where you can check the Omega 3:6 contents of food, and well as other useful nutritional data.

So *(calm understatement)* please do not forget to check the labels of your baby formula for Omega 3:6 content, long chain Omega 3 and 6, and medium short saturated fats, if you come to the conclusion this book may have a point. Fructose and sugar would, based on the above, be an additional issue to consider in your choice of baby foods.

I am not an expert, my aim is to inform debate, and I advise you to seek professional advice and do some research on fats in infant nutrition.

25.34 **A fat larder is for life**—If your bodyfat larder is high in Omega 6, your body will continue to draw Omega 6 while you lose weight. [500] High Omega 6 will increase inflammation pressures which Omega 3 intake will help counter.

Omega 6 release will continue to slow the metabolism. To counter this, it is necessary to increase the intake of the mother, and long chain Omega 3s on a regular basis. Gluteal fat takes years to change. Breast fat takes months. Changing the profile of fat stores is no quick fix and a long term project.

A low fat weight loss diet, lacking in long chain Omega 3, may ironically provide a worse Omega 3:6 ratio, than the less 'healthy' pre-weight loss diet. Trials suggest, even when weight is being lost, the inflammatory pressures will continue, in the absence of Omega Three in the diet. [501]

Alcohol in the absence of adequate Omega 3 would further worsen the situation by stripping the brain over time of long chain Omega 3 fats.

25.35 **Hunger or nutritional deficit**—Why do we feel hungry? What controls our urge to eat? Is it a simple search for energy? Is it a far more subtle combination to fill the tank, and to select the right fuels?

Hunger control systems are very complex. Amazing progress is being made, but I suspect that researchers are just scratching the surface. Interesting snippets included a recent discovery that rodents have taste buds that detect Omega Six. When they have enough Omega Six, the taste bud response declines.

So we too may be programmed to go out and search for food we need, as is evidenced in pregnant women. Some chemical pathways, and genes of hunger/ metabolic control, have been identified.

They, include leptin, serotonin, dopamine, and endocannaboids, which have been shown to respond to AA, ghrelin, and fat intake. [502] These hormones have roles all over the body, and in many of the body's activities. It is complex and not an area I have looked at or understand.

The question has to be asked, are food obsessives eating high fat food, looking for Omega 3s, which are often missing or low in processed industrial foods.

Omega Threes are deliberately, and actively, removed from the processed food chain, and low Omega 3 grains specially developed as Omega 3 has a short shelf life. Could an unsatisfied Omega Three craving, create a never fulfilled cycle of binge eating of processed foods. Does DHA help regulate appetite? It might.

Oxidation of fats in the liver, has been linked to reduction of hunger. DHA, short chain fats, and monosaturates, are all more effectively oxidised than Omega Six. DHA is the most highly oxidised of the long chain fats and increases available serotonin and dopamine. High serotonin and dopamine, have been linked to reduced appetite and consumption.[xi]

25.36 **Insulin and DHA deficit**—The ability to make long chain Omega Threes, DHA and EPA, and the long chain Omega Six, AA, from the mother Omega 3 and 6 depends on a process called desaturase 5.

Higher insulin levels produced higher enzyme desaturase 5. Higher Omega Six LA, and enzyme desaturase 5 activity, would lead to greater amounts of AA being made. Whammy - AA increases insulin driving a self increasing insulin loop. [See 25.26].

Children with higher levels of AA were more obese and had higher insulin levels.[503] Long chain Omega 3 has been shown to moderate diabetes. [See 29.30] Omega 3 is actively removed from processed foods. Omega 3 utilisation is at least as high as for Omega 6 and likely higher, as more reactive.[504] Omega 3 conversion to the long chain children is blocked by high Omega 6.

25.37 **Leptin**—Systems are interlinked and deeply complex. Leptin is a gauge of fat reserves. It is multifaceted. Trial results often point in different directions. If you are left scratching your head after reading this, so am I, after trying to make sense of leptin and fats. Leptin is an internally induced chemical and not an external agent like Omega 3 and 6, so cannot be the master factor.

This section is little more than a list of information that comes out of trials. It demonstrates the complexities of the body's systems and the difficulties in deciphering how they work.

Leptin is made by fat cells. Leptin interacts with both oestrogen and testosterone. Leptin is considered a long-term regulator of food intake, rather than a measure of immediate hunger. Leptin increases energy expenditure by possibly pushing down insulin levels. Leptin responds to sleep and waking cycles.

---

xi   Effects of dietary and pharmacological manipulations on appetitive and consummatory aspects of feeding in non-human primates. Appetite. 2005 Oct;45(2):110–20 Foltin RW. Division on Substance Abuse, Department of Psychiatry, New York State Psychiatric Institute, College of Physicians and Surgeons of Columbia University, New York, NY.

Leptin levels increase after puberty. There are leptin receptors in glands including the pituitary, ovary, adrenal, and pancreas. [505]

Leptin has a role in the control of the monthly fertility cycle. [506] Leptin causes the release of pro-inflammatory agents in adipose tissue and the placenta. [507]

Leptin in animals fed a high fructose diet is associated with increased fat cell size in a straight-line relationship. [508]

Women have a system that allows more leptin, presumably to take account of the need to accumulate fat, to support energy demanding processes, such as pregnancy, lactation, and puberty. Leptin follows the oestrogen cycle.

Leptin is reported to respond to fasting, re-feeding, and fat levels. [509] Leptin levels directly correlate with the amount of body fat. [510] The Omega Three–Six balance moderates leptin.

Higher Omega Threes compared to Sixes reduced leptin levels, [511] but leptin is reported as being increased by EPA. [512 528] Leptin may act as a signal modulating PGE2 release. [513] PGE2 administration doubled serum leptin. [514] PGE2 is produced in response to AA introduction. [515] Linoleic acid pushes up leptin. [516"] PGE2 in adipocyte cells pushes up leptin, [517] as does AA. [518]

Corn oil supplemented cattle had higher leptin levels. [519] How the relationship with PGE2 works, is recognised as a potential area of obesity research. [520] Omega Six pushes up PGE2, and PGE2 pushes up leptin. Safflower oil (high Omega Six) compared with tallow, perilla, fish oils, or a low fat diet, increased leptin significantly, but not simply as a function of weight. [521]

"In vivo, starvation or food deprivation, decreases plasma leptin concentrations, and leptin transcription in adipose tissue. [522"] "A high safflower oil diet, compared to a low fat diet, doubled the leptin mRNA level in white adipose tissue. However, high fat diets rich in n3 PUFA failed to increase it". [523]

Other trials also suggests Omega Threes reduce leptin. [524 525] Palmitic Acid suppresses insulin. Oleic and linoleic enhances insulin secretion. Leptin did not affect insulin secretion. [526] Long chain fats may suppress leptin. [527]

25.38 **Sucrose = half fructose half glucose**–Sucrose, common table sugar, is half glucose and half fructose joined together. The body separates it and then digests it. The digestion of fructose and glucose take different paths.

25.39 **Fructose**–Auto fructose body instruction; store it while you can, it is seasonal, and will not be about for long. Add to that the parallel auto instruction to store Omega Six, and you have a great team;Omega Six, and sugar to make fat, all in nature's pre-packed, fertility assisting, fruit.

Fructose provides a backbone for Omega Six, a filing cabinet to store fats. Fructose can also be broken down to make fats. [531]

"Hepatic metabolism of fructose favours de novo lipogenesis" [529 530] *or translated, the livers first choice with fructose is to make fat to store rather than energy.*

For thousands of years, it is estimated we consumed 16–20 grams a day of fructose, mainly from fruits. We now consume 85–100 grams a day.[532]

Fructose is the sweetest natural sugar. It is produced commercially from corn, and extensively used as a sweetener. These sugars are 'hidden'. We are seeing increasing use of 'natural' high fructose based sweeteners, and concentrated juice sweeteners. We are told they are 'natural' and so more desirable than sugar.

The reality is they probably increase fat deposition more than sucrose [table sugar]. Sucrose, common sugar, is half fructose. Some fruits, like sweet apples, contain much more fructose than sucrose.

We are also drinking far more soft drinks, fruit drinks, and juices. Trials suggest that sugars in drinks are more easily absorbed. Fructose seems to bypass the normal dietary controls. Brain mechanisms register glucose, and tell you that you have eaten enough, but this does not appear to apply to fructose.

Fruit, and so fructose was a scarce commodity. A permanent glut was never in the design specifications. Industrial production allows consumption to excess. The role of fructose in obesity is an ongoing debate.

25.40 Digestion jaw-dropping facts—Mr. Jordan Ruben, writing for the *Weston A Price Foundation*, made the following jaw-dropping observations.

"Thirty-eight million Americans are victims of digestive disorders", "The economic cost of digestive disorders is $123 billion per year[533].

Conditions included Crohn's disease, ulcerative colitis, diverticulitis, celiac disease, IBS, constipation, diarrhea, GERD, candida and food allergies. Elaine Gottschall in *Breaking the Vicious Cycle* writes clearly and persuasively. Digestive health is a subject on its own, but is so fundamental and indivisibly bound to the fat and sugar metabolism, that it cannot be left out.

The digestive system is functionally integrated with wider body systems. I make basic points, and refer you to the above, for background reading.

YOU ARE WHAT YOU DIGEST.

25.41 Digestion—Omega Three and Omega Six—Digestion is fundamental to health. Digestive disturbances are accompanied by low-level inflammation. Gut inflammation, is communicated, and indivisible, with wider body status and function. Excess Omega Six sets the scene for inflammation. Omega Threes moderate the production of Omega Six inflammatory chemicals.

When responding to any situation, the ratio of Omega 3 to 6 workers who turn out, reflects cell membranes fat content, which reflects what is in your body.

Too much Six and not enough Three, and your body's fire crew are permanently on high alert, expecting and waiting for a call out. The phone rings– everybody is stressed, the result is an overreaction. The same principle applies to threats to the digestive system, as to the body generally.

A key to sorting out your digestion, is to take the body off constant high alert, by getting your Omega Threes and Sixes into balance. This will for most mean supplementing with the mother, and long chain, Omega Threes, and balancing mother Omega Six intake with Mother Omega Three.

Intake recommendations vary but about 1 mother Omega 3 to 2 mother Omega 6 is a common recommendation, but we are all individual, and there are no trials I have seen looking at ratios round 1:1 to see what is best.

25.42 **Undigested food**—Poor digestion means food is not digested properly. This includes fats. So, digestive disturbances are a multiple whammy including disruption of fat absorption and metabolism. Constant diarrhoea strips the coalface of workers. Floaty loose greasy stool are a sign of fat malabsorption.

25.43 **Digestion and sugars**—It is a vicious circle of improper nutrition, poor digestion, bad bacteria, inflammation, and growing low-level long-term illnesses. Low-level inflammation due to excess Omega Six places the whole body on intruder alert.

Undigested sugars are a common source of digestive problems. It is often assumed it is due to a food allergy. In reality, the main culprit may be of excess sugar, and inflammation due to excess Omega 6.

One hears about gluten allergies and dairy allergies, but not sugar. Undigested sugars and starches do not pass quietly through the gut but putrefy. Putrefaction and bad bacteria lead to damage of the cellular coalface, which leads to improper digestion. Incomplete digestion leads to unfriendly bacteria, and to mucus. Mucus keeps the workers from getting to the coalface. This leads to undigested foods and putrefaction. Inflammation triggered by poor gut conditions sets in, fuelled by excess Omega Six, leading to protective mucus. And so the circle goes on. If Omega 3 is absorbed direct in the small intestine, good digestion may be even more crucial. [See page xxvii]

The whole body becomes much more sensitive to 'insults', and is exposed to higher inflammatory factors and immune activity. To get the gut back working, and stop the leaking of baddies into the body through the gut wall, means giving it the things it digests most easily, and balancing the Omega 3s and 6s to reduce the inflammatory pressures.

Foods that are not digested easily are complex sugars found in, sugar, milk, many grains, and some starchy things. Milk in hard cheese, or yoghurt, has reduced lactase, or lactose from fermentation, making them easier to digest.

Once digestion is again stabilised, the body will tolerate less easily digested food again in moderation. The key villains are likely to be refined sugars, processed and concentrated sugars, including fructose, excessive consumption of fruit juices, and particularly sweetened drinks. [See 25.40 and preface xxvii]

25.44 **Short saturated fats**–SMCTs, short medium chain triglycerides, are glycerol backbones (toast racks) with three fats, each less than 12 carbons long. Some call them short and some medium so I have used the term short medium. There seem to be strong arguments for including sensible amounts of SMCT fats in the diet. Trials to date would suggest the effect is stronger in men. Short chain fats have been shown to turn down several genes related with weight gain. SMCTs have been shown to promote weight loss.[534]

SMCTs have been shown to increase insulin sensitivity.[535] The body can use these fats immediately without too much digestive effort. Coconut fat is an SMCT and has a pleasant texture and flavour and goes well in milk form with fruit. It is an excellent addition in cooking. Trials suggest it is good at keeping hunger at bay.[536] SMCTs are reported as being more easily oxidised. SMCTs require less digestive processing. SMCTs are a good medium for carrying fat-soluble foods dietary supplements and vitamins into the liver. The SMCTs are absorbed direct into the liver without the need to process them first. Butter also contains a proportion of SMCTs and some of the very short fats.

I would emphasise I am talking about sensible amounts of these saturated fats, but on the variety principle, and the above evidence they would seem a useful dietary addition. Exclusion of SMCTs and very short chain fats may have unknown negative consequences. [See 11.31] Saturated fats are in fact essential to body structure and metabolism. Certainly, in moderation they are not the deadly enemy of humans, which is an impression one could be left with from media coverage.

25.45 **Longer MCT Palm fats**–This is complicated and requires very much more research. I simply raise the question. It has been suggested elsewhere that mid chain fats are the least efficiently oxidised. These fats are made in the body. The saturated forms are also found in quantity in some vegetable fats. Would a combination of oversupply of carbohydrate, and fats high in mid chain saturates, increase trends to obesity?[537][538][539]

25.46 **Recent Trials**–This is a recent trial finding;

"DHA AND EPA EXHIBIT "ANTI-OBESITY" EFFECT AS WELL AS IMPROVING INSULIN SENSITIVITY"[xii]

---

xii Anti-obesity effects of conjugated linoleic acid, docosahexaenoic acid, and eicosapentaenoic acid. - Li JJ, Huang CJ, Xie D. - Mol Nutr Food Res. 2008 Feb 28 - Institutes for Nutritional Sciences, Shanghai Institutes for Biological Sciences, Chinese Academy of Sciences, Shanghai, P. R. China.

26

OMEGA THREE-SOURCES, ENVIRONMENTAL IMPLICATIONS

26   **Environmental implications** – [Abbreviations listed at 1.1] Omega Three consumption is low, and even falling in the West. There is evidence falling Omega Three combined with excess Omega Six, may be a significant factor in chronic 'western' diseases. [540]

The mother Omega Three is common in greens, plants and some seeds. So, supply of the mother Omega Three is not a problem. Plants cannot and do not make the long chain fats. Long chain fats are only found in living creatures.

Supplementation of long chain fats, through fish or marine products, is a dietary necessity for many. Vegetable based equivalents from algae are coming on the market, but are expensive and limited.

Sadly, the best source of long chain Omega 3s is oily fish. Fish stocks are coming under increasing pressure. The long chain Omega 3 daughter fats, DHA, and EPA, and wider family, are only found in plenty in oily fish, and some eggs.

Conversion rates, of the mother fats, to the long chain fats, in humans can be poor. The supply of long chain Omega Three fats, will impact on our future development, brain size, neuron density, intelligence, aggression, social conscience and cohesion. These traits are fundamental to human survival.

Fish stocks are dependent on the health of the oceans. There are many unknowns ahead for climate and our oceans, including global warming and pollution, which are all inextricably linked.

Ocean acidity, rising temperatures, rising sea levels, higher carbon dioxide, rising ultraviolet levels, and over-harvesting, including the usage of vast amounts of small oily fish for fish food, are significant issues.

It does not look good if we continue to take our planet for granted. This chapter considers the sources of Omega Threes, and possible solutions.

26.1   Environmental implication—Where are we going to source the long chain Omega Three we arguably need? What are the environmental implications? Fish and marine animals, are the primary food sources of long chain Omega Threes.

We know we are over-fishing. Fish stocks are declining. Sea fish farming consumes four, and some claim more times as much fish as it produces. Sea fish farming accounts for 75 per cent of the world's fish oil consumption. The figure is expected to rise to 90 per cent.

26.2   Cost of fish farming on fish stocks—The statistics on our use of marine assets, to grow carnivorous farmed fish, are truly frightening. We are using a top quality, essential, natural, limited, wild product to turn into a lower quality product, in the sense that natural fish must be a better option. It is simply about taste and our palate.

Farmed fish are delicious I must admit, but not as good as their wild cousins. I am not against fish farming, if Omega Three sources can be produced from grain or algae, and without the overuse of a very precious resource, wild fish.

Currently, it takes four to five tons of wild fish, fed to farmed fish, to produce one ton of farmed fish. The sustainability of carnivorous fish farming is in question. There is little room for increasing production capacity, as the industry is highly reliant on fish processed as feed. [541]

There is concern as to increased pollutants in farmed fish. [542] Also farmed fish have higher fat levels than wild fish. Farmed fish, are dependent on being fed fish meal from oily fish, for their supply of Omega Three. As they are also fed grain, they have much higher Omega Six content than wild fish.

So farmed fish are a good source of Omega Three, which they get by being fed wild fish meal, but have high levels of Omega Six not seen in wild fish.

On the positive side, they make certain breeds of fish like salmon, available and affordable, and increase fish consumption. There are those that claim a more environmentally friendly niche by using by products from fish processing, off cuts etc., but in general terms the figures speak for themselves.

One of the main arguments put forward by proponents, is we will not eat the small oily fish used for fish farm food. The WWF said, "Marine fisheries in the world are under heavy pressure with many close to collapse. The FAO estimates that about 75 per cent of fisheries are over-fished, exploited to their maximum biological limits, or recovering. Most fisheries are under urgent need of management. The remaining biomass of our planet's large predatory fishes is only about 10 per cent of pre-industrial levels." [543][544]

The consumption of 4–6 tonnes of wild fish, for each tonne of salmon produced, not only means less food for humans, but also for the many ocean species that rely on these fish as part of their food chain. Currently, the continued expansion of salmon farming is not sustainable. [545]

26.3 **Fish farming—The good news**—There may be potential to satisfy fish demand, by farming more non-carnivorous fish. The Chinese layered pond model, using fish with different feeding habits to create a more complete mini ecosystem, is an area worth consideration.

Fish farming conversion per ton of grain, is far more effective than cattle. The Chinese are the world's largest fish farmers. Fish farming in China began more than 3,000 years ago. The Chinese accounted for 21 million tons, of the 31 million tons of world aqua cultural in 1998.

The Chinese farm vegetarian fish in mixed fish communities, including bottom feeders, and algae feeders, so as to create a mini ecosystem. Annual pond yield per hectare is about four tons. [546] Carp contain significant Omega Three, and are favourably viewed by consumers. [547] [548]

In terms of productivity per ton of grain, vegetarian fish would be a preferential food source to corn-raised livestock. Fish farming is far more efficient than intensive cattle rearing, based on theses figures.

Cattle need seven kilograms of grain, to add one kilogram of live weight. Fish can add a kilogram of live weight, with less than two kilograms of grain. Food efficiency, is likely to become increasingly relevant, with rising grain/corn prices, due to greater global consumption.

Rising oil prices, will change the viability and geopolitics of grain derived fuels, and may lead to further grain and corn price rises. Consumers may shift consumption habits, as meat prices rise in the wake of grain prices.

26.4 **Plankton and krill**—A report on krill made the following points. Plankton and krill may be one of the largest biomasses on earth, and a prospect for controlled harvest.

But a whole marine food chain relies on them. Numbers are reported as falling. If this is a reflection of the impact of global warming on ice melt and UV, it is worrying indeed. Krill, it is claimed, are dependent on ice to breed. [549]

A recent report on the declining number of Emperor Penguins in the Daily Telegraph [UK] 11/12/07 Paul Eccleston suggested that krill and fish in the feeding grounds may have declined by 80 per cent since the 1970s.

26.5 **ALA crops**—The mother Omega Three fat linolenic acid, ALA, is found in quantity in linseed [Flax], perilla, and other sources. The ALA market can be met, by changing crop emphasis from Omega 6 high sources, like sunflower, to Omega 3 high crops like flax.

Other crops might include purslane, perilla, chia, and possibly canola and hemp, etc. There is evidence that cannabinoids, active substances from hemp, can be present in oils, and may lead to positive results in tests for cannabis use. There are trials that suggest canola may have negative impacts. I do not have sufficient knowledge to do more than raise a flag that concerns exist over Canola and Hemp oils. [See westonaprice.org].

26.6   High Six livestock profile–We feed our livestock on grain, and limited grazing. They too have distorted Omega Three : Six fat profiles. A wild-fed chicken egg, has 8 to 10 times the DHA of a factory-farmed chicken.

Potential sources of balanced Omega Threes and Sixes, are lost through intensive farming, and grain diets. Commercial chicken meat, has high levels of Omega Six, and low Omega Three.

Imbalances also impact on livestock health, and reproduction. A lot of research is done into supplementation of livestock with Omega Threes. This includes Omega Three trials to improve animal fertility issues. By feeding animals with fish extracts, or algae (oils), the level of DHA is increased about 2–fold in beef, 7–fold in chicken, 6–fold in eggs, and 20–fold in fish salmon[550].

26.7   Feeding grass–Cattle with unrestricted grazing rights, have far better Omega Three and Six profiles. In nature, cattle will eat far more than grass. Wider meadow fodder has been lost, as has woodland grazing.

So, in terms of making decisions on milk and meat consumption, it is important to know how cattle are fed. Cattle fed organic high Six grain will still have high Six profiles.

Cattle that can graze more freely, with better pasture like alpine cows, have far better Omega Three–Six profiles.[551][552] Range-fed cattle are likely also to have better Omega Three–Six profiles.

26.8   Egg farming–Chicken fed with higher levels of flax seed, develop eggs with a higher Omega Three profile, and a lower level of saturated fats. Feeding flax seed to laying hens increases the Omega Three fatty acid in the egg by six to eight times, and reduces saturated fats and cholesterol.[553]

26.9   Algae and plankton production–There are a number of products on the market, or coming to the market. It is clearly an area of great potential. Algal DHA may be an important future source. Marine algae produce a wide range of fats. The economies of production are improving.[554]

26.10   Genetic engineering– Genes are being inserted into plants and animals, which enable them to make long chain Omega Threes.

Genes from worms have been inserted in pigs, mice, and fish that enable them to make their own DHA.[555][556] The potential unseen dangers are significant, but DHA and EPA are essential to human health.

So if you were off on a space voyage, or the world was facing a food crisis, and it was a matter of survival, you might be prepared to look at inserting genes into humans, that allowed us to make Omega Threes and Sixes.

We would no longer be linked to the fecundity of nature. Who knows what the consequences might be in the long-term. If we had a constant supply of Omega Three would we see increasing brain sizes in the long term? Would we be more intelligent cooperative beings?

What is the future for those genetically altered, Omega Three making, mice and pigs who can make their own DHA ...? Might they rule the world one day? Interestingly the Omega Three–Six profile, of the modified Omega animals, was autonomously adjusted towards a 1:1 Omega Three–Six ratio.

26.11   **Bioengineering–Plants**–Scientists are looking at putting genes from algae into plants to make DHA. Trials have suggested it is possible.[557] Algae are a good sources of long chain Omega Threes.

Recent media coverage suggests that viable plants may be available in three years. What would be the impact of putting a long chain Omega 3 plant source, into the land environment.

Ramifications, good or bad, are likely to be enormous in the long term. Land creatures, like humans, are likely to use the current lack of availability of a supply of EPA and DHA in the plant world, as part of their behavioural and operating control mechanisms. Animals have evolved in a world, where there is no land based plant supply of DHA and EPA.

Hibernation is one example of a consequence. *The long term ramifications of any plant DHA/ EPA/ AA supply, viable in the wild, could be Ginormously significant, unforeseen, and of huge long term significance at a global design/ evolutionary level.* Modified crops and algae capable of producing DHA and EPA, may be a simple case of necessity, in the not too distant future.

Long chain fats are essential to health. Nations will compete to find sources. Very limited reading on the subject of genetic modification, suggests there are significant risks in some of the genetic technologies such as seed terminator genes, if they were to get into other plants.

IF long chain Omega 3s do have the wide ranges of benefits suggested then a stable future supply other than fish could be of significant importance. I am simply seeking to raise the matter, and not to future guess the arguments, or preform any judgement on future supply sources, and the impact of the commercial imperative.

27

SLEEP, OMEGA 3, AND 6

27   Sleep, fat, and the eicosanoid pathway—[Abbreviations at 1.1] This section on sleep is based on my own thoughts, and trying to join the dots of the work of others. I looked for trials on DHA, EPA, and sleep in adults and found none. I found limited sleep trials on babies and children.

Since I have balanced my Omega 3s and 6s, and taken fish oil, I sleep far more soundly, and deeply. I also awake feeling more refreshed than I used to. That is it in a nutshell. I again try and bring a glimpse through the mist.

Reducing excess Omega 6, and increasing long chain Omega 3, should improve sleep. Infants, whose mother's have a high DHA profile, sleep far more soundly. This is a summary list of mechanisms and factors;

- ☞ A lack of melatonin is consistent with poor sleep.
- ☞ A lack of Omega 3 DHA inhibits melatonin creation and function.
- ☞ Melatonin is a COX2 blocker, but does not block COX1. Melatonin switches down Omega 6 AA activity, and so indirectly influences steroids and hormones including cortisol [Fig. 23.11b], and Omega 6 inflammation.
- ☞ Melatonin inhibits release of Omega 6 from the fat stores.
- ☞ Melatonin is a very powerful antioxidant including of AA, and EPA.
- ☞ Melatonin levels link to cortisol, serotonin, dopamine, immune function, sex hormones, fat pathways, insulin, and leptin, in a day night rhythm.
- ☞ Melatonin increases long chain fat production of EPA, AA and DHA.
- ☞ DHA increases melatonin levels.
- ☞ Many inflammatory western conditions involve sleep degradation, and connect to a lack of EPA, DHA, and excess Omega 6.
- ☞ Lack of sleep causes stress. Stress causes lack of sleep.

☞   Coronary heart disease links to lower melatonin, and higher cortisol[i].

☞   Stress increases the level of immune and inflammatory markers.

☞   In animals with no pineal gland mitochondrial formation was impaired.[ii]

☞   Shift workers may have a higher risk of breast cancer.

☞   Melatonin levels are reported as lower in Alzheimers and Cancer.

Poor quality sleep, and sleep deprivation, are common in western conditions. Balancing the Omega Threes and Sixes, and ensuring a supply of the long chain fats EPA and DHA, has made a big difference to the quality of my sleep.

I have not seen it suggested by anybody else, that the Omega 3:6 balance, and DHA, are central to sleep. This is a theory, and no more.

27.1   **Omega Three and Six and sleep**–I suggest sleep, melatonin, and the long chain Omega 3s and 6s, are intimately linked. Sleep involves closing down Omega 6 pathways, and opening Omega 3 pathways. If the Omega 3 and 6 pathways, are excessively out of balance, the body will be difficult to put to sleep.

Melatonin closes down Omega Six COX2 activity directly. Melatonin increases fat conversion desaturase activity. Melatonin closes the Omega 6 chemicals by increasing Omega 3, EPA and DHA levels. EPA and DHA close down the Omega 6 pathway. Melatonin shuts down COX2, but not COX1. Melatonin prevents the release of Omega Six from fat stores.

Melatonin increases DHA, enhancing serotonin production. Serotonin is essential to make melatonin. Rising DHA, and melatonin, may create a self fuelling cycle of melatonin, so more DHA, more serotonin, more melatonin etc.

Melatonin has multiple mechanisms for sleep. Melatonin is a powerful antioxidant. It switches fat pathways activity at night from inflammatory Omega 6, to repairing Omega 3. *If there is a lack of Omega 3, not enough melatonin will be made to put the body into deep sleep.* If fat conversion pathways are blocked, this will inhibit the function of melatonin by restricting DHA production. If there is excess of Omega 6, melatonin has more difficulty in closing the Omega 6 pathways. Excess Omega 6 connects to western conditions. Western conditions including diabetes, asthma, CHD, and obesity, connect to poor sleep.

A lack of Omega 3 and excess Omega 6, you will not sleep, at or at least not deeply and fully. Without the Omega 3, the sleep raw material, melatonin will not be made, and cannot work it's sleep magic.

---

i   Human Melatonin and Cortisol Circadian Rhythms in Patients with Coronary Heart Disease Biological Rhythm Research, Volume 29, Number 2, April 1998 , pp. 121-128(8) Brugger P.; Herold M.

ii   Ultrastructural clues for the potent therapeutic effect of melatonin on aging skin in pinealectomized rats fundamental & Clinical Pharmacology 20 (6), 605–611. Mukaddes Eşrefoğlu, Mehmet Gül, Muammer Seyhan, Hakan Parlakpınar Department of Histology and Embryology and Department of Dermatology , Faculty of Medicine, Inonu University Malatya, and National Hospital, Malatya, Turkey.

27.2 **When we sleep?**– What happens in sleep. A guess is repair and renewal, rubbish removal, some filing and organisation in the brain, and a bit of tidying up. Melatonin regulates immune function, metabolism, interacts with the hormones and steroids, and is a very powerful antioxidant.

Cytokines, immune signalling agents, are observed to have day/night rhythms, indicating changes of emphasis in immune function between day and night. White blood cell numbers peak at night. T cells are highest in the morning, and B cells in the evening. [iii] Cholesterol production has a cyclical pattern, and is at it's highest about six in the morning. Cholesterol is the raw material of the sex hormones, and steroids including cortisol [23.11b].

Cortisol is an example of a cholesterol child. Cortisol regulates the immune system. Stress instructs cortisol to be made. Many people have high cortisol levels. Cortisol falls at night, and rises to its highest level around wakening. Growth in the young requires sleep. Lower cortisol permits bone and connective tissue growth. Night time cortisol levels increase with age, and REM sleep declines.

The body normally has routines for a reason. Melatonin interacts with progesterone, prolactin, oestrogen, dopamine, serotonin, steroids, and other hormones. Dopamine levels fall at night as does serotonin activity.

Omega Six products are reduced by melatonin. Melatonin blocks PGE2 production. Omega 6 PGE2 falls at night. Omega Six PGE2 is need to make the sex hormones, steroids, brain chemicals, immune agents, and other chemicals.

This joining of the dots would suggest Omega Six/COX2/PGE2 products have a day night cycle, and trials hint they do. *In animals Omega Six chemical PGE2 has been linked with wakefulness.*[iv] It is complicated and I struggle with it. This is only a an outline of a possible shape in the mist.

27.3 **Sleep, melatonin, DHA, and serotonin**– Melatonin is produced by the pineal gland, and increases in quantity with darkness. The body is aware of light and dark, through various receptors. Melatonin is essential to sleep.

Omega 6 emergency repair crews are based round the inflammatory Omega 6 chemicals. They are high energy, day time, here and now, wakeful, watchful, ready for everything, insults, intruders, malfunctions at a moment's notice.

Omega 3 crews are gentler, more night time people, concerning themselves with long-term repair and maintenance. Melatonin puts frenetic day-time inflammatory Omega 6 activities into background mode, switches down the alarm reactions, sets the body up for repair, and patrols to minimise disturbances.

iii Content of T and B lymphocytes in healthy human peripheral blood V. P. Lozovoi, M. Shergin and A. A. Povazhenko Department of Clinical and Experimental Immunology, Institute of Clinical and Experimental Medicine, Siberian Branch, Academy of Medical Sciences of the USSR, Novosibirsk.
iv Evidence that brain prostaglandin E2 is involved in physiological sleep-wake regulation in rats. Proc Natl Acad Sci U S A. 1989 July; 86(14): 5666–5669. H Matsumura, K Honda, W S Choi, S Inoué, T Sakai, and O Hayaishi Department of Neuropsychiatry, Osaka Medical College, Japan.

A number of mechanisms are involved. Melatonin puts many of the Omega Six, COX2 chemicals, the day workers, fire, police officers, emergency crews, and everybody else, apart from a few night-watchmen, to bed. It calls out extra night-time Omega 3 repair crews, and allows COX1 maintenance crews to continue.

How does melatonin do this so neatly and yet so simply? "In a nutshell there seems to be a relationship between the level of sleep you are getting and how much melatonin you produce," Malow said.[v] Low levels of melatonin are linked with poor sleep, according to a trial [Nov 2007] on poor sleep and autism.

I suggest the following mechanisms may help explain sleep;

☞ Melatonin rises towards sleep time.

☞ Melatonin blocks COX2, so reducing Omega 6 inflammatory chemicals.

☞ Melatonin blocks fat cells from releasing Omega 6. Brown and white fat cells have melatonin receptors.

☞ Melatonin does not block the COX1 pathways. Omega Six COX1 based chemicals can continue normal housekeeping activities at night.

☞ Melatonin increases desaturase activity [Enzymes to make long chain fats]. More DHA is made. DHA helps shut down the Omega Six COX2 inflammatory chemicals, steroids and hormones.

☞ Rising melatonin, causes DHA to rise, which encourages the signalling pathways to make serotonin. Serotonin is needed for melatonin to be made. More serotonin, means more melatonin is made; more melatonin pushes more DHA to be made, so creating a loop boosting melatonin, its friends serotonin and DHA.

☞ Melatonin an antioxidant damps down remaining Omega Six day workers on overtime, by blocking the Omega 6 oxidative cascade, and keep them away from work, until time to go back in the morning.

☞ Melatonin also works with hormones[558] and steroids. Switchover from the Omega Six, to the Omega Three pathway, reduces the production of Omega 6 chemical PGE2. PGE2 is associated with wakefulness. Reduced PGE2 results in lower aromatase, and related enzymes in the cholesterol pathways, reducing hormones and steroids. Cholesterol falls at night. Progesterone has to go through less Omega Six dependent steps [Fig. 23.11b]. The reduction in onward conversion of progesterone to hormones and steroids, due to lower PGE2 based enzymes, would probably increase progesterone levels. Progesterone rises, and cortisol falls at night, which would be consistent with melatonin acting as a COX2 blocker. Increased progesterone, and falling cholesterol means less raw

---

v   Nocturnal urine 6-sulfatoxymelatonin levels are related to sleep parameters in children with autism B. A. Malow, L. Beydman, E. J. Botzolakis ; Dept Neurol, Vanderbilt Univ. Med. Ctr., Nashville, TN.

material for conversion to the steroids and hormones. On this basis, sleep would produce a cycling hormone and steroid pattern over 24 hours, with lower levels of cortisol, oestrogen, testosterone, and higher levels of progesterone at night. The process by which cholesterol, is transported into the mitochondria also has a daily cycle. Trials suggest that the hormones steroids and immune function have a day night cycle.

☞ Melatonin directly or indirectly interacts with leptin and insulin to regulate energy in sleep. Leptin has a peak in the very early hours.[vi] Leptin encourages heat production [23.52]. Insulin levels fall at night which may assist in increasing metabolism.

☞ More mitochondrial membrane DHA may influence oxidation, and so metabolism. Mitochondrial metabolism at night changes, and results in higher basal metabolism [23.52]. CoQ10 and cholesterol drop.[vii] What is the source of energy? Is DHA protected by melatonin as an antioxidant, and for how long? Is DHA oxidised as night passes?

☞ Melatonin, and the fat conversion enzymes desaturase 5 and 6 are enhanced by calorie restriction. Increased intake may inhibit long chain fat manufacture, and so sleep.[viii] Sleep degradation connects to obesity.

☞ To sleep less when there is Omega 6 to eat and store as fat for breeding reserves, and daylight to see by, makes sense as a survival strategy.

Melatonin is not generally stored by the body. A fresh supply is made each night. Melatonin is a very powerful antioxidant. The exhaustion of melatonin as a 'one use only' antioxidant, and reduction in production and usage of DHA, as night passed, would allow the Omega 6 chemicals to come back on line, as melatonin is oxidised, so restarting the Omega 6 day time routines.

These chemical reactions, and pathways, form the basis of a virtuous sleep circle. More DHA means more Omega Three chemicals, and less Omega Six chemicals. This all depends on melatonin, which in turn depends on DHA being available.

---

vi   Diurnal and Ultradian Rhythmicity of Plasma Leptin: The Journal of Clinical Endocrinology & Metabolism Vol. 83, No. 2 453-459 Effects of Gender and Adiposity Mohammed F. Saad, Maggy G. Riad-Gabriel, Arshad Khan, Alok Sharma, Ragui Michael, Sujata D. Jinagouda, Rima Boyadjian and Garry M. Steil.

vii Coenzyme Q10 concentration in plasma and blood cells: What about diurnal changes? BioFactors Issue: Volume 28, Number 1 / 2006 Petra Niklowitz , Werner Andler, Thomas Menke Vestische Kinderklinik Datteln, University Witten-Herdecke, Datteln, Ge.

viii A defect in the activity of Delta6 and Delta5 desaturases may be a factor predisposing to the development of insulin resistance syndrome. Prostaglandins Leukot Essent Fatty Acids. 2005 May;72(5):343-50 Das UN. UND Life Sciences, 1083 Main Street, Walpole, MA 02081, USA.

THE BIG BUT–*You can only get mother Omega 3s from food. IF you do not make DHA, or eat DHA, you don't have DHA.*

Poor old melatonin simply cannot work its magic, if there are no Omega 3 raw materials, because you have not eaten them. Whammy -No Omega 3, and excess Omega 6 makes more Omega 6 chemicals as melatonin levels rise.

Excess Omega 6 AA means more PGE2 inflammatory chemicals, and immune agents to switch off. Excess Omega 6 would create high levels of undesirable oxidation for melatonin to control, before the sleep processes can start. Early exhaustion of melatonin as an anti oxidant, by excess LA and AA oxidation products, and lack of Omega 3 raw material to assist melatonin, would contribute to poor and shortened sleep, as the DHA cycle would not happen.

No DHA raw material, and the whole sleep and repair cycle is compromised. With incomplete or partial sleep, there is a lack of proper repair downtime, and incomplete shutdown of inflammatory, immune, and stress systems at night. Exhausted cellular staff, working the wrong hours, are less effective.

Stress due to lack of proper shutdown mounts, leading to inflammation and heightened immune response, increased stress, lower basal metabolism, higher fat stores, creating a self-fuelling sleep degradation cycle. It all takes it's toll.

Melatonin levels start falling at puberty, and some but not all studies suggests it continue to decline into old age.

27.4 **Melatonin–Us and algae–**Melatonin is deeply linked to body function, at an early design and evolutionary level. Melatonin is found in all living creatures. Single cell algae, have eyes, and melatonin. They use the same chemical, rhodopsin, in visual receptor membranes, as we do.

SAD (seasonal affected disorder), an emotional imbalance due to lack of light, underlines the importance of being able to turn light into electrical impulses in the body. DHA is a key chemical in the process.

Inadequate DHA, and the retina does not turn light efficiently into electrical signals. Light moderates melatonin production. The body processes are deeply interconnected, a lack of DHA, has fundamental consequences.

High DHA levels are needed for visual receptors to function properly. If light received by the eye is not effectively converted to chemical signals, this could impact on melatonin, and so wakefulness, sleep, repair and wider function.

27.5 **Melatonin - light, dark, and artificial day–**The amount of melatonin produced by the body varies in a daily cycle. The timing of the cycle is controlled by our ability to sense light. [559] Before electric light, melatonin provided an activity control mechanism, to the seasons, and the day night cycle.

Quality artificial light sources have dramatically changed our behaviour, and sleep pattern. Bright lighting may have much deeper consequences than we realise. Even bright light of short duration, can alter melatonin rhythms.

We are not going to abandon the electric light. Melatonin is key to sleep. Sleep is key to health. It is a question of trying to understand the body's functions, so we can so far as possible minimise any negative impact.

27.6   Melatonin–Heap powerful, all areas pass–Melatonin is a heap powerful factor in the body. Its roles include a very powerful antioxidant, immune regulator, a role in delaying puberty, oestrogen regulation, manipulation of the fats and the fat chemical pathways. Melatonin is able to increase and regulate DHA, and long chain Omega Three production. Melatonin is a COX 2 blocker but does not inactivate the COX1 pathways.

Melatonin gets about, which is be essential to such an influential hormone and antioxidant. "The data prove that melatonin can easily pass through the cell membrane and bath every part of the cell". [560]

27.7   Melatonin and adipose tissue–Melatonin talks to fat cells, which have melatonin receptors. Melatonin blocks the release of Omega Six, linoleic acid, from fat pads in animals. [561]

This is another way melatonin, tips the balance, from the Omega 6 chemical pathways, to Omega 3. In cancer cells, Omega Six uptake was lowest, 75 per cent reduced, during the mid-dark phase.

The uptake of Omega Six in cancer cells cyclically followed the melatonin cycle. When melatonin was blocked, the reduction in Omega Six uptake is no longer seen, so there is no question the effect is due to melatonin.

27.8   Inadequate melatonin sleep and health–Melatonin is a 'once only use' antioxidant. If the melatonin supply is exhausted in its antioxidant role, by excess inflammatory oxidation, trying to put the emergency workers to bed, it will not have sufficient numbers to call out the Omega Three, and Omega Six COX1 one, workers to perform their night-time repair work, close down the fat cells stores, change the immune function status, and put the body into deep sleep.

Worse, if the body has reached permanent low-level inflammation, with many more Omega Six emergency workers, than Omega Three workers, in the cell membranes, it is like a house of ill-disciplined over-excited children, who will never go to bed, and allow the parents to get on with those other things that need doing. In the end, this leads to long-term breakdown somewhere.

If the body's fats are seriously out of balance, the brain and pineal gland, simply may not have the Omega Three raw materials available, to allow sufficient melatonin to be made. The electrical and chemical signals from the retina may be diminished by lack of DHA.

There may be a point where high Omega Six and low Three, simply make it impossible for melatonin to do its work. My experience, is that my quality of sleep has significantly improved since rebalancing my Omega Three and Six intake.

27.9 **Melatonin and the immune system**—Melatonin is reported as having a variety of effects on immune function. An explanation for a part of melatonin's role in the immune system, is the blocking of the COX 2 pathways, and the upgrading of desaturase 5 fat conversion pathways, that produce AA, EPA, and DHA. Melatonin blocks the release of the Omega Six fats from fat stores.

This would cut down the inflammatory/daytime immune chemicals in the body on a nightly basis, to allow repair. In sleep, some immune systems appear to be upgraded, and some downgraded. Interestingly, hibernating squirrels appear to shut down the immune system, which restarts on waking.[ix]

This re-engaging of the Omega 6 inflammatory pathways, with awakening, is consistent with melatonin acting as a COX2 blocker. As usual it is complex and multifaceted. Cortisol is seen as an immune supressant, suggesting immune function is higher at night. Cortisol[x] is at its lowest in the early hours of the morning, rising to its highest levels at about 6am with waking.

Cortisol blocks some cytokines, and promotes others. IL1, 6,10,12 and TNA are highest in the early morning.[xi] Il1 and IL6 are connected to the fever response. IL10 is an anti inflammatory cytokine. Il12 is involved in T cell production, and killer cells. Melatonin, and quality sleep, are a very important integral cyclical parts of regulating the body's sleep immune and repair system.

27.10 **Melatonin and the pineal gland**—DHA is essential to the pineal gland. DHA has been shown to increase the pineal gland's production of melatonin. A key job of the pineal gland is to produce melatonin.

In an Omega Three deficient diet, or if DHA is not available, then the body substitutes DHA with the nearest Omega Six 22:5n6 DPA. [562 563]

Trials in Omega Three deficient animals have shown significant DHA deficiency, increased DPA, and a decline in melatonin production. Fish oil replaces DPA, with DHA, and normalises melatonin levels. [564]

27.11 **Melatonin up rates DHA**—Melatonin has been reported as uprating delta 5 desaturase, a step in the conversion of mother fats Omega 3 and 6 to DHA and AA. Long-term melatonin supplementation restores delta 5 desaturase activity. Melatonin may increase the number of mitochondria over time. Mitochondria produce energy, hormones, steroids, chemical manufacturing capacity, and fat conversion.

---

ix Immune System Turned Off During Hibernation in squirrels Jeff Grabmeier Ohio State Research.

x   Endocrinology Physiology of the Adrenal Gland www.lib.mcg.edu/edu/eshuphysio/program.

xi Diurnal rhythms of pro-inflammatory cytokines: regulation by plasma cortisol and therapeutic implication. Cytokine Volume 10, Issue 4, April 1998, Pages 307-312 Nikolai Petrovsky, Peter McNair and Leonard C. Harrison Walter and Eliza Hall Institute, Post Office, Royal Melbourne Hospital, Parkville Victoria 3050, Australia.

Increased long chain fat conversion, combined with a COX2 blocking effect, would reinforce the production of Omega 3 EPA chemicals. Melatonin helps normalise levels of long chain fatty acids, by increasing levels of long chain fats, presumably DHA produced through activation of delta 5 desaturase,[565] so improving diabetic status [25.21]. Blocking of melatonin in rats produces "severe hyperinsulinemia and accumulation of triglycerides in the liver".[566]

More DHA may contribute to high efficiency mitochondrial oxidation at night, working synergistically with leptin and insulin. The greater availability of high energy DHA oxidation products, might be used in the destruction of faulty cells, changes in metabolism in sleep, production of body heat, rebuilding processes, and thyroid function. Thyroid function increases at night. [23.52]

27.12 Melatonin inhibits COX2,–Melatonin is a selective Cox 2 inhibitor, that does not inhibit the COX 1 pathway. The COX1 pathway is concerned with the running of the body, rather than emergency response. The current finding corroborates a role for melatonin as an anti-inflammatory agent. These anti-inflammatory actions seem not to be exclusively mediated by the free radical scavenging properties of melatonin.[567][568]

27.13 Melatonin reduces oxidation–Melatonin acts as a once only use antioxidant. Melatonin was reported as 20 times more powerful than vitamin C. Many oxidants can be reprocessed for reuse, but melatonin cannot.

Melatonin scavenges free radicals, stimulates antioxidant enzymes, augments the effect of other antioxidants, and increases the efficiency of mitochondrial oxidation, thereby reducing electron leakage, and so uncontrolled oxidation.

Melatonin protects fats including EPA and AA[xii] from oxidation. Protecting AA from oxidation would reduce AA chemicals. AA oxidation needs less energy than EPA oxidation, so oxidation blocking may favour AA. Melatonin initiates a cascade of antioxidants, which may explain the high efficiency of melatonin.[xiii]

Melatonin may increase the number and structural integrity of mitochondria. The reverse if applicable, a relative loss of mitochondria with declining melatonin, might be a factor in metabolic slowdown observed in obesity, and old age.

Sleep deprivation is a symptom of obesity and western inflammatory conditions. Lower melatonin, would result from high Omega 6, lack of 3, stress, inflammation and overactive immune function.

[xii] Melatonin preserves arachidonic and docosapentaenoic acids during ascorbate-Fe2+ peroxidation of rat testis microsomes and mitochondria. - Int J Biochem Cell Biol. 2003 Mar;35(3):359-66 -Gavazza M, Catalá A.Facultad de Ciencias Veterinarias, Cátedra de Bioqui;mica, Universidad Nacional de La Plata La Plata, Argentina.

[xiii] Melatonin as an antioxidant: biochemical mechanisms and pathophysiological implications in humans Russel J. Reiter, Dun-xian Tan, Juan C. Mayo, Rosa M. Sainz, Josefa Leon and Zbigniew Czarnocki Department of Cellular and Structural Biology, University of Texas Health Science Center, San Antonio, Texas, U.S.A.; Department of Chemistry, Warsaw University, Warszawa.

Melatonin is a highly efficient free radical scavenger in the central nervous system, and yet at the same time promotes mitochondrial respiration, with possible benefits against Alzheimer's and Parkinsonism.[569] Increased DHA may be a factor in increased cellular respiration [21.7]. Reconciling melatonin's role as an antioxidant with increased basal metabolic rate requires clarification.

A trial suggested that melatonin lowers killing power against bacteria.[570][571] Other trials suggest DHA assists immune function. [See 22 and 29.2].

At *very high* doses melatonin inhibits lutenising hormone.[xiv] Different countries hold different positions on the sale of melatonin over the counter.

Melatonin's powers as an antioxidant, may reduce factors that underpin stress, so again assisting with the sleep process. Control of body mechanisms by melatonin through fats, and in response to fats, would connect to the necessary processes for a step change in body function in the form of sleep.

27.14 **Melatonin reduces oestrogen production**–Melatonin blocking COX2, would reduce night-time oestrogen, and sex hormone production. Trials suggest oestrogen has a daily cycle and is lower at night. Melatonin, is an effective inhibitor of oestrogen-based breast cancer, in animals,[572] and a possible treatment agent in hormone-based cancers.[573] Melatonin may prevent DNA damage and act synergistically with oestrogen against lipid oxidation.[577]

There are melatonin receptors in the ovaries.[xv] Melatonin acts at several levels including as a selective oestrogen modulator.[574][575] Progesterone is increased by melatonin. Increased progesterone, may follow reduced conversion of Omega 6 and lower enzymes meaning less gets used. [Fig 23.11b]. [The role of AA in the hormones involves an enzyme cytochrome 450. It is complex, and I struggle.]

27.15 **Melatonin–Gastrointestinal cancer, and weight loss**-Melatonin and DHA, taken together, stabilised weight loss in 63 per cent of patients with advanced gastrointestinal cancer not amenable to standard treatment.[576]

27.16 **Melatonin–Shift work and cancer rates**–An increase of cancers has been noted in those on shift work. A loss of melatonin production in shift workers, poorer high Six diets, and asynchronicity with the day night signals might lead to lower levels of DHA production, and melatonin. Lower DHA and melatonin may link to more risk of inflammatory conditions and some cancers.

---

xiv The Journal Of Clinical Endocrinology & Metabolism; Voordouw, BCG; 74(1): 108-117 (1992).

xv Direct Action of Melatonin in Human Granulosa-Luteal Cells The Journal of Clinical Endocrinology & Metabolism Vol. 86, No. 10 4789-4797 Michelle M. M. Woo, Chen-Jei Tai, Sung Keun Kang, Parimal S. Nathwani, Shiu Fun Pang and Peter C. K. Leung Department of Obstetrics and Gynecology , University of British Columbia, Vancouver, Canada V6H 3V5; and Department of Physiology, University of Hong Kong, Hong Kong, China.

27.17   Melatonin delay of puberty – Higher levels of melatonin are noted pre-puberty. The pineal gland is large in children, but shrinks at puberty. [578] Melatonin is highest between 1-10 years, starting to fall significantly in early to mid teens with puberty, and then declining continuously with age.[xvi] [23.44]

Higher melatonin equates to higher DHA levels, lower Omega 6, and maybe lower sex and steroid hormones. Melatonin suppresses cholesterol [23.11.b].

DHA is essential for brain formation, growth of neurons and brain components. A new period of brain growth and reorganisation, key to development of language and mathematical thought, is reported in puberty, ages 6–13.

Higher oestrogen levels will increase conversion to DHA in girls after puberty, [23.3, 23.4] so providing DHA for continued brain formation. In males, what happens to DHA levels after puberty, and does reduced DHA production, adversely effect brain growth and reorganisation? Brain formation may slow dramatically between 11 and 15.[579] This is a key time for language development.

Does this explain, in part, better communication skills of women? What is the impact on brain function in this crucial period, of low Omega 3 DHA, and high Omega 6, with possible low level inflammation? High melatonin pre-puberty may protect DHA/EPA levels[580] in both sexes, and so brain neuron formation.

Omega 3 / DHA dietary deficit, excess Omega 6, melatonin decrease post puberty, poor long chain fat conversion, Omega 6 inflammatory pressures, high PGE2, and hormone increases, may adversely impact on brain function and formation, and jointly account for behavioural issues in teenage males.

Melatonin acts independently as a COX2 pathway blocker. The combination of higher Omega 3 conversion to DHA, due to melatonin, with the blocking effect by Omega 3 DHA on Omega 6, and the COX blocking effect of melatonin on PGE2 and aromatase, would reduce or delay hormone production levels.

Lower hormones would result in later puberty. Later puberty, could allow more time for brain growth, with the necessary DHA supplies, through better conversion rates. Blockages of the fat conversion pathways, and lack of supply of Omega 3 ALA, may negate the effects of melatonin, and bring on early puberty.

Early puberty has been linked with higher levels of Omega Six, obesity and related conditions. [581] In girls, central adiposity, and early age at menarche increases the risk of being overweight in late adolescence. [582]

Leptin does not look like it is the controlling factor in the time of puberty. [583]

Fats, hormones, sleep, growth, and puberty are clearly very interdependent. Low DHA is a factor in, ADHD, brain function, cognitive skills, sleep, impulsiveness, aggressiveness, behaviour, hormones, western inflammatory conditions, and early puberty.

---

xvi   Melatonin the "light of night" in human biology and adolescent idiopathic scoliosis Scoliosis 2007, 2:6doi:10.1186/1748-7161-2-6 Theodoros B Grivas and Olga D Savvidou Orthopaedic Department, "Thriasio" General Hospital, G. Gennimata Avenue, Magula, 19600 Greece.

27.18 **Loss sleep ability in young**–Higher levels of melatonin in the young, would be consistent with a higher sleep need. Between the ages of 1-3 95 per cent of brain growth occurs. There is a second major spurt between about 10-12. Between 13-20 the brain is being pruned and organised.

DHA is fundamental to brain formation and neuron growth. Melatonin promotes DHA production. Lower melatonin, due to high Omega 6, would also be consistent with poorer sleep, disturbed sleep patterns, etc.

High levels of Omega 6s, and imbalances with Omega 3, would result in the multiple effects of excess Omega 6, including higher hormone levels, lower melatonin, higher oxidation, greater aggressiveness, loss of cognitive function, less self-restraint, greater levels of depression, and earlier puberty. It appears to be another self reinforcing down ward spiral. Inflammation reduces sleep. Sleep deprivation increases inflammatory factors.

"The biological consequences of sleep deprivation in young adults include metabolic, systemic inflammatory and immune changes that are similar to those of aging and age-related disorders".[584] High PGE2 has been noted in Alzheimers.

High Omega Six, low Omega Three, disruption of melatonin, less time for growth and maturation of the brain, could account for a number of the social behaviour changes we are seeing in the young, as well as early puberty.

Sperm is high in DHA [23.17], 25% in monkeys and rams, and important to fertility. Whilst it has always been 'an old wives tale', maybe 'old wives' were right this time. Excessive masturbation could reduce DHA levels, if DHA was in very short supply [E.g. famine] and so conceivably diminish brain function and eyesight. DHA is key to brain and eye function. This is a male issue.

27.19 **Melatonin–Diabetes, metabolic syndrome, and fats**–The blocking of melatonin in diabetic rats produced "severe hyperinsulinemia and accumulation of triglycerides in the liver."[585] The impact of melatonin, on the fats pathways and metabolism, reduction of quality sleep, and close-down of the inflammatory pathways, could be a contributing factor to reducing obesity. Basal metabolic rate increases in sleep. DHA may assist increased basal metabolism in sleep [23.53]. Longer puberty through better sleep, and increased BMR, might help reduce obesity and so in a self reinforcing cycle, further delay puberty.

27.20 **Melatonin may improve sexual drive and fertility**–Both male and female West African goats, showed enhanced sexual behaviour, after melatonin supplementation.[586] Melatonin blocks oestrogen in cats, but oestrogen increased immediately after treatment.[587] Turn activity down in sleep, repair and maintenance followed by increased output? Melatonin increases progesterone, and may reduce the other hormones.[588] In ewes, melatonin increased fertility, and increased progesterone. Rising hormones would be consistent with PGE2/P450 coming back on line, and cholesterol rising in the early morning.

28

OMEGA SIX – ULTIMATE HORMONE CONTROLLER, AND LINK TO NATURE

28   **Ultimate hormone controller**—Omega Six is natures ultimate fertility controller of humans. Omega Six alters the chemistry of the brain and body. It involuntarily alters behaviour through brain chemicals. It alters the physical structure of the brain. Omega 6 with the opposing effect of Omega 3 controls hormones and steroids. [23.11.b].

Omega 3 and 6 are external agents. Without Omega 3 and Omega 6, there is no life. Without adequate Omega 6, reproduction does not occur.

The body was designed or evolved to work within certain Omega 3:6 balances. Excess of Omega 6, and lack of Omega 3, is pushing human metabolism and behaviour into unknown territory.

Our global increase in Omega Six consumption primarily through vegetable oils is a vast experiment. Vast excess of Omega Six, and lack of Omega Three, likely makes us all, women and men, more male, more aggressive, acquisitive, impulsive, and less cooperative, by manipulation of hormones, steroids, and brain chemicals like serotonin, and dopamine.

What would be the future of a crowded world, full of more aggressive, impulsive, and less cooperative people?

Humans start life as essentially 'brain female'. The central nervous system starts life as female. In boys the 'female brain', at the end of pregnancy is turned to a 'male brain', by the influence of hormones. [589]

By likely making the world more male, we are moving away from our natural emotional and physiological state. What will be the result of a world that is more male in outlook, and can the world survive it?

The continuing lack of recognition of the importance of Omega Three and Omega Six in shaping human behaviour, could at worst be the seeds of human self-destruction.

28.1   Nature's autonomous control system–It would make sense as a design constraint, or evolutionary strategy, to have an 'autonomous' control system linking us to the environment, controlling breeding and related behaviour, to optimise survival of the species.

It makes sense to programme species to reproduce, when conditions are suitable, and discourage them when breeding conditions are poor. It makes sense to build in different behaviours dependent on food status. Population density, and location, reflects environmental fecundity, food type and timing.

There is no guarantee that education, and support, from peers will always be available. Survival of a species requires innate programming, and inbuilt responses to various environmental conditions.

High Omega 6 foods seeds, nuts, fruits, and berries, grow in particular areas and territories. Land which produced high Omega Six sources was valuable, and essential for breeding, to the individual, and the group or tribe. To defend territory when there was sufficient food to settle, or occupy a 'grazing' range would require more aggression, and bigger stature, etc.

Aggression is linked to testosterone and low levels of serotonin.[590] Testosterone production requires Omega Six based chemicals. Serotonin requires Omega Three, and is reduced by high Omega Six. Aggression is linked with predation, defence, and acquisition of females.

Good Omega 6 territory would attract males. Good territory for both sexes, reduces the need for cooperation and encourages, selfishness, acquisitiveness, propensity to gather, and impulsiveness. Omega Six produces behavioural characteristics that optimised the likelihood of holding onto high Omega Six producing territory. Hunter gatherers may have migrated between marine and land environments on a seasonal basis, as is reported in Aboriginal peoples.

If you lived by the shore, mud flats, or inter-tidal area, and Omega 3 was plentiful in shore-based food, cooperation would have conferred a greater survival advantage, than aggressive defence.

Behaviour at a water hole, or bears feeding on salmon are examples of recognition that in some instances, territorial defence is not always the best option. The sharing of marine/fresh watershore resources would be consistent with the higher Omega Threes available in food sources downgrading aggression, and upgrading the female attributes of cooperation.

28.2   The behavioural impact–In a world where excess Omega Six is predominant, we are seeing increasing aggression, selfishness, greater acquisitiveness, less cooperation, impulsiveness, lack of self-control, increase in stature, and hormonal behavioural issues.

The Omega Three Six content of the cell membrane, is dependent on levels of dietary intake. Omega Three and Omega Six must be obtained from external food sources.

Both the absolute, and relative, levels of consumption of Omega 3, and Omega 6, have the ability to modify behaviour, in significant and fundamental ways. In evolutionary terms, behaviour based on the availability and territorial nature of food supplies, would be a good survival strategy. Omega 6, and 3, are available in different amounts, and types, in different locations.

More Omega 6 and less Omega 3 DHA in food sources would lead to more aggression in the men of the society. Aggression has been linked with lack of serotonin. Serotonin deficiency links with low levels of EPA, and DHA. [591] Lower DHA and higher Omega 6 upgrades the production of arachidonic acid AA, and so testosterone. [592] Testosterone reduces serotonin. Aggression is linked with high testosterone and low serotonin. [6.8]

Higher DHA from marine sources would lead to more cooperative behaviour. DHA is associated with the more feminine virtues, lower aggression, more cooperation, better communication, lower impulsiveness.

A society with better access to marine food would have a higher DHA intake. More DHA would lead to sounder sleep. Melatonin production requires and increases DHA and serotonin. Better food availability with more DHA would lead to, less aggression, ability to settle, more cooperation and sharing of resources, and a more settled organised society. Different Omega 3 and 6 food balances would shape different types of behaviour and societies.

28.3 Environmental fecundity and population control—A pregnancy unlikely to result in a successful outcome, placing a parent at risk of death, is not a good survival strategy. It is an evolutionary or design advantage to have a control system to limit breeding, based on environmental conditions.

We were designed or evolved from a simpler beginning. Even now, with all our technological advances, humans on a global basis have not intelligently, and cooperatively, found a mechanism to limit population, to take account of available resources. Nature has mechanisms to limit population to resources.

Omega Six arguably provides the core fertility and behavioural control mechanism. Humans have at least temporarily bypassed the natural population control mechanism, by agricultural production of high Omega Six sources. Omega Three and Six control many aspects of the human body, including, structural elements, hormones, steroids, chemical messengers, long and short-term fuel reserves, and storage regulators.

Omega Three, and Six, are the raw materials for two of the most fundamental families of chemicals in the body, the eicosanoids. [20 Carbon long chemicals Fig 1.19] The eicosanoid pathways are crucial to many functions, including the immune function, levels of cellular oxidation, tissue breakdown and repair, fertility, fat storage, sleep, and the reproductive cycle.

As a hunter gatherer, Omega 3 intake balanced with Omega 6 unless you lived by water, with more constant, and higher access to Omega Three. High Omega Six would be available to both groups only in the fruiting season.

The scarcer and more environmentally dependent resource for humans is Omega Six. Omega Six controls the reproductive pathways. Omega Six controls steroid and hormone production, including androgens and oestrogens.

The weather ultimately regulates land based plants setting seed, and reproducing. Seeds and nuts are the primary land based source of high levels of Omega Six. This makes Omega Six the land based Master-controller. The oceans were less weather sensitive, a more stable environment, and food source, than the land. Life in the oceans is skewed to Omega Three. Omega Three underlies everything, and relates to humans being essentially female at their core, reflecting our likely ocean origins. Omega 3 is the Mistress. Omega 6 the master.

28.4 **Primary regulator and precursor of hormones** – Hormones, and steroids, are produced from cholesterol. Cholesterol is a fat, and is used as a structural element in the cell membranes. PGE2 is a product of Omega 6. PGE2 with P450 controls many of the enzymes, which make the hormones and steroids, from cholesterol.

Omega Six up-regulates oestrogen, and testosterone. DHA down-regulates them, by counter balancing the production of Omega Six. Omega Six chemicals are required to allow production of hormones, and steroids. Once the body has sufficient stores of Omega Six, it can breed. As the body's Omega Three–Six balances shift to Omega Six, the breeding pressure would increase. Hormone levels would rise.

There is a dance between the eicosanoid derivatives of Omega Three and Omega Six. Increases in Omega Six derivatives light the fires, and Omega Three damps them down. This is achieved by creating self-regulating cycles between the Omega Six and Omega Three families. Push up the creation of DHA and EPA, or AA, and you push up the delivery of the Omega Three or Omega Six eicosanoid 20 carbon family [Fig 1.19] chemicals. For instance, higher levels of AA, through the prostaglandin PGE2, and aromatase P450 push up oestrogen and testosterone. [593] On the other hand oestrogen pushes up DHA/EPA. DHA/EPA down-regulates the production of AA, so pushing oestrogen back down.

28.5 **The Cycle is broken** – *The body was designed to work in a world, where the Omega 3 and 6 mother fats are in balance, within reasonable amounts subject to seasonal variation. If there is large excess of Omega 6, the system breaks down, and Omega 3 is unable to balance Omega 6 based processes.*

The cycle is broken. The monthly fertility cycle does not close down properly. The body becomes confused, trapped by low DHA, and high hormone levels, leading to system breakdown. PCOS is an example of the consequence of failure to properly close the monthly cycle. This problem is compounded as the body expects Omega 3 supply to equal, or exceed 6, except for limited periods.

The body is not equipped to deal with large long running excess, of Omega Six, over Omega Three.

Low intakes of the mother Omega 3, and DHA / EPA sources, with blockage of the conversion pathways, are compounding the imbalance caused by excess Omega 6. The body does not work off a recipe book; the quantities of fat used for chemicals are strictly in proportions to what is in the store, the cell membrane.

The body cannot tell a 20 carbon Omega 3, from a 20 carbon Omega 6. The amounts of Omega 6, and 3, available in the cell membranes, rather than any plan, determine the chemicals made. The chemicals made influence the body's behaviour.

That is the point. Omega Six is the controller. Omega Three is a presumed 'constant'. The cell membranes and intracellular spaces, [including specialised cells like adipocytes (fat cells)] will contain a mix of ingested fats, elongated ingested fats, and fats made from scratch in the body. We are only concerned here with the Omega 3s and 6s, and the balance in the cell membranes.

The key fact is, unlike all other fats, the body cannot make Omega Threes and Sixes from scratch. It has to select from what is available, which reflects what has been ingested, or stored. Omega Three is oxidised in preference to Omega Six. Omega Six is actively stored. Very little Omega Three is stored.

The body actively stores Omega Six to build up sufficient reserves of Omega Six, and ensure a constant supply of the sex hormones, steroids, chemicals, and energy reserves, necessary to complete a successful pregnancy cycle.

The chemical cascades are simply based on the available Omega 3s, and 6s, stored in the cell membranes. With excess Omega 6, and lack of Omega 3 in the cell membranes, and the whole chemistry of the body is radically changed, to the point of operating outside design parameters.

28.6   **Fats, hormone regulation**–The balances of the Omega fats change through the menstrual cycle.[595] Ovarian function is subject to lipid availability.[597] Increased androgens in PCOS, are accepted at least in part as being due to fat levels.[598] The Omega 6 inflammatory chemicals are recognised as having a role regulating, ovulation, endometrial physiology, reproductive tract pathology, including dysmenorrhoea, endometriosis, menorrhagia, and cancer.[599][600]

There is no question that fats, reproduction, hormones, and steroids are inextricably linked, with very fundamental implications. In a trial the oestrogen estradiol, increased DHA 42 per cent, in male to female transsexuals. Testosterone reduced DHA by 22 per cent in female to male transsexuals.[594]

The hormones influence conversion of the mother Omega 3 and 6, to the long chain fats.[601][602] Excess Omega 6 LA suppresses conversion of Omega 3s.[603] Long chain fat conversion is lower in post-menopausal women.[604] Dietary fat content significantly alters the rates of conversion of fats.[605][606] Hormones are made in the adipose fat, as well as sex organs. Men with more fat have higher androgens.[596] Levels of hormones reflect the amount Omega 6 stored in fat.

28.7   **Women oestrogen and DHA**—The female fertility cycle is immensely complex. It is undeniable that Omega Three and Omega Six are key factors, in the control and operation of the fertility cycle. The hormones and fats are inextricably linked in a dance in time through the monthly cycle.

The Omega Three and Omega Six fat pathways, and the hormones, give rise to a series of self, and inter-regulating mechanisms. Exactly how it all fits together is not clear. It is clear a balance and adequate supply of Omega 3 and 6 is essential, to allow the delicate monthly dance of the fats pathways to happen.

I list below, some of the links between the fat pathways and hormones that I have seen. For me, as described above, they contain the possible ingredients of a control system for the monthly cycle, viewed from an Omega Three and Omega Six perspective. I suggest shapes in the mist and no more. This is a huge complex subject. It is a lifetime's of work on its own and the detail is largely beyond me.

28.8   Fat and hormones a dance in time–

- ➤ ALA   Linolenic acid the mother Omega Three 18:3 n3
- ➤ LA   Linoleic acid mother Omega Six 18:2 n6
- ➤ AA   Arachidonic acid long chain Omega Six 20:4 n6
- ➤ DHA   Docosahexaenoic acid long chain Omega Three 22:6 n3
- ➤ EPA   Eicosapentaenoic acid long chain Omega Three 20:5 n3
- ➤ PGE2   Prostaglandin–a chemical made from AA
- ➤ P450   Aromatase, a chemical that needs PGE2 to make it
- ➤ Estradiol   A form of oestrogen production, depends on aromatase P450

  ☞ **AA stimulates oestrogen production via PGE2**–The Omega Six matriarchal fat LA, is made into AA by elongation and desaturisation. AA is the raw materials used by the COX2 enzyme. COX2 gives rise to PGE2. PGE2 facilitates aromatase P450 which gives rise to estradiol, a key oestrogen in the reproductive cycle, and primary oestrogenic product of the ovary.[607] PGE2 supply in the uterus is increased by the supply of AA.[608] PGE2 also controls other key enzymes, in the chemical tree, in which cholesterol is converted to sex hormones and steroids. PGE2 has a very significant role in reproductive function and behaviour [See 23.11.b].

  ☞ **Estrogens stimulate the production of DHA**–"Estrogens cause higher DHA concentrations in women, than in men, by up regulating synthesis of DHA from vegetable precursors by desaturase 5.[609][610]" "The synthesis of AA and DHA from precursors may be enhanced through an oestrogen receptor-dependent pathway."[611] HRT significantly increased EPA and DHA.[612] A foetus needs high levels of DHA for the creation of the brain, eyes, and cell membranes generally. A baby is a DHA sponge. Absorption by a growing baby of the extra DHA, consequent on higher oestrogen, would stop DHA shutting down the Omega Six AA production. High AA would keep the hormones high. On the other hand, if there is no fertilisation, DHA would not be need to make a baby, build the womb lining, or placenta. With no fertilisation, DHA would rise shutting off AA, so significantly reducing hormone production, and closing the cycle.

☞ **Estrogens stimulate AA**–Oestrogen also stimulated AA and DGLA production. [613][614] Up-rating the desaturase 5 would increase both Omega Three and Omega Six products, subject to imbalances and blockages by excess Omega Six, sugar, trans fats, etc. Higher AA would stimulate hormone production, unless shutdown by higher DHA. The body would equate lack of DHA to successful fertilisation and usage of DHA for cell building, rather than a DHA shortage.

☞ **AA stimulates production of testosterone**–"AA alone stimulated testosterone production by increasing cAMP production, but the effects of other PUFAs alone were marginal" [615].

☞ **EPA, DHA inhibited testosterone**–"EPA and DHA inhibited gonadotropin-stimulated testosterone production in a dose-related manner." [616] DHA regulates estradiol and testosterone in pregnancy. "Oestrogen level during pregnancy may be regulated by dietary polyunsaturated fatty acids, and mediate their effects on foetal growth." [617] DHA reduced testosterone in Japanese men [I guess oestrogen too].

☞ **AA stimulates egg maturation**–In fish, AA, PGE2, or PGF (2alpha) induced egg maturation and were blocked by COX inhibitors. DHA and EPA slowed maturation [618].

☞ **Progesterone and AA**–AA affects progesterone [619] in ovine material. "Progesterone at concentrations of $10(-7)$M and $10(-8)$M inhibits release of [3H]–arachidonic acid from stimulated, perfused, endometrial cells. The effect is independent of the mechanism of stimulation. [620]" Progesterone rises at night. This would be consistent with close down of Omega 6 pathways by melatonin and DHA.

☞ **Testosterone**–Testosterone may inhibit Delta 5, Delta 6 and Delta 9 desaturase activities. "We concluded that testosterone modifies the fatty acid pattern of cultured Sertoli cells, and this hormone is involved in polyunsaturated fatty acid biosynthesis, modulating Delta 5 and Delta 6 desaturases activity. [621]" So if this is the case more widely, then testosterone is working in the opposite direction to oestrogen.

☞ **Estriol**–Estriol is made from estrone or estradiol. Levels increase very significantly in pregnancy. Obese women, produce more estriol than lean women do. Heavy prolonged cycles have been linked to elevated estriol and estrone. [622] No trials have been found on estriol and Omega 3 and 6 metabolisms. Estriol has profound effects on lipid metabolism [623].

Much is unknown. These systems are exceptionally complex and interlinked and very much beyond me. The above is only intended to demonstrate the complexity and extent of the links between reproductive pathways and fats.

29

OMEGA THREE, OMEGA SIX, AND 'WESTERN' CONDITIONS–OVERVIEW

29   **Omega Three, Omega Six, and 'western' conditions–Overview**–I am not a doctor. I am a person with no specialist knowledge. This book is not intended to be a substitute for medical advice.

I am not professing any expertise in any disease on this impressive list. I have simply noticed in hours of unconstrained wandering, that many of the 'western' conditions involve inflammation, and have common elements. I bring you a glimpse into the work of others from an Omega 3 : 6 perspective, gathered in a way I hope is thought provoking.

Trails suggest Omega 3 intake may assist in auto immune conditions generally. Some genetic conditions have been included, cystic fibrosis, sickle cell anaemia, and macular dystrophy, as supplementation has been shown to be of possible benefit. Autism whilst not a 'western' condition has been included as trials show some promise.

Trials with fish oil supplementation have included rheumatoid arthritis, Crohn's disease, ulcerative colitis, psoriasis, lupus erythematosus, multiple sclerosis and migraine headaches. Many of the placebo-controlled trials with fish oil showed significant benefit. [624][625]

Please find below a list of conditions that have responded to various extents, to Omega Three/DHA supplementation.

Omega Six is readily stored in body fats, and Omega Three is not. Omega 3s need taking on a regular consistent basis, BUT start having some effect quite quickly.

Short-term drops in Omega 6 intake will be compensated for from Omega 6 in fat stores, so you won't see changes in Omega 6 levels over night. Fat profile takes 2 years to change by half. Omega 3s, in contrast, are not stored significantly.

This section mainly deals with the Omega 3s, as trials are conducted using Omega 3s. Relatively few researchers look at Omega 6 alone, or when looking at Omega 3. I suspect it is very hard to 'sell' a trial, that has a 'negative' as a conclusion. It is difficult to envisage how you get a marketable, drug, or supplement product, from a recommendation of "do not eat so much Omega 6".

29.1   A growing global crisis–The most serious health issues are partially or wholly due to diet. The threat to global health of excess mother Omega 6 and lack of Omega 3 is significant. Edible oils are often high in Omega Six or have very little Omega 3. Global oil consumption is rising rapidly. [3.26, p.287].

The medical conditions affected by DHA, and fatty acids, are not minor. They include some of the most prevalent 'western' conditions. These are some historic figures I found. They are for the USA simply as because they were easier to find.

More than 64 million Americans, have heart disease of one sort or another, 38.5 per cent die of heart conditions, 50 million are hypertensive, and 11 million have type 2 diabetes. 7.2 per cent of postmenopausal women over 50 have osteoporosis, and 39.6 per cent have low bone mineral density. One-third of all cancer deaths are due to nutritional factors, including obesity. [626]

29.2   Growing recognition in the medical industry–The *Journal of Human Nutrition and Dietetics* said,

> **"Medical doctors ought to have a sound knowledge of nutrition, but it is clear that most do not.** [627]**"**

A Medscape doctor's continuing educational training module, 19th October 1995, included recognition that long chain Omega Threes, have a part to play in pregnancy, including gestational length and birth weight, pre-eclampsia, recurrent miscarriages, maternal depression, eyesight, heart disease, and mental conditions including depression, schizophrenia, and aggression.

An excellent book I have only found fairly recently *Omega 3 Fatty Acids in Clinical Nutrition* edited by Axel R Heller, S N Stehr, T Koch, looks at Omega 3 in clinical nutrition from a practical perspective. I humbly suggest this book is a definite recommended read for Medical Professionals, and particularly those involved in surgery and hospital management. It contains absolutely fascinating, and potentially very exciting, observations on the potential practical impacts of enteral and parenteral administration of Omega 3, on post operative patient care. Their results show significant reduction in ICU and hospital stay times.

> **"Supplementation with Omega-3 FA improves survival and accelerates recovery. These substantial effects were shown in different diseases to a variable extent".**

Conditions considered included peritonitis, abdominal sepsis, and trauma. Results noted included, reduction of complications, reduction of length of stay, and reduction of infections.

29. 3   **Autoimmune and inflammatory disease, general**–As set out in the overview, Omega Three and Omega Six are yin and yang, inflammatory and anti-inflammatory. Disturb their balance and you have a problem.

Most people have an excess of Omega Six over Three. Excess Omega Six tips the body's raw materials and chemical production gauges towards inflammation. Omega Threes are associated with lower pro-inflammatory markers, and higher anti-inflammatory markers [7.13];

☞ DHA and EPA, reduce the amount of long chain Omega Six fat, AA, made from the mother Omega Six fat LA, by blocking the conversion process, and *competing for the conversion enzyme desaturase 5*. So there is *less Omega 6 AA raw material made,* for conversion to Omega 6 chemicals by COX2, and more Omega 3 DHA and EPA fats produced.

☞ DHA and EPA, *block COX2 pathways* from making inflammatory chemicals from AA Omega Six, *and so the Omega Six oxidation cascade* [Ch. 22.], by competing for COX2 production line capacity, so making more DHA and EPA chemicals [286].

☞ DHA and EPA, produce chemicals called resolvins and protectins that *close down inflammatory reactions*.

☞ DHA and EPA, act through gene expression, to *reduce inflammatory immune response agents* such as IL6, and TNF-alpha.

☞ DHA is *essential to mitochondrial and peroxisomal oxidation*, for defence, and key high energy chemical reactions, E.g. iodine conversion

☞ DHA and EPA *alter cell function*, like calcium and electrical pathways.

☞ DHA and EPA *alter the physical characteristics*, fluidity organisation and fat contents of the cell membranes [1.36].

☞ DHA and EPA *link to melatonin production*. Melatonin controls sleep function in part by shut down of the inflammatory pathways.

Omega 3 may be beneficial in diseases that are characterised by active inflammation. [628] DHA and EPA have the most potent positive effect. Mechanisms are complex and multiple, and change may take time. Trials on inflammatory conditions with fish oil supplementation have shown benefit. [629] [630] [631] Men on six grams a day of DHA, increased DHA in blood from 2.3 to 7.4 wt. per cent, and decreased AA from 19.8 to 10.7 wt. per cent.

Omega 3 reduces inflammatory chemicals and agents like LTB4. Decreased Omega Six AA, also reduces inflammatory products, including IL6 and LTB4.

Coronary heart disease, major depression, ageing, cancer, arthritis, Crohn's disease, ulcerative colitis, lupus erythematosus, are diseases characterised by a high IL1, and the pro-inflammatory leukotriene LTB4.

Psoriasis, migraine, atherosclerosis, IgA nephropathy headaches, are also inflammatory conditions. [632] [633]

In the DHA supplemented men, prostaglandin PGE2, and leukotriene LTB4, production, in response to a stimulant fell by 60–75 per cent. [634]

DHA is a more effective COX2 blocker than a number of NSAIDS [Drugs used to block inflammatory pathways]. Usage of DHA and EPA, does not carry the same long list of side effects as NSAIDS. Inflammatory cytokines such as TNF alpha and IL1 are also downgraded by fish oil. In contrast it is suggested that NSAIDS increase TNF-alpha synthesis[i].

An article *Fish oil; what the prescriber needs to know* [www.pubmedcentral. nih.gov Article no 1526555] looks at supplementation from a doctors perspective. The article is about arthritis, but considers other conditions.

The article deals with common questions, dosages, side-effects etc. The article suggests, that for supplementation with EPA and DHA to be effective, dosage needs to be in the order of 2.7 grams combined. This concurs with a trial suggesting utilisation in women drops off at about 2 grams of DHA a day. Smaller doses may be effective, where Omega 6 intake and stores are low, which is not common in the West. Optimal intake recommendations for EPA and DHA vary from 300mg to 3500 mg [See preface *Fish Oil The Natural Anti-Inflammatory*].

As well as ensuring adequate long chain Omega Three intake, the aim is to balance the Omega Threes and Sixes, and replace excess Omega Six fats where necessary, with monosaturates, or saturates. Fat intake should be moderate.

29.4   **Acne vulgaris**–Acne is a big problem in the West. 79–95 per cent of the adolescent population are affected. 40–54 per cent of men and women over 25 are affected. Our skin is a barrier between the environment and us. Skin is made of cell membranes. Membranes are made of fats. Studies show rates of acne are much lower in other societies.

The qualities of the membrane is dependent on the fats it is built from. Chemicals used to defend the skin, are made from the fats in the membrane. For skin to function effectively, it must contain the correct fatty raw materials.

In Kitavia, Papua New Guinea, of 1,200 Kitavan subjects examined (including 300 aged 15–25 years), no case of grade 1 or grade 2 acne was observed. From 115 subjects in Ache, no case of active acne was observed. [635] A number of trials suggest acne may benefit from Omega Three/fish oil supplementation. [636]

Acne can be an indication of PCOS. [637] Fat elongation pathways may be blocked to such an extent, or functioning so poorly due to medical conditions or inherited factors, that for a few, Omega 6 AA deficit may also be an issue. Fish oil contains mainly Omega Threes, and some Omega Six AA depending on source.

You might like to discuss testing of lipids with your medical practitioner, and determine if there might be possible causes of blockages of lipid conversions.

---

i   Fish oil: what the prescriber needs to know Arthritis Res Ther. 2006; 8(1): 202. Leslie G Cleland Michael J James, and Susanna M Proudman Rheumatology Unit, Royal Adelaide Hospital, North Terrace, Adelaide, Australia.

29.5   **ADHD**–[Also see 24.6, 23.44] ADHD and behavioural problems, including aggression in children, are frequently reported in the media. In the U.S., (2002) it is believed that between three and five per cent of the population has ADHD. That is about 17 million people. It is primarily seen in males.

Depression, sleep issues, impulsiveness, allergies, and poor vision are reported as symptoms of ADHD, all of which relate to DHA. Fatty acid treatment for ADHD, was also noted to reduce asthma, eczema, and hives. A number of trials, suggest that ADHD is linked to the type of fats consumed.

Fatty acid composition of red blood cells in those with ADHD, differs from that of normal children. [638] Absence of DHA is reported as causing neural problems. Adequate DHA is essential to brain formation, and visual function (See Chapter on brain function 24).

The loss of Omega 3 DHA, and higher Omega 6 DPA in the brain and retina, are associated with loss of nervous system, neural, and visual, function. Lower levels of DHA link to vegetable oil consumption. Vegetable oils generally are high in Omega 6 [P.287]. High Omega 6 intake blocks Omega 3 conversion to DHA.

Improvements in mood, complex cortical processing, increased energy, reduced anger, reduced anxiety, hyperactivity, depression rates, brain function including neuroplasticity, and synaptic function, have been reported with increased Omega Three intake. [640] Omega Three supplementation reduces the Omega Six–Three ratios.

The addition of DHA to the infant diet has resulted in improved neural function, including visual acuity, cognitive, visual recognition, memory, and means-end problem-solving tests. [639]

Research has linked a number of genes involved in the fatty acid pathways with ADHD. Research also suggests that the fat pathways of Omega Six are disturbed and distorted, with more DPA Omega 6 in the brain, and less AD (adrenic acid AD 22:4 n6) and AA.

Low Omega Three, with disturbed Omega Six ratios, would be consistent with imbalance in supply, conversion and utilisation issues. This would be consistent with diets high in fat pathways conversion blockers, and low in Omega Threes [11.13]. Some may lack the ability to effectively convert the mother Omega 3 and 6 to the long chain fats for medical or genetic reasons.

ADHD is less evident in breast fed children, which raises issues as to formula AA and DHA content, which can be almost totally absent in some formula feeds. [25.33]. DHA and AA are essential to brain formation in babies [24.19-24.27] [23.24-24.30].

Dr. Jacqueline Stordy and Malcolm Nicholl reported, that just as many positive outcomes, are seen from fat supplementation, as Ritalin.

Dr. Jacqueline Stordy and Malcolm Nicholl wrote *The Remarkable Treatment for ADHD, Dyslexia and Dyspraxia*, which is a very useful specialist book on the subject, and the source of some of the above.

29.6   Age-related mental degeneration–Ageing brains have lower Omega Threes, and particularly DHA and EPA. A study suggests the Omega Threes help protect the brain from ageing. [641]

29.7   Allergies in babies–There have been a number of trials, linking allergic hypersensitivity conditions in children, to lower mother Omega 3 and long chain Omega 3 levels. There is controversy over the issue.

Mothers of allergic children had lower EPA and DHA. Breast milk reflected the fat levels in the mothers. [642] Formula feeds can be very low in EPA and DHA [25.33]. Atopic conditions did not relate to allergen exposure in the mother. [643]

A trial suggested, there is not strong evidence, to support avoidance of the common allergens, by the mother. Preliminary data suggests more Omega 3s may help protect against some childhood allergies. More trials are required. [644]

29.8   Alzheimer's–The long chain fats, are key, and fundamental, to brain function. Sixty per cent of the brain is made of fat. IF you have a DHA deficit, your brain cannot form or function properly. It is as simple as that (See Ch. 24).

There are a number of trials, suggesting a link between low DHA Omega Threes and Alzheimer's. Elderly subjects, and Alzheimer's sufferers, have lower DHA levels in the brain. [645] Omega Three deficits generally, and lower fish intake, have been associated with depression and Alzheimer's. [646]

DHA is suggested to be protective against amyloid production, accumulation, and toxicity. [647] DHA is reported as assisting brain function generally, and may reverse functional decline. [648] DHA can reduce levels of an enzyme linked to Alzheimer's disease [10.1523/JNEUROSCI.3593-07.2007].

DHA in the brain influences, dopamine and serotonin function, [6.8] signalling, reduction of Omega 6 inflammatory chemicals, protection of neural cells from death, cell membrane fluidity, and regulation of neuron size. [649] *In a trial involving 131 participants, those who consumed fish once a week or more, had a 60 per cent less risk of Alzheimer's.* [650]

29.9   Arthritis–(Greek artho = joint, itis = inflammation). Osteo and rheumatoid arthritis are inflammatory conditions. Trials suggest that Omega 3s, and particularly the long chain fats, may assist arthritis. [651 652 653 654]

DHA is a more effective COX2 blocker than a number of NSAIDS, drugs used to block the inflammatory pathways. DHA and EPA do not come with a long list of potential side effects. Inflammatory cytokines such as TNF alpha, and IL1, are also downgraded by fish oil.

In contrast it is suggested that NSAIDS increase TNF-alpha synthesis. TNF-alpha and IL1 are reported as being involved in cartilage degradation. Omega 3s reduce cartilage degradation.[ii] DHA and EPA also reduce bone loss.

---

ii   Fish oil: what the prescriber needs to know Arthritis Res Ther. 2006; 8(1): 202. Leslie G Cleland Michael J James, and Susanna M Proudman Rheumatology Unit, Royal Adelaide Hospital, North Terrace, Adelaide, Australia.

DHA and EPA also reduce pain, by blocking the inflammatory effects of the PGE2 pathway. Fish oil may alleviates symptoms of rheumatoid arthritis.

Conventional treatment has a very valuable role, and provides almost instant results, but should prevention, so far as possible, not be the starting point?

29.10   Atherosclerosis—Atherosclerosis is a chronic inflammatory response in the walls of the arteries. *Atherosclerosis is seen in the coronary arteries of 50 per cent of young humans between 10 and 14 years of age (late 1980s).* [655] A traditional Mediterranean diet, with Omega 3 supplementation, reduced deaths after a first myocardial infarction by 70 per cent (*Lancet* 1994; 343:1454–9).[656]

Omega Six high diets, have been linked to greater plaque formation in the arteries [See graph in preface]. Omega Three, and particularly DHA and EPA, prevent plaque build-up. EPA and DHA combined at about three grams a day, were noted to reduce plasma triacylglycerols, blood pressure, inflammation and platelet aggregation, and are associated with decreased cardiovascular death. [657]

29.11   Arrhythmia—Fatty acids, and particularly DHA, are essential to the electrical and mechanical function of the heart. In mice and marmosets taking fish oil, no deaths from arrhythmia were recorded. [658] [659]

Studies suggest a diet high in Omega Threes may prevent sudden cardiac death. [660] A diet high in Omega Six, causes mitochondrial damage, and cardiac dysfunction. [661] Trials suggest Omega 3 levels are a predictor of heart disease. [662]

DHA is critical to the function of the mitochondria. DHA is a critical component of cardiolipin, an essential fat, in the inner mitochondrial membrane. The mitochondrial membrane, is very sensitive to DHA in the diet. DHA alters the fluidity of the membranes, and modulates the calcium channels controlling the heart's electrical functions. [663]

29.12   Asthma—Asthma is an inflammatory-linked condition. It is also linked with allergic response. The number of asthma sufferers continues to rise, despite increasing numbers of treatment options.

A diet high in Omega Six, and low in Omega Threes, sets the scene for inflammation in the body. Omega Six pro-inflammatory chemicals are made from long chain AA. Other inflammatory chemicals are also made in response to high AA. Omega 3:6 ratios in the West of 20–25:1[664] have been noted.

Fish oil (Omega Three PUFA) supplementation reduces airway hyper-responsiveness and pro-inflammatory factors [665] after exercise, and medication use. Concentrations of markers [LTB4, LTC4–LTE4, PGD2, IL1beta, and TNF-alpha] were lower before and after exercise, where fish oil is in the diet.

A mother's nutritional status, may put the infant at higher risk of asthma, through breast milk fat deficits. [666] Fats in breast milk reflect the mother Omega 3 and 6 fat intake, long chain fat intake, and the conversion ability to make long chain fats. Consumption of fish links to lower airway hyperreactivity among children and better lung function in adults. [667] [See 25.33 re formula milk].

29.13 **Atopic eczema**—Skin is made of cells. Cell membranes are made largely of fats. The shapes and types of fats in the cell membranes, determine the cell wall characteristics and function, flexibility, porosity etc. It also determines how the skin cells react to invaders or threats.

The Omega Three mother fat is essential to skin function. Omega Threes are oxidised before Omega Sixes. When fats are oxidised, the by-products are used to make the defence weapons, and chemicals, necessary to skin function. Imbalance in the cell membranes results in structural stress, change in permeability, and immune response. [668]

Improved Omega Three intake may play a role in allergies (Atopic conditions). Trials suggest low levels of Omega Three may link to atopic conditions. Atopy was made worse by saturated fats [which and how much ?], low levels of PUFAs, and higher AA. [669]

29.14 **Autism**—Autism is not a 'western' condition, in the sense of having a recognised connection through inflammation, although some are proposing links to inflammation and oxidative stress. [670]

An adequate, balanced fat supply is essential to the immune function, as it to brain function. (See chapter 24 on the brain) Long chain fats are generally essential to brain function and structure.

A number of trials have reported possible benefits from fat supplementation in Autism. A trial looking at aberrant behaviour (which includes tantrums, aggression and self-injury) suggested that Omega Threes might assist with autism. [671] Other trials suggested autistic children had higher levels of Omega Sixes and DHA and low EPA, and looked at supplementing with high EPA fish oils. [672] As usual, it is a case of more research required.

29.15 **Bipolar disorder**—A paper looking at Omega 3 intake globally, claimed a very strong inverse link between bipolar disorder, and Omega 3 intake, 99.9 per cent. [673] However, trials using Omega Threes have had mixed results.

Longer-term studies in animals, suggest Omega Three deprivation, does increase the AA COX2 based chemical cascades. Anti-manic agents seek to control AA COX2 based activity. [674] So, increasing Omega Threes and reducing Omega Sixes, may assist treatments.[iii]

The difference between the trials, and the statistical population overview, may be that fat reserves have long-term impact, and changing the fat composition of the brain is a slow process. Many trials fail to account for Omega 6 intake or Omega 6 fat reserves, and some use low doses of Omega 3 for short time frames, or use the mother Omega 3 ALA which may be subject to conversion blockages.

---

iii   Addition of Omega−3 Fatty Acid to Maintenance Medication Treatment for Recurrent Unipolar Depressive Disorder Boris Nemets, M.D., Ziva Stahl, Sc. and R. H. Belmaker, M.D. Am J Psychiatry 159:477−479, March 2002 © 2002 American Psychiatric Association.

29.16   **Bone density**–Bone density BMD connects to the inflammatory and hormonal Omega Six pathways, and fat content in the bone. High levels of Omega Six, and low Omega Three, are associated with lower BMD at the hip in both sexes. The relative balance of Omega Three and Sixes, appears to play a vital role in preserving skeletal integrity in older age. [675] (See also Osteoporosis)

29.17   **Brain disorders**–[See ch. 24.] The brain is more than 60 per cent fat. The structural materials, the bricks of the brain cells, are fats. Fats are released from the membrane cell walls, to make brain operating chemicals, and used as messengers. Fats control cell membrane physical and electrical properties [1.36]. Neuropsychiatric and neurodegenerative diseases, link to decreased Omega 3 PUFA. [676] [See Alzheimers]

Higher Omega 3s are associated with better brain function into old age. [680] Higher Omega Three counters amyloid production seen in Alzheimer's. [681]

DHA is a key fat for visual function, cognitive function, receptor activities, gene expression, chemical cascades, energy metabolism, mitochondrial function, and neurotransmitter mechanisms.

Astrocytes grown with DHA, functioned better, and were very sensitive to Omega 3/6 balances. [678] Lack of Omega Three is associated with abnormalities of cerebral structure, particularly the frontal cortex and pituitary gland.

The sense of smell, vision, and taste, are dependent on adequate brain function, and loss of taste has been linked to high Omega Six. [679] Lack of DHA leads to impaired brain and eye function. [677]

In gliomas and tumours, DHA was reduced and the Omega Six mother fat and AA [682] [683] increased, compared with 'normal' brains. [684]

The brain can make long chain fats from the mother fats, but largely relies on conversion by the liver to supply long chain fats. The Omega Three and Omega Six mother fats, can only be got from food. The body can turn the mother fats into long chain children DHA, EPA, AA, etc., but cannot make the mother fats.

It is equally essential, to reduce mother Omega 6s, to a point of near balance, with mother Omega 3 intake, remove conversion blockers, and ensure a supply of long chain fats. Brains in wild animals all have a 1:1 Omega 3:6 ratio.

29.18   **Breast cancer**–Mechanisms of breast cancer are recognised as being multiple, various, and complex. Trials suggest, the risk of breast cancer, is lowered by reduction of Omega Six intake, and increased Omega Threes, including both the mother fats and long chain children. [685] [686] [687]

Put another way, high levels of Omega Six and low Omega Three, may be contributing to breast cancer risk. A trial linking lump excisions, to breast fat make-up, showed women with the highest levels of long chain Omega Threes in the breast fat, had a 70 per cent less chance of the excised lumps being invasive.

A number of possible mechanisms have been identified, including reduction of inflammatory factors, moderation of new vessel growth, impact on the hormone pathways, function of lipid rafts, mitochondrial function, etc.

Trials suggest that reduction of inflammation factors by blocking the COX2 pathways, has a potential therapeutic role. [688] COX2 products are made from Omega Six AA. Reduction in long-term supply of AA, should reduce the availability of COX2 products. PGE2 aromatase is key to controlling oestrogen levels. [689] PGE2 is a product of AA. AA is a product of Omega Six [p. 286].

Lower long-term AA levels may moderate PGE2 production, and so control oestrogen levels. [690] [691] DHA/EPA also reduces the amount of AA products produced, and has a more immediate effect, than reducing Omega Six intake.

The tissue degrading products, MMPs, which are key to inflammation and tumour invasion, are also reported to be moderated by Omega Three. [692] Melatonin also links, to DHA, the hormone pathways, and breast cancer. [27.3]

A consequence of oestrogen blockers, or ovarian removal, may be that the increased levels of DHA conversion, caused by higher oestrogen in women, will not occur. IF conversion is already poor, this may further increase DHA deficiency in women on oestrogen blocking strategies. It appears low DHA /Omega 3s are a risk factor, in breast cancer and other cancers.

This would make it sensible that women receiving anti-oestrogen treatments, consider their Omega 3:6 profile, in consultation with their medical advisors, and look at long chain Omega 3 supplementation, and the wider risks and benefits. A trial demonstrated that 10 grams a day [About 2 tps.] of fish oil with a low fat diet, produced a significant change in fat profiles of both circulating plasma and breast fat tissues.[iv]

29.19 **Cancer**–Imbalances in Omega Threes and Sixes, and lack of ALA, EPA, and DHA, have been linked in trials, to a number of cancers, including breast, prostate, melanoma, lung, and ovarian.

In a multinational European case control study, in four of five cases, the ratio of Omega 3 to 6 was inversely associated with breast cancer [693] (Higher n3, less breast cancer). Risk differentials for women with high DHA in breast tissue biopsies, have been reported as 70 per cent lower, than those with low DHA. [694]

Omega 3 and 6 influence inflammatory factors, hormone levels, membrane structure, oxidative potential, energy availability, antioxidant availability, etc. Balancing Omega 3 and 6, may reduce risks, for some cancers.

29.20 **Cardio-vascular conditions in children and adults**– Increasing obesity in children, is accompanied by diseases only previously seen in adults. It is a cause of significant concern. Low Omega 3, and high Omega 6, may be factors. [695] [696] Trials in children and adults have shown that DHA may help. [699]

---

iv   Dietary modulation of omega-3/omega-6 polyunsaturated fatty acid ratios in patients with breast cancer D Bagga, S Capone, HJ Wang, D Heber, M Lill, L Chap and JA Glaspy Department of Medicine, School of Medicine, University of California at Los Angeles, 90095-6956, USA.

"Overweight and obesity in children and adolescents should no longer be regarded as variations of normality, but as diseases with an extremely high risk for the development of atherosclerosis and cardiovascular complications in adulthood. Knowledge of these complex associations implicate even the young in the need for intervention". [697]

"Cardiovascular risk factors were frequently present in a large collective of overweight European children and adolescents. They occurred mostly independently of age, gender, and degree of overweight. Therefore, screening for cardiovascular risk factors seems meaningful at any age and degree of overweight in childhood". [698]

"These new epidemics in chronic health conditions among children and youth will translate into major demands on public health and welfare in upcoming decades" [James Perrin, MD, of the Center for Child and Adolescent Health Policy, Mass General Hospital for Children.]

29.21   **Cataracts**–Cataracts have been linked to general factors of ageing, including oxidative stress. Lipid consumption could have a part to play. Limited trials were found, one positive and one leaving a question. More trials are required. Higher Omega Threes were suggested as reducing the five-year risk of cataracts [700].

29.22   **Crohn's disease–IBS**–Poor digestion = poor health. Inflammation links to poor digestion. IBS is an inflammatory condition. Inflamed guts produce mucus, which stops digestion, by preventing contact between the food and cells [25.40-25.43]. Poor digestion has fundamental long-term impact.

No matter how good the food you eat, if your digestion is not working well it is wasted. It is key you absorb those foods supplied in limited quantities like Omega 3s. Omega 3 may be digested direct in the small intestine.

Changes are so gradual, that they are viewed as 'normal'. Remember, the easy, solid stool of youth. If you no longer have them, your digestion is compromised. Excess Omega 6 creates a permanent low-level all-body inflammation alert.

Adequate Omega 3 (mother and long chain) improves IBS. [701][702] A high level of PGE2 [Omega 6 product] may exacerbate the inflammatory process[v]. Food allergy may worsen the situation. Medical treatments include anti-inflammatory and immune suppressors which block downstream Omega 6 activity.

Balancing the mother Omega Three and Six, and ensuing supplies of the long chain fats, should assist in reducing digestive issues, by reducing inflammatory pressures. My own experience is they do. Stored fats are a long-term source of Omega Six so this is a long-term project. More trials are needed.

---

v   The proinflammatory effect of prostaglandin E2 in experimental inflammatory bowel disease is mediated through the IL–23––>IL–17 axis. J Immunol. 2007 Jun 15;178(12):8138–47 Sheibanie AF, Yen JH, Khayrullina T, Emig F, Zhang M, Tuma R, Ganea D. Department of Physiology, Temple University School of Medicine, 3420 North Broad Street, Philadelphia, PA 19140, USA.

29.23 Colon cancer—Colon cancer is a disease of the West. It is the second leading cause of cancer death in the U.S.. Levels may reach as high as 10 per cent of the population.

There have been a significant number of trials looking at DHA, Omega 3, and colon cancer. Omega 3 appears to reduce the risk of colon cancer. Higher Omega 3, and lower Omega 6, have been shown to be beneficial. [703]

Fibre has been implicated in colon cancer but results of fibre trials are mixed. A combination of fibre and fish oil [704] has been shown to be beneficial. [705]

29.24 Chronic obstructive pulmonary disease—COPD is the fifth-leading cause of death worldwide. COPD is an inflammatory condition. Omega Three, is suggested as a safe and practical method of treating COPD. [706] LTB4, TNF alpha, IL8 levels were reduced with Omega Three supplementation. Dietary change must be discussed with your doctor.

29.25 Chronic fatigue–(CFS)–The severity of chronic fatigue, aches, pains, and failing memory, were correlated to LA, AA, and oleic acid levels. Results of a trial suggested that patients with CFS should respond positively to treatment with Omega Threes including DHA and EPA. [707]

29.26 Cystic fibrosis—This is a hereditary and not a 'western' condition. It has been included, as research suggests, a lipid metabolism element. There are a number of trials suggesting potential positive impacts from Omega Three supplementation.

Given the difficulty of treatment, and the importance of nutrition, lipid testing might be a worthwhile area of investigation. As usual, more trials are required. Long-term EPA plus DHA supplementation (eight months), has been shown to reduce inflammation, in cystic fibrosis. [708]

29.27 Dementia—Higher levels of DHA are associated with a 50 per cent reduction in dementia risk, based on the Framingham Heart Study. [709]

29.28 Depression—Readers interested in this section may like to read chapter 24 on brain function. Long chain Omega Three and Omega Six balance is key to brain function. [710] [711] [712] Lack of Omega Three [713] and excess Omega Six leads to the use of an Omega Six substitute, DPA, that simply does not work as well. There are a large number of trials on DHA and depression.

Several trials suggest DHA and/or EPA may improve depression. [714] [715] Depression is linked with high AA and low EPA [716] and a low ratio of Omega Three to Omega Six. [717] It is better predicted by levels in adipose tissue than blood serum, which underlines the importance of stored fats in body function.

New Zealand had an annual depression rate of 5.8 per cent (40 lbs. fish a year), Korea 2.3 per cent (100 lbs. + fish a year) and Japan 0.12 per cent (150 lbs. fish a year). [718] Patients with major depressive disorder exhibit lower levels of DHA in the orbitofrontal cortex. [719] Further trials are required.

29.29   **Diabetes Type 1**—Type 1 diabetes is one of the most common chronic childhood illnesses affecting 18—20 children per 100,000. Increasing rates, and diversity of incidence, give it the hallmark of a 'western' condition.

Rates in Europe, are increasing at three to four per cent annually, and most commonly in 0—4 year old children. [720]

A Finish child is almost 40 times more likely to develop type 1 diabetes than a Japanese child, and almost 100 times more likely than a child from Zunyi, China. Finland is reported as having very high incidence of heart disease.

The Japanese, in general terms, are reported as having a lower incidence of 'western' conditions. As always, it is only being suggested that fat management is on the average, a risk reduction strategy, and not a panacea.

It is believed that the genetic susceptibility is not a prime factor. Diet, environmental factors, and viral infections, are considered possible factors.

Omega Threes may reduce the risk of type 1 diabetes. A trial in September 2007, by Jill M Norris of the University of Colorado suggested a 55 per cent risk reduction, in diabetes type 1 occurrence in high risk children [a diabetes type 1, parent or high risk typing] with higher consumption of Omega Three fatty fish.[vi]

Omega 6, and inflammatory factors, may increase the risk.[721] Elevated inflammation markers, including CRP, are seen before the onset of type 1 diabetes, and may prove a risk marker. [722] CRP, an inflammatory marker, features in many conditions [7.13]. A search on NCBI for CRP produced 13,000 entries.

A degradation of the fat conversion mechanisms has been noted in type 1 diabetes. [723] [724] Lower long chain fats, have been suggested as explaining the lower cognitive performance, in type 1 diabetes patients. (See Chapter 23).

29.30   **Diabetes type 2**—Diabetes is a metabolic disorder. There is an inheritance pattern for the condition. Care must be taken, in assuming genetic inheritance, being the sole inheritance factor.

Environmental inheritance, in terms of diet, etc., could also be a big factor. Fats certainly play a part in diabetes. Altered levels of fatty acids, and fatty acid metabolic disturbances, are regularly seen in diabetics. Relative to other fats in diabetics Omega Six AA levels are high.

Here, we have the common thread to many of these conditions. Higher AA levels, low Omega 3, and poor conversion, puts the body into a low-level inflammatory state. AA has significant influence in controlling activity of fat cells.

INTERESTINGLY IN ANIMALS, REMOVAL OF THE MOTHER OMEGA 6 FROM THE DIET, PREVENTS DIABETES.

---

vi   JAMA. 2007 Sep 26;298 (12):1420—8 17895458 Omega—3 polyunsaturated fatty acid intake and islet autoimmunity in children at increased risk for type 1 diabetes. Jill M Norris, Xiang Yin, Molly M Lamb, Katherine Barriga, Jennifer Seifert, Michelle Hoffman, Heather D Orton, Anna E Barón, Michael Clare-Salzler, H Peter Chase, Nancy J Szabo, Henry Erlich, George S Eisenbarth, Marian Rewers.

Essential fatty acid (EFA) deficiency, has a striking protective effect, in several animal models of auto-immune disease [725] presumably due to lack of Omega 6.

DHA encourages oxidation of fats. Omega 3s are oxidised in preference to Omega 6s. Storage, oxidation and obesity are intimately linked in diabetes. [726]

Omega Threes are potential anti-diabetes agents. [727] Consistent with other groups with Omega Three deficiency, and excess Omega Six, diabetics have a higher rate of heart disease, [728] and lower neural and visual function. A trial in India showed a very striking straight-line relationship between diabetes and Omega Six intake.

29.31   Dyslexia and dyspraxia—Reports suggest that improved Omega 3, and AA, profile has a part in dyslexia, dyspraxia, and ADHD [29.5, 24.6]. Many ADHD symptoms are common to Omega Three deficiencies. These include sleep deficiency, rough dry skin and hair, soft or brittle nails, cracked skin, etc. [729]

29.32   Dry eye syndrome—(DES)—Fats are used as lubricants. A higher dietary intake of Omega Threes, is associated with a decreased incidence of DES in women. These findings, are consistent with anecdotal clinical observations, and suggested biological mechanisms [29.58]. [730]

29.33   Eye conditions—DHA makes up a very high proportion of the rods in the retina membrane. The shape, position, and number of double bonds, give DHA unique, electrochemical, and mechanical properties. [See 29.42 macular degeneration] DHA may 'only' be a fat but it is hugely influential.

DHA related chemical mechanisms in the eye, include eicosanoids, angiogenic factors, matrix metalloproteinase [MMPs], reactive oxygen species [ROS], cyclic nucleotides, neurotransmitters and neuromodulators, pro-inflammatory and immunoregulatory cytokines, and inflammatory AA products.

Eyes require adequate DHA to function properly. If there is insufficient DHA, the body uses Omega Six DPA, with only five double bonds in different positions, instead of six. It is very much a second rate substitute.

There is consistent evidence, that Omega Three long chain children (EPA, DHA, etc.), are protective against ischemia, light, oxygen, inflammatory, and age-associated damage of the vascular and neural retina. [731] [732]

29.34   Fertility—Female—(See chapter 23 on female issues, and chapter 28). As explained in the introductory chapters, Omega Six is nature's fertility controller of humans. The Omega Six long chain fat, AA, is used to make a whole family of 20 long carbon chemicals [Page 286, Fig 1.19]. These Omega Six chemicals, and particularly PGE2, control enzyme production, which indirectly controls oestrogen, androgen, and steroid production [23.11b].

Excess Omega Six in body fat, combined with low Omega Three intake, results in imbalances, and failure to properly shut down the menstrual cycle. Inflammation is a key part of cell creation, destruction, and repair. High stored Omega Six puts the body into a permanent state of low-level inflammation.

The combination of hormone imbalances, low-level inflammation, and DHA shortages, means the monthly cycle may not shutdown properly. Several studies show fats impact on fertility. In sheep it altered sizes and numbers follicles, progesterone, and length of gestation. [733] The Omega 3:6 mix in cell membranes, and adipose fat, is fundamental to the monthly cycle, and fertility. [23.11a]

29.35 **Fertility–Male**–DHA is a key fat in sperm. DHA is almost the only Omega Three in sperm. DHA levels rise greatly in sperm at the onset of puberty. In monkey sperm, DHA content was 24 per cent of total fatty acid. DHA is an important element of various lipids in sperm. [734] In human trials, EPA 810 mg, and DHA 2100 mg, increased sperm count, DHA weight, and quality. [735] DHA high sperm swim better and straighter in animal trials. [736] [23.17]

29.36 **Glaucoma**–Patients with glaucoma, had reduced EPA, DHA, and Omega Three fats. [737] Patients supplemented with DHA, vitamin E, and B complex, showed improvement in Glaucoma. [738]

29.37 **Gums gingivitis**–A number of trials suggest Omega Threes may assist in maintaining bone, following gingivitis. [739] Periodontal disease, is associated with obesity, and cardiovascular disease. [740] Cardiovascular disease and obesity are inflammatory conditions.

Gingival tissues had higher levels of AA, DPA, and the mother Omega Six, LA. [741][742] In rats fed a high Omega Three diet, compared to a high Omega Six diet, AA was reduced by 56 per cent, and PGE2 by about 80 per cent. [743] Omega Three fatty acid, significantly reduced the gingival tissue levels, and inflammatory factors [E.g. PGE2, LTB4], in experimental periodontitis. [744]

29.38 **Heart disease**–A report said 64 million-plus Americans, have one or more types of cardiovascular disease (CVD), which accounts for 38.5 per cent of all deaths. Patients with heart disease, had consistently and significantly reduced DHA. Omega Threes are viewed as cardioprotective. [745] Omega Threes from fish oil, are rapidly incorporated, at the expense of AA in heart fats. [746]

Omega 3 in prescription form has been approved for high triglyceride levels. [747] Cardiac societies, recommend using one g/day of EPA and DHA, for cardiovascular prevention, after a myocardial infarction, and for prevention of sudden cardiac death. [748][749] The Omega 3 index, compares very favourably with other risk factor identifiers, for sudden cardiac death [750][vii] [See graph preface]. "Pericardial administration of n-3 PUFAs could represent a novel approach to treating or preventing myocardial infarctions.[viii]"

---

vii Omega3 Fatty acids for cardioprotection. - Mayo Clin Proc. 2008 Mar;83(3): 324-32.- Lee JH, O'Keefe JH, Lavie CJ, Marchioli R, Harris WS. - Kansas City, MO

viii Pericardial Delivery of Omega-3 Fatty Acid: A Novel Approach to Reducing Myocardial Infarct Sizes and Arrhythmias. - Am J Physiol Heart Circ Physiol. 2008 Mar 7 - Xiao YF, Sigg DC, Ujhelyi MR, Wilhelm JJ, Richardson ES, Iaizzo PA. - Medtronic Inc.

29.39 Kidney—The eicosanoids, are the chemical families generated from Omega Three and Omega Six. When not properly controlled, trials suggest they can play a significant part contributing to vascular injury, and end stage renal disease. [751] Omega Threes may be protective.

29.40 Liver fibrosis—Liver fibrosis is a common and rising problem in society. More alcohol, and falling Omega 3 consumption are factors. Trials on animals, suggest the effect of alcohol, is exacerbated by a lack of Omega 3s.

In two groups of monkeys taking identical amounts of alcohol, the group with adequate Omega Three intake, developed no liver lesions, while the deficient group developed fibrotic lesions. [752] The risk of liver lesions is increased where Omega Three / polyunsaturates intake is low. [753] [1.30]

Adequate Omega Three consumption, may offer some protection, against some potentially damaging effects of alcohol consumption. This simple observation, may help explain the increasing levels of liver disease, in the young.

29.41 Lung cancer—Trials suggest that increased Omega 3s, and balancing the Omega 3s and 6s, reduces the invasion potential of lung cancer. [754]

A 78-yr-old man with malignant fibrous histiocytoma, with multiple lesions in both lungs, declined conventional chemotherapy, and elected for nutritional intervention under medical supervision increasing intake of Omega 3, and lowering intake of Omega 6. Serial computed tomography scans, and pulmonary x-rays, revealed remarkably, a slow and steady very significant decrease, in the size and number of bilateral nodules. [755]

Oleic acid OA, and DHA, significantly inhibited lung metastasis in the lab. [756] In mice, a combination of EPA and DHA markedly decreased tumour growth (45 per cent), reduced AA content by 50 per cent, and increased EPA/DHA 3–5 fold. Interestingly, prostaglandin E2 levels were reduced by a factor of 7.4. [757]

Lupus—Please see 29.62.

29.42 Macular degeneration—Macular degeneration, is the main cause of vision loss and blindness in Americans aged 65 and older. In 2004, it was estimated 1.75 million U.S. residents suffered symptoms. Numbers are expected to rise to three million by 2020. [758] Macular degeneration is considered to be caused at least in part by oxidative damage.

The retina has one of the highest rates of metabolism and oxygen utilisation in the body.[ix] Adequate blood supply is very important.

Omega 6 is less effectively oxidised than Omega 3 in the mitochondria, and peroxisomes. Does oxidation of Omega 6 produce damaging oxidants [21.3].

Excess Omega Six may contribute to greater oxidative stress, poor circulation, and disturbed sleep. DHA is key to retinal function, and forms a high proportion of the fats in the retina.

---

ix   Environmental Stressors in Health and Disease. Jurgen Fuchs and Lester Packer.

There is consistent evidence suggesting Omega 3s, may act in a protective way against damage to the retina. [759] Photoreceptors and synaptic membranes, have the highest levels of DHA of all membranes. Photoreceptor membranes contain 60 per cent DHA. The higher the DHA, the higher the visual sensitivity.

When DHA is lacking, it leads to use of Omega 6 DPA as a substitute. DPA is a second rate substitute, and simply does not function as well. [760]

DHA is a key factor, in eye health. DHA supports cell membranes in the lens, retinal receptors, nerve fibres, conjunctiva, and retinal blood vessels. [761]

29.43 Macular dystrophy–This is an inherited condition, but a study suggests that dietary factors can influence the severity of the condition. Low levels of DHA, and EPA, in red blood cells, correlate to the severity of the condition. [762]

29.44 Melanoma–There are a number of trials on DHA, and melanoma, several as an adjunct to treatment. Malignant melanoma is dramatically increasing, in light-colour skinned people around the world. U.K. rates have risen by 43 per cent in 10 years. Omega 6 consumption is increasing. Omega 3 consumption is falling. Treatment prognosis is reported as poor. Epidemiological studies, and experimental data, suggest Omega 6s stimulate, and Omega 3s inhibit development and progression of a range of human cancers, including melanoma. DHA inhibits growth of cultured melanoma cells. [763] AA and Omega 6, increased invasiveness, and DHA and EPA, inhibited invasion in brain-metastatic melanoma. [764] ALA, the mother Omega Three, reduces UVB skin damage.

29.45 Multiple sclerosis–MS, is categorised in the auto-immune inflammatory category, and so may be amenable to Omega 3 intake, and reduction in Omega 6[765] MS patients show significant reductions in EPA and low DHA. [766]

29.46 Osteoporosis–See chapter [23.48] [25.30].

29.47 Polycystic ovary syndrome–See chapter [23.46].

29.48 Postnatal depression–See chapter [23.35].

29.49 Pre-eclampsia–See chapter [23.34].

29.50 Prostate cancer–Prostate cancer is one of the most commonly diagnosed U.S. conditions. As many as half of all men of 70 years and older in the U.S., have latent prostate tumours, according to figures cited in Campbell's *The China Study*. In the U.K., it represents 23 per cent of all cancers in men, and 31,900 were diagnosed in 2003. The rate is increasing. [767] Evidence suggests high Omega 6 increases prostate cancer (PCa) risk, and Omega 3 decreases risk. [768]

Fish oil, is linked with a reduced rate of prostate cancer [769]. Improved Omega 3:6 ratio, may reduce the 'bad' metabolites, and slow down or even inhibit the risk of prostate cancer. [770] Prostate cells in the lab, proliferate more vigorously, when AA was provided. [771] PGE2 levels rise within five minutes of the addition of AA.

29.51 **Psoriasis** – Psoriasis is another condition that connects to inflammation. It is suggested it may have a genetic component. Trials suggest, increased Omega Three intake, may help moderate the inflammatory response, and treatment of chronic plaque-type psoriasis.[773][774][775] Patients respond far more effectively, to fish oil intravenous infusion, by orders of magnitude, over oral supplementation.[776]

29.52 **Obesity** – See chapter 25.

29.53 **Reproductive** – See chapter 23.

29.54 **Sepsis** – Sepsis is a whole-body inflammatory state. Sepsis and septic shock are major causes of death in intensive care, at rates of 30 to 60 per cent.

The Omega 3:6 balance, impacts on the balance between pro- and anti-inflammatory cytokines and inflammatory factors. For views on Omega 3 and 6 and sepsis see *Omega 3 Fatty Acids in Clinical Nutrition* edited by Axel R Heller, S N Stehr, T Koch.

Oral supplementation needs to be long-term. Intravenous, or enteral supply of fish oil produced significant reductions in infectious complications, and septic events. Intravenous provision in patients with skin disease, and bowel disease, showed rapid changes in the membrane constitution.[777]

Systemic inflammation, and sepsis, are accompanied by severe metabolic alterations. Orogastric DHA, may protect the nutritional status of neonates with sepsis.[778] Omega 3 appears to have beneficial effects on cellular immunity and helps prevent hyper-inflammatory complications.[779]

Increased mortality with sepsis, is associated with Omega 6. Fish oil protected against increases of TBX2 and PGF1 in sepsis.[780] Omega 3 infusion pre or post abdominal surgery, may reduce post-operative infection.[781][782]

29.55 **Sickle cell** – Sickle cell is a genetic disorder. It has been included as supplementation was reported to be of possible benefit. Sickle cell patients, show a 40 to 50 per cent reduction in the proportion of total Omega 3 fatty acids. Administration of Omega Threes, has been shown to reduce anaemia, and confer clinical benefit, to sickle cell patients.[783][784]

29.56 **Schizophrenia – see chapter on brain function** – Levels of EPA, and DHA were significantly lower in schizophrenic patients.[785] Studies suggest Omega Three may support treatments for schizophrenia.[786] Patients with schizophrenia exhibited lower levels of DHA in the orbitofrontal cortex.[787]

29.57 **Sinusitis** – Patients with asthma, and allergic rhinitis may benefit from hydration and a diet low in sodium, Omega Six, and trans fatty acids, but high in Omega Three, onions, fruits, and vegetables.[788]

"Cod liver oil and a multivitamin-mineral with selenium, as adjunctive therapy for children with chronic/recurrent sinusitis, is an inexpensive, non-invasive intervention that clinicians can use for selected patients, pending the performance of definitive, large, well-controlled studies."[789]

29.58 **Sjogren's syndrome**—See also dry eye syndrome above [29.32]—Sjogren's syndrome is an auto-immune condition. It is commonly associated with rheumatoid disorders. The condition is associated with low DHA levels. Trials suggest supplementation with Omega Three, and reduction of Omega Six, may help alleviate the condition. [790] [791]

29.59 **Skin ageing**—EPA is a potential agent for the prevention of skin ageing. "In conclusion, our results demonstrate that EPA can inhibit UV-induced MMP-1 expression . . .Therefore, EPA is a potential agent for the prevention and treatment of skin ageing". [792] Omega 3s reduce damage from UV [See 29.44].

29.60 **Suicide**—Lower DHA and higher Omega Three:Six ratios were predictive of suicidal behaviour in depressed patients over a two-year period. [793] Low DHA is associated with major depression. A trial in Belgium linked seasonal variation in Omega Three intake to depression and suicide. The trials link both depression and suicide to serotonin disorders. [794] DHA is necessary for serotonin production. In China, comparing 100 people who attempted suicide, to control patients, showed those who attempted suicide, had much lower EPA levels. The quartile with the highest EPA was eight times less likely to attempt suicide, than the quartile with the lowest EPA. [795]

29.61 **Zellweger's syndrome**—(Inherited Condition) DHA deficiency, could be a contributing factor, to lack of development of cognitive and visual function, in peroxisomal disorders. [796] [797]

29.62 **Lupus**—I apologise that Lupus is at the end. I realised at the very last moment there was no section for it. Trials suggest Omega 3 helps. To finish, some quotes, with many thanks to the authors;

"Many of the placebo-controlled trials of fish oil in chronic inflammatory diseases reveal significant benefit, including decreased disease activity and a lowered use of anti-inflammatory drugs." [x]

"Therefore, the use of n-3 fatty acids can be recommended to the general healthy population, not only to prevent atherosclerosis but possibly also to reduce the risk of autoimmunity." [xi]

---

[x]   Omega-3 fatty acids in inflammation and autoimmune diseases.- J Am Coll Nutr. 2002 Dec;21(6):495-505. - Simopoulos AP. -The Center for Genetics, Nutrition and Health, Washington, DC 20009, USA

[xi] n-3 fatty acids and the immune system in autoimmunity. -Isr Med Assoc J. 2002 Jan;4(1):34-8. - Ergas D, Eilat E, Mendlovic S, Sthoeger ZM. - Department of Internal Medicine B, Kaplan Medical Center, Rehovot, Israel.

TERMINOLOGY

30.1 Adipokines–Adipokines are cytokines. Cytokines are signalling compounds. They are involved heavily in immune function, and activate, and are activated by the steroids.

Adipokines are produced from the fat tissue, as against other organs [but not directly from Omega 3 and 6]. The quantities produced appear to relate to the amount of fat carried. Omega 3 and 6 change gene expression, and lipid raft activity, which change protein production. Cytokines are proteins.

It is suggested the Omega Three–Six balance can indirectly control the levels of cytokines. Observations would suggest they do, as Omega Three appears to reduce several inflammatory factors including Il6 and IL8. It is complex.

30.2 Arachidonic Acid AA–20:4 n6– Arachidonic acid is a member of the Omega Six family. It is 20 carbons long. It has four double bonds. It is a very influential fat. AA is the only raw material for the Omega 6 eicosanoid 20 carbon COX2 inflammatory chemicals, and related downstream products.

The Omega 3 equivalent raw material is EPA [30.14]. AA is made from the mother Omega Six, by adding carbons, and double bonds. AA is found in limited quantities in some animal-based foods, but not in vegetable matter.

High levels of arachidonic acid AA are linked with inflammatory conditions. High arachidonic acid levels, are a consequence of high Omega Six intake.

30.3 Alpha Linolenic acid ALA–18:3 n3 Alpha linolenic acid is the mother fat of the Omega Three family. It is made in the chloroplasts in green plants from the mother Omega Six. Animals eat green plants, and turn the mother fat into the long chain children. Animals and humans are unable to make the mother Omega Three. It is 18 carbons long, with three double bonds. ALA is found in high quantities, in a relatively small list of foods. High ALA sources include flax and perilla.

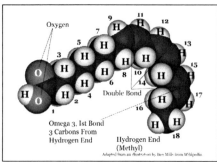

Fig. 30.3 Linolenic Acid Omega 3. The Carbon Has a Bend at Each Double Bond.

30.4   **Cis fats**–'Cis' describes the position of the double bonds in a carbon chain. A carbon has four attachment points. They are called 'bonds'. A carbon can link to another carbon, with one or two attachment points, 'bonds'.

A carbon must use all four attachment points. When a carbon atom forms a link to its neighbour, using two of these four bonds, it is called a double bond. The two spares of the four links, when a double bond is formed, can either be adjacent to each other, or opposite.

If the spare links are adjacent to each other, the bond is called a Cis bond. Cis bonds produce a noticeable kink in the carbon chain. Trans bonds produce a carbon chain that is more or less straight. The shape of the carbon chains is important for a number of reasons.

The shape dictates how well the carbon fits, and interacts to other compounds. The shapes also dictate how neatly the fats are ordered in the cell membranes. The neatness of the fats in the membrane [Figs 30.27] determines its properties, rigidity, permeability, electrical function, etc. More chaotic membranes are more permeable and flexible.

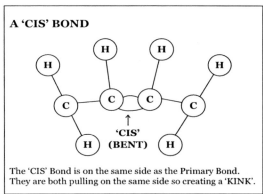

A 'CIS' BOND

'CIS' (BENT)

The 'CIS' Bond is on the same side as the Primary Bond. They are both pulling on the same side so creating a 'KINK'.

Fig. 30.4 CIS Bonds give Fats the same shape as saturated Fats.

30.5   **COX1**– COX1 is an enzyme. COX1 products are not shown on the chart p.286 for clarity. COX1 controls a second Omega Six based family of chemicals, made from DGLA. COX1 competes with COX 2 for DGLA. Blockage of the conversion will prevent DGLA being made. Some plants supply GLA.

The products of the COX1 pathway primarily maintain body function, rather than responding to 'situations' by inflammatory response, as COX2 does. It is always present in cells, at the same concentration, unlike COX2 which responds on a call out basis. Melatonin [Ch. 27] blocks COX2 at night, but not COX1.

30.6   **COX2**– [See COX1] [See chart Page 286 'Making the Children from the Mother Fat'] COX2 [cyclooxygenase] is a very important enzyme. COX2 makes the Omega Six and Three based families of chemicals. The exclusive Omega Six raw material is AA, arachidonic acid. COX2 converts AA to the prostaglandins. These chemicals include PGE2, PGI2, and PGH2.

PGE2 indirectly controls the levels of the sex hormones, and steroids. Many inflammatory chemicals are made in the COX2 pathways [Fig.1.19]. COX blockers NSAIDs are drugs that block onward conversion of AA. NSAIDs can work on both or either the COX1 or COX2 pathways. NSAIDs have a number of side effects.

Pain is a result of inflammation. Aspirin is a NSAID, a COX blocker.

A reduction of Omega 6 in the diet and stored body fat, with the balancing of Omega 3 and 6 intake, will reduce Omega 6 chemical COX2 products over time, reducing need for NSAIDs.

The COX2 enzyme also makes the Omega 3 family of chemicals. Omega 3 products of COX2, connect more with long term repair. Less Omega 3 COX2 than Omega 6 COX2 is made. [*Fish, Omega-3 and Human Health* Lands]

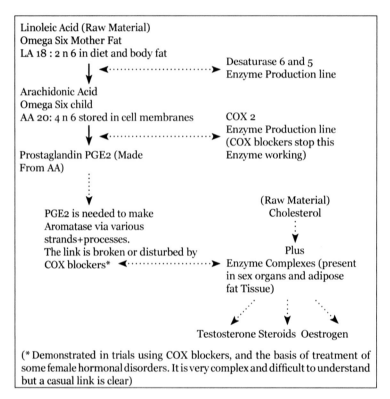

Linoleic Acid (Raw Material)
Omega Six Mother Fat
LA 18 : 2 n 6 in diet and body fat

Desaturase 6 and 5
Enzyme Production line

Arachidonic Acid
Omega Six child
AA 20: 4 n 6 stored in cell membranes

COX 2
Enzyme Production line
(COX blockers stop this
Enzyme working)

Prostaglandin PGE2 (Made
From AA)

PGE2 is needed to make
Aromatase via various
strands+processes.
The link is broken or disturbed by
COX blockers*

(Raw Material)
Cholesterol

Plus
Enzyme Complexes (present
in sex organs and adipose
fat Tissue)

Testosterone Steroids Oestrogen

(* Demonstrated in trials using COX blockers, and the basis of treatment of some female hormonal disorders. It is very complex and difficult to understand but a casual link is clear)

Fig. 30.6 The amount of Sex Hormones Produced Depends on the Balance of Omega Six, and Three, and Consequent Levels of PGE2 and COX2 Products.

Omega 3 and 6, compete for the COX2 production line. This competition for resources keeps the system in balance. For the body to work properly, there has to be a balance of Omega 3 and 6 mother fats. Shortage of either causes a problem. The COX2 products are very influential in the body's biology.

30.7   Cytokines—(See also adipokines)—Cytokines are small secreted proteins, with important roles, in innate, and adaptive immune responses [Ch.22] They are chemical messengers in the defence against inflammatory and infectious diseases, and have a part in baby making.

They signal that a problem, or need, exists, to draw other agents into the area. Omega 3 and 6 levels, significantly alter production of some inflammatory cytokines. Cytokines are not direct products of Omega 3 and Omega 6.

Omega 3, and 6, work through mechanisms such as gene expression alteration, and lipid raft manipulation, to communicate with cytokines. It is complex, and I have great difficulty in understand how it all fits.

I simply seek to communicate that these mechanisms exist. Omega 3 and Omega 6 influence cytokine levels, and so immune and inflammatory responses, through the balances of Omega 3 and 6 in the cell membranes.

30.8   Desaturase—A desaturase is an enzyme, that removes two hydrogen from an organic compound. This is part of the process of the creation of a carbon to carbon double bond. There are a number of different desaturases.

The desaturase work on different bonds in the chain. Desaturase are used in the making of longer carbon chains. Omega 3 and 6 compete for the use of desaturase 5 and 6. There is a limited supply of desaturase.

30.9   Docosanoids—Docosanoids are chemical children of Omega Three and Six family, made from fats [E.g. DHA] that are 22 carbons long.

30.10   DHA—22:6 n3—Docosahexaenoic acid is the long chain Omega Three, DHA. It is 22 carbons long. It has six double bonds. The first double bond is found three carbons from the hydrogen [methyl] end.

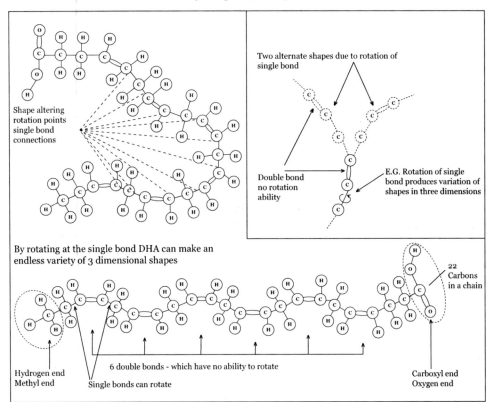

Fig. 30.10   DHA 22:6 n3 Docosahexaenoic Acid, Structure and Shapes.

It gets confusing. Most numbering describing where double bonds sit in the chain of fats is by reference to the oxygen end (carboxyl). But the family identifiers of fats, the Omega 3, 6, 7, and 9s, are described by counting back, to the first double bond, from the hydrogen end. (Methyl).

DHA is a unique and fundamental fat. There is no Omega Six equivalent. Six double bonds give DHA a particular and unique shape making ability. The nearest Omega Six, DPA, has five, and not six double bonds.

Omega 6 DPA is a poor substitute. It has one less double bond to make shapes. Single bonds are capable of rotation, DHA is capable of forming a huge number of shapes. Now imagine the joints of DHA are in constant motion at very high speed - a crazy articulated hyperactive worm.

DHA is used in the structure of cell membranes, and as a raw material for day-to-day production of chemicals required by the body. DHA is used at high levels in the brain, eyes, and reproductive organs. If adequate DHA is not supplied, the function of the brain, eyes, and reproductive organs is seriously degraded. Low levels of DHA, are connected with a wide range of conditions.

30.11 Double Bonds and shape—Much is not known about life in the cell membrane. The general impression is that these molecules are fixed in shape. However some suggest, that they are very flexible and in constant motion within the membrane. Single bonds can rotate, double bonds cannot. The bend at a double bonds creates a 'cranked' motion. Then an infinite variety of shapes is possible as the links are rotated at the cranks produced by the double bonds.

Susan Allport, described fats in the membrane, as more like dancers at a rave. For me this question was clarified in a Web lecture, by William L. Smith, Ph.D., Professor and Chairman of Biochemistry, Michigan State. [www.efaeducation.nih.gov] This fascinating short video. http://videocast.nih.gov/ram/crii01c303202000.ram examines how reactions occur in the cell membrane.

The shapes of the molecules, are based on x-ray viewing.

For a chemical reaction to take place, the fat must fit very precisely into a defined space. Imagine a ruler 5 cm long, split into 7 joined segments [Fig 30.10]. Imagine bending it to a shape, to fit in between a random fixed pile of dried spaghetti. A DHA ruler with one less link like DPA may not fit. Shapes are important in determining if chemical reactions happen.

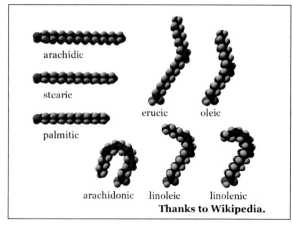

arachidic

stearic

palmitic

erucic   oleic

arachidonic   linoleic   linolenic

Thanks to Wikipedia.

Fig. 30.11 A selection of fats which demonstrates the variety of shapes that they form

30.12 **Eicosanoids**—Eicosanoids are chemical children of the Omega Three and Six family, made from fats that are 20 carbons long [E.g. EPA and AA].

30.13 **Elongase**—Elongase, is an enzyme used by the body, to add carbons to make carbon chains longer. Elongase works in conjunction with desaturase.

Shorter fats are turned into longer fats, for instance, ALA mother Omega 3, 18 carbons long, is turned to DHA that is 22 carbons long, by a series of steps adding carbon bonds. The process can be reversed to shorten chains too. Omega 3 and 6 compete for the elongase enzyme.

30.14 **EPA—20:5 n3**—Eicosapentaenoic acid is an essential fatty acid, 20 carbons long, with five double bonds. EPA is the Omega 3 equivalent of AA.

EPA is made from the mother Omega 3 ALA. Omega 3 mother fat ALA competes with Omega Six LA, for the desaturase 5 and 6 enzyme production lines, which allows EPA to be made in steps, from the mother fat ALA [p.286].

EPA is the unique raw material used to make the Omega 3 family of 20 carbon long chemicals, eicosanoids. EPA competes with Omega 6 AA, for access to the COX2 enzyme production line. COX2, is used by both Omega 3, and Omega 6. By competing for the production lines, EPA counteracts the Omega 6 AA pathways. EPA slows the processes to make AA Omega 6 products five of more times.

Oxidation in the Omega 6 chemical production cascade pathways, takes place more furiously and faster, than Omega 3 reactions in the Omega 3 pathways which need more energy [Lands *Fish, Omega-3 and Human Health*]. Would restraining Omega 6 chemical cascades reduce unwanted oxidation?

EPA importantly reduces inflammatory Omega Six pathway activity, by keeping COX2 busy, reducing conversion of AA onward to Omega 6 chemicals. The Omega 3 chemicals are less aggressive and connected more with repair.

Some EPA is found in the membranes, but the body uses EPA mainly for day-to-day activities rather than cell structure. EPA has the same chain length as AA. The body when taking AA, or EPA, from the membrane, cannot tell them apart.

The body is indifferent, if AA, or EPA, is collected from the cell membrane. The body simply takes as many units of fat as are needed, and puts them into the production processes. The fats get processed by defined production lines into defined products. The products are controllers of function and behaviour.

30.15 **Essential fatty acids EFA**—Essential fatty acids are also known as EFAs. The EFAs are fundamental to health and life. The body cannot make the mother EFAs, Omega Three and Omega Six. They must be obtained from diet.

The body can make daughter EFAs [AA DHA EPA etc.], provided it has the raw materials in the form of the mother fats, and the conversion pathways are not blocked. The long chain EFAs in food, are only found in animal sources.

No Omega 3s and 6s in your diet, and you do not have them in your system.

30.16 **Fat**—Fats are carbon chains. A carbon atom has four bonds. The bonds are equally spaced on the surface of the carbon. They form up as carbon daisy chains. Just add carbon and hydrogen, in the daisy chain, to make longer fats.

The ends stay the same. At one end is a carbon, with three hydrogen attached, the methyl group. At the other, there is always a carbon with two oxygen and a hydrogen, the acid carboxyl group.

This is acetic acid (vinegar) the simplest 'fat', if defined by structure, although it is only with three carbons in the chain, that you first see fat like qualities. So acetic acid looks like a fat but does not behave like one. (Does the ability of vinegar, to turn fat into an emulsion, give it a special synergy with fats, and particular properties?) The word fat is used to describe a wide family, and includes fats joined together, for example a triglyceride [30.38]. Fats usually do not mix with water. They can be solid, or liquid, at room temperature. Fats often have a greasy feel.

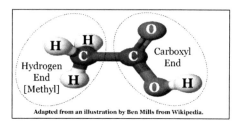

Adapted from an illustration by Ben Mills from Wikipedia.

Fig. 30.16 Acetic Acid has the Chemical but not Physical Characteristics of A Fat.

31.17 **Hydrogenation**—Hydrogenation, is a manufacturing process removing one of the bonds in a double bonds [30.11] to make a single bond, by adding hydrogen. Refining, may "remove" more naturally reactive Omega 3s, by partial hydrogenation, in the sense of making a fat the body may not recognise.

Hydrogenation, turns an unsaturated fat, saturated, or partially saturated. Partial saturation, changing only some of the double bonds, and full saturation, changes the shape of fats, and alters interaction with other chemicals. Unfamiliar fats to the body may be created. In addition some single cis [30.6] bonds may have their shape changed to become trans bonds [30.37].

The body likely has no established processing facility for these new fats. Hydrogenation of fats, changes the shape, fluidity, and properties of the cell membranes [1.36]. Partial hydrogenation, links to heart and circulatory disease.

30.18 **IL6 is a cytokine**—Interleukin 6, [IL6] is a signalling agent. It is an inflammatory marker, involved in many conditions, including fever and response to foreign pathogens, diabetes, heart disease, obesity, and depression.

The fat matrix produces a significant portion of the body's IL6. Other organs can produce IL6 as well. IL6 levels link to Omega Six and Omega Three [See adipokines and cytokines]. IL6 is one of a big family of interleukins. IL17 is the highest I have seen reference to.

Each IL has a family of its own. It is frighteningly, wondrously, vastly complexly subtle, and interlinked. Each IL is a subject on its own. Look up IL17 on Wikipedia, and you will see what I mean. I do not understand most of it. The point is the mechanisms dependent on, and related, to fats are wondrously complex interlinked and influential.

30.19 **Interestification**—Food manufacturers are replacing hydrogenated fats with interesterified fats. Interesterified fats can be used to prolong shelf life. Interesterification can also be used to change the physical properties of fat. A liquid fat at room temperature, is chemically altered into a semi-solid, or solid for use in the food industry.

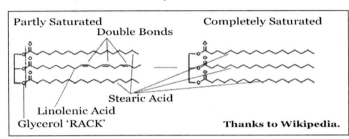

Partly Saturated
Double Bonds
Completely Saturated
Stearic Acid
Linolenic Acid
Glycerol 'RACK'
Thanks to Wikipedia.

Fig.30.19 Interestification of a Triglyceride, Linolenic acid is removed and replaced by Stearic Acid so saturating the Triglyceride

One leg of the triglyceride is removed, and a polyunsaturated fat replaced with a saturated fat. In the diagram above are two triglycerides. A triglyceride is a chemical comprising three fats. The fats looks like crinkle cut chips.

The 'E' shaped bit is a glycerol, and is the rack that holds the fats. The triglyceride on the left, has the mother Omega Three linolenic acid, as its middle leg. On the right, the mother Omega Three linolenic acid has been removed, and has been replaced with stearic acid.

Linolenic acid has three double bonds, stearic acid has no double bonds. The result is more solid, and has a longer shelf life. There are questions as to the health impact of these products. Interesterified fats may not be as easily metabolised, or may have adverse consequences in the body. Like trans fats, history will probably tell if they have a wider health implication. The jury is 'out' at the moment.

I am puzzled why the industry does not use traditional vegetable and animal fats, if it needs more solid fats with a longer life for baking. If the point, is to swop non-saturated fats, for artificially saturated fats, why not simply use naturally more saturated fats in the first place?

30.20 **LA Linoleic Acid**—18:2 n6 linoleic acid the mother Omega Six, is an 18 long carbon chain with two double bonds. The first double bond starts at the sixth carbon from the hydrogen end, so it is called an Omega 6.

It is found in all greens plants. We and other animals cannot make it in our body. Omega Six, 18:2 n6, can only be got from diet. Seeds nuts and grains are high in linoleic acid.

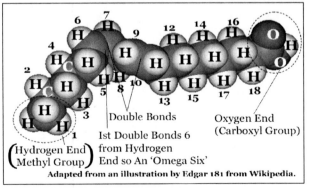

Double Bonds
Oxygen End
(Carboxyl Group)
Ist Double Bonds 6 from Hydrogen End so An 'Omega Six'
Hydrogen End
Methyl Group
Adapted from an illustration by Edgar 181 from Wikipedia.

Fig. 30.20 Linoleic Acid – Mother Omega 6 has two double bonds. The first double bond in all the Omega Six fats is six from the Methyl end.

Before agriculture, access to high levels of Omega Six would have been seasonal. There would have been competition for high Omega Six food sources. Now the Omega Six fat from vegetable oils [p287] is everywhere.

In the last 200 years, intake of linoleic acid has increased considerably, and continues to increase. [3.26]. Excess mother Omega 6 fat, the consequent excess AA [30.2], and inflammatory chemicals, is arguably a basis for ill health. [See also 30.3]

30.21   LTC4–[p286] A chemical made from Omega Six fat AA. LTC4 stimulates mucus production in the lung, and produces contraction of some muscles.

30.22   LTD4–[p286] A chemical made from the Omega Six fat AA. LTD4 increases vascular permeability, and stimulates muscles.

30.23   LTB4–[P286] A chemical made from the Omega Six fat AA. It is involved in inflammatory reactions in the body. It is regarded as a measure of inflammation. There is also a series 5 LTB that relates to the Omega Threes.

30.24   Lipid Raft–Fats in the membrane attach to a mix of chemicals. The mix of chemicals and fats, gives cell membranes their properties. Chemicals and fats gang up in units. Changing the fat mix changes the cell membrane properties.

Some rafts will specialise, just like in an ordinary factory. Imagine the cell membrane is the factory. Within a factory, you have engine fitters, maintenance men, press operators, etc. The body cells have specialist production units called lipid rafts. Each specialist unit will produce and do different things with different raw materials, and send out different protein signals and activity information.

Lipid rafts are too small to image. They are ordered and sober in behaviour. They contain more trans and saturated fats, and cholesterol. They like to stay away from the disorganised zany high energy DHA gangs. Think formal cocktails for saturates, and carnival for DHA, each in its own cell membrane space. [1.36]

This is an image of from Wikipedia. Do I understand much of its implication? No! Does it help give an idea what a membrane might look like? Yes! Does it give an idea as to how complicated the body and all this is? Yes!

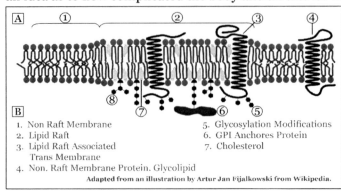

Fig. 30.24 Cell Membrane – Lipid Raft - Note the Fats in The Membrane are Different Lengths, the Fats in the Raft are Longer.

1. Non Raft Membrane
2. Lipid Raft
3. Lipid Raft Associated Trans Membrane
4. Non. Raft Membrane Protein. Glycolipid
5. Glycosylation Modifications
6. GPI Anchores Protein
7. Cholesterol

Adapted from an illustration by Artur Jan Fijalkowski from Wikipedia.

30.25 LCPUFA—LCPUFA is an acronym for Long Chain Polyunsaturated Fatty Acid. LCPUFA refers in general terms to unsaturated carbon chains, of 20 or longer.

30.26 Lipoxins—Lipoxins, LOX are chemical products of AA, the Omega Six fat [p286]. Lipoxins are also made from the Omega Three EPA. They play an important part in inflammatory reactions and body processes.

30.27 Membranes—A wonder of nature and a subject on its own. Cells are tiny wondrous mini worlds. The outer wall of a cell is a twin-layered bubble. The composition of the outer wall, is not necessarily the same as the inner wall. The bubble walls are made largely of fats. One of those fats is cholesterol. Cholesterol is the raw material for the sex hormones and steroids.

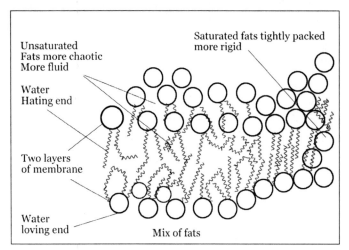

Unsaturated Fats more chaotic More fluid

Saturated fats tightly packed more rigid

Water Hating end

Two layers of membrane

Water loving end

Mix of fats

Fig. 30.27(a) The Fats are in constant motion. Saturated fats pack more tightly and make a more rigid membrane. Unsaturated fats are more loosely packed.

The fats are held in pairs. The chemical that clips the fats in pairs, likes water. The tails of the fats don't like water. Fats form a pair of layers, water loving parts facing outwards, and water hating parts facing inwards.

The membrane wall, allows chemicals, and supplies, to pass in and out of the cells. The type of fats determines the properties of the membrane. Membranes contains proteins, carbohydrates, protein channels, and a wide range of other wonderful things, as shown in the diagram from Wikipedia [See next page].

The fats in the membrane are not permanent they come and go. The fats 'magic bricks,' are used as the raw materials for the membrane and for a host of chemicals, including the inflammatory Omega Six chemicals.

The cell walls, reflect your dietary intake of Omega Threes and Sixes, and fat store content. When the membrane fats are used for chemical reactions, the body is indifferent if the fat is an Omega Three or Omega Six, provided it is the desired carbon chain length [E.g. a 20 or 22 long carbon chain].

The balance of Omega Six, and Threes, influences other processes less directly through gene expression, lipid rafts, fluidity, porosity of the membrane, and electrical function. The balance of Omega 3 and 6 fats you eat, control the balances of chemical reactions in your body.

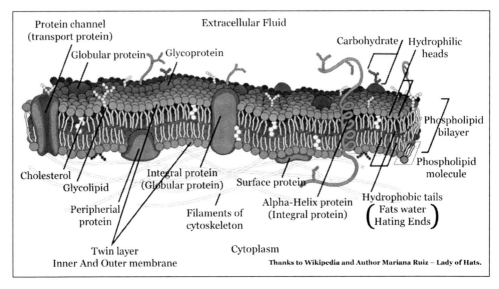

Fig. 30.27(b)   Detailed Diagram of Cell Membrane

30.28 **Mitochondria**—Mitochondria are the body's power plants, furnaces fat fabricators, and miraculous mini chemical factories. Mitochondrial function, is essential to health, at the most fundamental level.

They have their own DNA, and are in effect symbiotes. The inner membrane of the mitochondria, is very sensitive to levels of DHA, and LA, in the diet. DHA is much more effectively utilised as a fuel than LA. DHA changes the characteristics of the membrane.

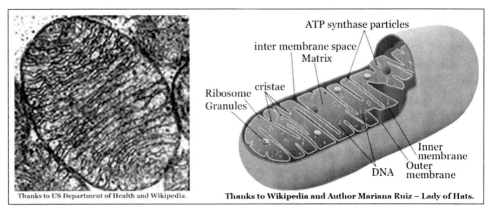

Fig. 30.28(a) Image of Mitochondrion

Fig. 30.28(b) A Diagram of the Mitochondrial Cell part of our complex wondrous inner world

DHA produces much greater levels of oxidation products, but does DHA produce a 'cleaner burn'? The function of the mitochondria is very dependent on the balance of supply of the Omega 3 and 6 fats, and particularly DHA.

30.29 **Monosaturate MUFA**—A mono saturated fat has one double bond in the chain, the rest of the bonds are single.

The bond is normally a Cis bond [30.4] and so the fat will have a bend in it. An example is Oleic acid 18:1 n9, which makes up about 70 per cent of the fats in olive oil. Mono saturates are less sensitive to heat than polyunsaturates. They are therefore more stable when used for cooking. A trans mono saturate would be straight and not kinked, as a trans double bond has no bend

30.30 **Myristic acid**—Myristic acid was named after nutmeg. It is 14 carbons long and saturated. Saturated fats are more rigid, and have their own properties. As it has no double bonds it is nearly a straight line in shape.

Saturated fat are incorporated into the cell membranes, where they perform particular functions. When it is realised, that these saturated fats have particular

uses in the body, it raises questions, as to why we harbour such prejudice against them.

Eaten in excess, they are a problem, but in the right amount, they are essential to the body's functions, and are made by the body.

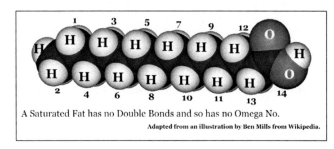

A Saturated Fat has no Double Bonds and so has no Omega No.

Adapted from an illustration by Ben Mills from Wikipedia.

Fig. 30.30 Myristic Acid–A Saturated Fat with 14 Carbons

30.31 **Omega Three**—The Omega 3s are a family. The mother fat is alpha linol**enic** acid, ALA [5.2]. The family is made by adding more carbons and double bonds. The first double bond is three from the hydrogen end [Fig 30.10].

Well-known Omega 3s include DHA and EPA. Omega 3s are called essential fatty acids, because they are fundamental to the body's structure, function, reproduction, metabolism, brain function, and general health

The Omega 3 mother fat can only be got from diet. It cannot be made in the body.

The body can make the long chain Omega 3 children, from the raw material the mother fat, ALA, if conversion pathways are not blocked.

The Omega 3s moderate the effect of the Omega 6s. Omega 3s have one more double bond than Omega 6s, which is 3 carbons closer to the end of the chain.

Omega 3 intake in the West, is falling. Omega 3s are less chemically stable than Omega 6s. The food industry tries to breed low Omega 3 grains and oils and remove the Omega 3s, by hydrogenation and esterification. We feed livestock with grain, which is high in Omega Six and increases their Omega Six levels.

These factors worsen already falling Omega 3 intakes. DHA in breast milk in the West is much lower than in the East.

The Omega Three family includes, with thanks to Wikipedia:

Common name		Lipid name	Chemical name
α-Linolenic acid	ALA	18:3 (n−3)	Octadeca−9, 12, 15−trienoic acid
Stearidonic acid		18:4 (n−3)	Octadeca−6, 9, 12, 15−tetraenoic acid
Eicosatetraenoic acid		20:4 (n−3)	Eicosa−8, 11, 14, 17−tetraenoic acid
Eicosapentaenoic acid	EPA	20:5 (n−3)	Eicosa−5, 8, 11, 14, 17−pentaenoic acid
Docosapentaenoic acid	DPA	22:5 (n−3)	Docosa−7, 10, 13, 16, 19−pentaenoic acid
Docosahexaenoic acid	DHA	22:6 (n−3)	Docosa−4, 7, 10, 13, 16, 19−hexaenoic acid

A limited number of plants have seeds that contain moderate or high levels of the mother Omega Three ALA. Some contain quite high levels of Omega Six which must be factored into dietary consideration. (Thanks to Wikipedia for the table) .

Common name	Alternate name	Linnaean name	% ALA
Chia	Chia sage	*Salvia hispanica*	64%
Kiwi	Chinese gooseberry	*Actinidia chinensis*	62%
Perilla	Shiso	*Perilla frutescens*	58%
Flax	Linseed	*Linum usitatissimum*	55%
Lingonberry	Cowberry	*Vaccinium vitis-idaea*	49%
Purslane	Portulaca	*Portulaca oleracea*	35%
Sea Buckthorn	Seaberry	*Hippophae rhamnoides L.*	32%
Hemp	Cannabis	*Cannabis sativa*	20%
Rapeseed	Canola	*Brassica napus*	10%
Soybean	Soya	*Glycine max*	8%

30.32 Omega Six—The Omega 6s are a family of EFA fats. The mother fat is called linol**eic** acid. Children are made from the mother fat, by adding more carbons and double bonds. Well known Omega 6 children include AA, GLA, and DGLA [5.1]. The 1st double bond is 6 from the hydrogen end.

The Omega 6 mother fat cannot be made in the body, it can only be obtained from diet.

The body makes long chain omega 6s, if conversion paths are not blocked.

The mother Omega 6 in large quantity is a scarce resource in the wild. It is found in all green plants, roots and fruit flesh, in small amounts. It is found in seeds grains and nuts in high quantities. It is essentially seasonal.

The body places a premium on storing it. Linoleic acid is the master fat. Omega 6 is essential to the body structure, metabolism and reproduction.

Where Omega 6 is present in excess of Omega 3, the body uses the nearest Omega 6 [E.g. DPA n6] to substitute for Omega 3s DHA and EPA. These Omega 6 substitutes are very second best, and lead to degradation of body function.

Omega 6 sits at the top of a family of highly inflammatory chemicals. Excess Omega 6 in the diet, results in excess Omega 6 in the cell membranes, which leads to excess inflammatory chemicals, disturbed hormones, reduced sleep, obesity, and a greater risk or disposition to a whole range of 'western' illnesses.

The Omega Six family includes, with thanks to Wikipedia:

Common name		Lipid name	Chemical name
Linoleic acid	LA	18:2 (n−6)	9, 12−octadecadienoic acid
Gamma-linolenic acid	GLA	18:3 (n−6)	6, 9, 12−octadecatrienoic acid
Eicosadienoic acid		20:2 (n−6)	11, 14−eicosadienoic acid
Dihomo-gamma-linolenic acid	DGLA	20:3 (n−6)	8, 11, 14−eicosatrienoic acid
Arachidonic acid	AA	20:4 (n−6)	5, 8, 11, 14−eicosatetraenoic acid
Docosadienoic acid		22:2 (n−6)	13, 16−docosadienoic acid
Adrenic acid	AD	22:4 (n−6)	7, 10, 13, 16−docosatetraenoic acid
Docosapentaenoic acid	DPA	22:5 (n−6)	4, 7, 10, 13,16−docosapentaenoic acid

30.33 Omega Seven−The Omega Sevens, are a family of fats like the Omega Threes, and Sixes. The mother fat is palm**itic** acid. The difference is the body can make Omega Sevens from scratch. The body can elongate Omega 7s in the same was as it elongates Omega 3 and 6. The first double bond is at position 7, from the hydrogen end. It is found in palm oil, dairy products and meat.

Palmit*oleic* acid is 16 carbon monosaturate, made in the body using the enzyme desaturase 9. It is a common constituent of fatty tissue. Palmitoleic acid occurs in Macadamia and Sea Buckthorn oil.

Vaccenic Acid, 18 carbons is the next longest Omega 7. Vaccenic acid naturally occurs as a trans and cis fat, and is found in dairy products. Trials suggest natural trans fats [11.28] are often beneficial to health.

30.34 Omega Nine−The Omega Nines, are a family of fats in the same sense that the Omega Threes, and Sixes are. The difference is the body can make Omega Nines. The first double bond is at position 9 from the hydrogen end. The body, as with the Omega 3s and Omega 6s, can elongate the Omega 9s by adding carbons and double bonds.

Oleic acid is about 70 per cent of the fat in virgin olive oil. In times of shortage of Omega 3, and Omega 6 [e.g. famine], the body will use the nearest Omega 9 as a substitute. As can be easily imagined, a 22 carbon chain fat with one double bond [Omega 9 22:1 n9], will have very different effects to one with six double bonds like DHA [Omega 6 22.6 n3] [Fig 30.10].

Common name		Lipid name	Chemical name
Oleic acid	OA	18:1 (n−9)	9−octadecenoic acid
Eicosenoic acid		20:1 (n−9)	11−eicosenoic acid
Mead acid		20:3 (n−9)	5, 8, 11−eicosatrienoic acid
Erucic acid		22:1 (n−9)	13−docosenoic acid
Nervonic acid		24:1 (n−9)	15−tetracosenoic acid

30.35 Prostaglandins PGE2−PGF2−PGH2−PGI2−Prostaglandins are made by oxidisation of fatty acids by the COX enzymes. They are made from the 20 carbon chain fats, Omega 6 AA and Omega 3 EPA [Page 286.].

Prostaglandins indirectly control sex hormones, and steroids [Fig 23.11b]. Each has its own properties. The Omega 6 family are the most aggressive.

The prostaglandins are found in almost all tissues and organs, and have many roles. [1.19]. Treatment of conditions, due to high prostaglandins, are by drugs that block the COX enzymes, NSAIDS. Much is not known. The type of prostaglandins produced depends on the quantities of the raw materials in the membranes. [E.g. The amount of AA, or EPA]. The amount of AA and EPA in the membranes depends on dietary intake, conversion rates, fat stores, and the blocking effect of DHA. High levels of Omega 6 are stored in the fatty tissue deposits. In contrast, only small amounts of Omega 3 are stored.

The diagram in the appendix page 286, and Fig 1.19 give an inkling of the complexities of the pathways involved. Some COX blockers are general, some are selective. On a long-term and gradual basis, reduction of Omega Six, and increase of Omega Three, in the diet should reduce the level of Omega Six AA prostaglandins. Fat balancing, as a starting point, is a cheaper and safer long-term prevention option for common inflammatory conditions, than seeking to chemically block very complex far-reaching interlinked sophisticated pathways.

There will always be a need for COX blockers, which provide immediate relief, but given the complex areas in which COX blockers operate, and the long-term risks, prevention so far as possible and practical has to be a first line option.

Aspirin is an example of a COX blocker. Even aspirin intervenes at a very low level in the sex hormone pathways. Painkillers may be having very much wider impact than you realise; some are suggested to impact on fertility.

30.36 Saturated fats−Saturated fat carbon chains have no double bonds. They are more stable and less susceptible to damage by heat. They are more rigid and almost straight in shape. [See 11.19, 30.30 and following].

Saturated fats are made by the body. Saturated fats are essential to health. Some saturated fats have antibacterial properties. Saturated fats are an essential part of cell membranes.

30.37 Trans fats–[See also Cis fat above and sections 11.28 and 11.29] Trans fats use opposite carbon connections, [bonds] to make the link. In consequence, the bond is straight. The trans fat bond has no ability to make shapes, other than a straight line, with a bit of wiggle room.

The double bond may not be able to get into position to react, because the chain is the wrong shape. Straight fats make cell membranes more rigid, and less flexible.

There are natural trans fats and artificial trans fats. The body has no experience of artificial fats, and so no processes for them. Trans mother fats, can be elongated and have been found in the brain. Trans fats have been associated with a number of medical conditions.

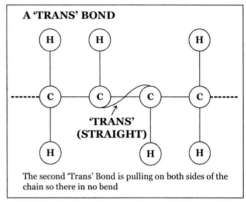

The second 'Trans' Bond is pulling on both sides of the chain so there in no bend

Fig. 30.37 Trans Bonds give Fats the same shape as saturated Fats.

30.38 Triglycerides–Triglycerides are the storage racks of fats. [See 30.19]. Triglycerides are used for storage and transport, but NOT in the cell membranes. The fats are assembled, and disassembled, from the storage racks as needed, to transport them across cell membranes, and into blood vessels, etc. The storage rack comprises a backbone and three legs. The legs are the fats. The fats most commonly stored are 16, 18 and 20 carbons long. The mix of fats determines the melting point and properties of triglycerides. There are some common patterns, but a huge number of variations are possible. The middle leg in nature is generally unsaturated.

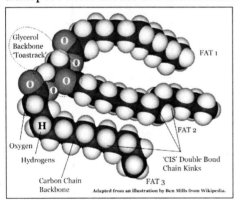

Fig. 30.38 A Triglyceride

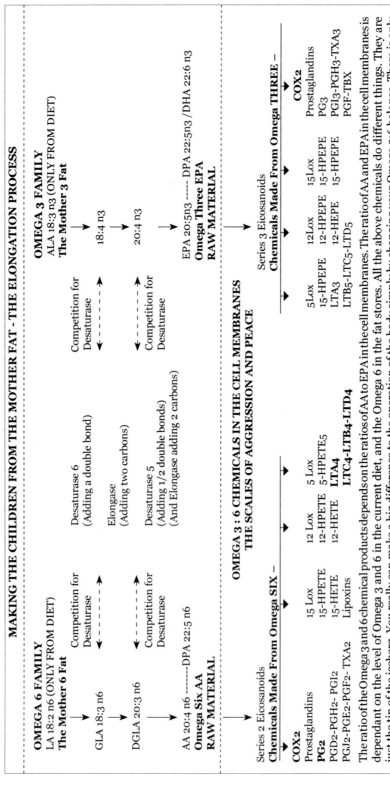

MAKING THE CHILDREN FROM THE MOTHER FAT - THE ELONGATION PROCESS

OMEGA 6 FAMILY
LA 18:2 n6 (ONLY FROM DIET)
The Mother 6 Fat

Competition for Desaturase

GLA 18:3 n6

Desaturase 6 (Adding a double bond)

Elongase (Adding two carbons)

Competition for Desaturase

DGLA 20:3 n6

Desaturase 5 (Adding 1/2 double bonds) (And Elongase adding 2 carbons)

Competition for Desaturase

AA 20:4 n6 ——— DPA 22:5 n6
Omega Six AA RAW MATERIAL

OMEGA 3 FAMILY
ALA 18:3 n3 (ONLY FROM DIET)
The Mother 3 Fat

Competition for Desaturase

18:4 n3

Competition for Desaturase

20:4 n3

EPA 20:5n3 ——— DPA 22:5n3 / DHA 22:6 n3
Omega Three EPA RAW MATERIAL

OMEGA 3 : 6 CHEMICALS IN THE CELL MEMBRANES
THE SCALES OF AGGRESSION AND PEACE

Series 2 Eicosanoids
Chemicals Made From Omega SIX –

COX2	12 Lox	5 Lox
Prostaglandins		
PG2	12-HPETE	5-HPETE5
PGD2-PGH2- PGI2	12-HETE	**LTA4**
PGJ2-PGE2-PGF2- TXA2	15 Lox	
	15-HPETE	**LTC4-LTB4-LTD4**
	15-HETE	
	Lipoxins	

Series 3 Eicosanoids
Chemicals Made From Omega THREE –

5Lox	12Lox	15Lox	COX2
15-HPEPE	12-HPEPE	15-HPEPE	Prostaglandins
LTA3	12-HEPE	15-HPEPE	PG3
LTB5-LTC5-LTD5	LTC5-LTD5		PGI3-PGH3-TXA3
			PGF-TBX

The ratio of the Omega 3 and 6 chemical products depends on the ratios of AA to EPA in the cell membranes. The ratio of AA and EPA in the cell membranes is dependant on the level of Omega 3 and 6 in the current diet, and the Omega 6 in the fat stores. All the above chemicals do different things. They are just the tip of the iceberg. You really can make a big difference to the operation of the body simply by changing your Omega 3:6 balance. There is only a limited amount of desaturase. When both Omega 3 and 6 are adequately supplied it is a constant delicate jostle for dominance of the desaturase pathways. The raw materials levels and desaturase pathways control the levels of Omega 3 and 6 eicosanoid chemicals.

Chemicals referred to in the book, or listed in the terminology section are highlighted. Other products are included to give an idea as to how very complex and extensive the fats pathways are. Much is still unknown. This is only a glimpse of the links and complexities. Each pathway and product is a specialism and a life's work. Only the highlighted items are considered. The other pathways are beyond the scope of this book, and me. [Fig.1.19]

TABLE OF FATS AND OILS APPROXIMATE

| Approximate fatty Acid Composition | | Saturated Fats | | | | | Omega 9 | Omega 6 | Omega 3 | |
Oil or fat	n6/n3 Ratio +	Capric % C10:0	Lauric % C12:0	Myristic % C14:0	Palmitic % C16:0	Stearic % C18:0	Oleic % C18:1	Linoleic % C18:2	Linolenic % C18:3	DHA % C22:6
Almond	17:-	-	-	-	7	2	69	17	-	-
Beef Tallow	3:1	-	1	3	25	19	36	3	1	-
Butter	2:~	3	3	7	21	10	17	2	~	
Canola Rapeseed	2:1	-	-	-	4	2	55	20	10	-
Coco Butter	3:-	-	-	-	25	32	32	3	-	-
Cod Liver	1:20	-	-	4	10	3	20	1	Total 9*	11
Coconut	1:-	6	44	17	8	3	6	1	-	-
Corn	53:1	-	-	-	11	2	27	53	1	-
Flaxseed	1:4	-	-	-	5	4	20	13	53	-
Grape Seed	70:~	-	-	-	7	3	16	70	~	-
Lard	10:1	-	-	1	24	14	41	10	1	-
Olive	10:1	-	-	-	11	2	71	10	1	-
Palm	10:~	-	-	1	44	4	37	9	~	-
Palm Kernel	2:-	4	47	16	8	3	11	2	-	-
Peanut	32:-	-	-	-	10	2	45	32	-	-
Safflower + 6	75:-	-	-	-	4	2	14	75	-	-
Sesame	45:-	-	-	-	9	5	39	41	-	-
Soy	7:1	-	-	-	10	4	23	50	7	-
Sunflower + 6	69:-	-	-	-	6	5	20	66	-	-
Walnut	5:1	-	-	-	7	2	22	53	10	-

Figures vary according to source. ~ = Under 0.5%. - = None detected. + = Variety selected where a high Omega 6 or 9 variety * Inc EPA
[Figures can change significantly with varieties - Figures cited are from www.nal.usda.gov]. - See also Nutritiondata.com -

INDEX

A

E

Early adolescence 173
Early puberty 48, 73, 124, 161-2, 173, 242-3
East Africa 68
Eating, food obsessives 222
E.Coli bacteria 139
Eczema 21, 255
EFAs (Essential fatty acid) 29, 45-7, 53, 59,
    77, 95, 111, 122, 128, 146, 160-2, 164, 173,
    216, 264, 275
Eggs 10, 40, 61, 69, 77, 81, 83, 87, 105, 107,
    123, 145, 147, 154, 156, 230
  fertilised adhesion 124
  fertilised developing 154
  wild-fed chicken 230
Egyptians 5
Eicosanoid pathway 56, 127, 168, 232-3,
    235, 237, 239, 241, 243
Eicosanoids 11, 34-5, 46, 48, 116, 217, 246-
    7, 264, 266, 270, 275, 286
Elaine Gottschall 103
Electrical function 52, 106, 257, 271, 279
Electron transport efficiency 136
Elevated inflammation markers 263
Elongase 275, 286
Emergence of placental land animals 123
Endometrial physiology 159, 248
Endometriosis 160, 175, 248
Enig 90, 93, 95
Environmental conditions 54, 68, 123, 173,
    177, 245-6
Environmental factors 7, 37, 65, 73, 263
Environmental Implications 227-9, 231
Enzymes 28, 67, 69, 74, 85, 97, 99, 114,
    139, 143, 145, 155, 192, 212, 235, 271-3
EPA oxidation 240
Eskimos 82, 87, 119, 129, 181
Estriol 250
Europe 4, 68, 164, 188, 197, 263
Evolution 6, 7, 29, 66-7, 69, 71, 73-5, 104,
    123, 173
Evolutionary advantage 72, 215
Evolutionary discord 75
Evolutionary fertility controller 147
Excess
  alcohol 40, 183, 195
  antioxidants 135
  body fat 8, 55
  hormone levels 8
  mucus 206
  sugar 85, 225
Exercise 136, 202, 207-8, 214, 257
Eye retina 117, 169

F

Factories
  chemical 34, 102, 112, 211, 280
  fat processing 89
  mini, cells 33, 156
  supersize, cells 150
Famine 24, 62, 74, 114, 123, 209, 243, 284
Farmed fish 15, 77, 83, 228
Farming 117, 229
  industrial 68, 125
  objectives 107
Faroe Islands 168
Fat
  absorption blockers 62
  burn 77, 204
  cell matrix 102, 156
  cells 6, 7, 17, 32-3, 55, 102, 111, 114, 150,
      153, 156, 176, 203, 205-6, 215-6, 218
    bigger 32, 150, 196, 201, 209, 211 218
    inactive 209
    melatonin blocks 235
    size of 205, 209, 220
  content 23, 34-5, 55, 79, 80, 92, 181, 205,
      218, 253, 259
    linoleic acid body 218
  conversion 10, 105, 116, 167, 186, 204,
      220, 239, 248
    blockers 70, 125
  deposition 103, 214, 224
  deposits 69, 205, 207, 219
  factories 30, 35, 111, 198
  imbalances 21, 31, 34, 53, 108, 159, 161,
      169-70, 175, 182-3, 219
  insulates 32
  intake 18, 23, 53, 63, 81, 112, 143, 167,
      173, 176, 209, 219, 221, 254, 257
    saturated 90, 93, 96, 122, 207
  levels 58, 61, 223, 228, 248, 256
  malabsorption 225
  matrix 111, 153-4, 156, 276
  metabolism 43, 91, 165, 169
  oxidation rates 203
  pathways 41, 56, 170, 176, 232, 249, 255
  profiles 18, 83, 87, 107, 129, 167, 218,
      230, 251, 260
    animal's 77
  ratios 92, 181
  reserves 9, 55, 109, 160, 197, 209, 222,
      258
  storage 34, 64, 83, 116, 124, 141, 196-8,
      201, 209, 212, 219, 246
  stores
    low cyclical 55
    softer 149
  switch 7

[Created by the author based on TExtract
    www.Texyz.com and the patient
    assistance of Quadrant in setting]

ENDNOTES

1 Healthy intakes of n–3 and n–6 fatty acids: estimations considering worldwide diversity – Joseph R Hibbeln, Levi RG Nieminen, Tanya L Blasbalg, Jessica A Riggs and William EM Lands · Laboratory of Membrane Biochemistry and Biophysics and the National Institute on Alcohol Abuse and Alcoholism, National Institutes of Health, Bethesda, M D · American Jnl. of Clinical Nutrition, Vol. 83, No. 6, S1483–1493S, June 2006.

2 Production of eicosapentaenoic and docosahexaenoic acid-containing oils in transgenic land plants for human and aquaculture nutrition. – Robert SS · Food Futures National Research Flagship Division of Marine and Atmospheric Research, Commonwealth Scientific and Industrial Research Organisation (CSIRO), Hobart, Tasmania · Mar Biotechnol (NY). 2006 Mar–Apr;8 (2):103–9. Epub 2006 Jan 1. Pubmed 16372159.

3 Developmental programming of obesity in mammals. · D. Taylor and L. Poston Division of Reproduction & Endocrinology, King's College London, UK. · Experimental Physiology 92.2 pp 287–298 DOI: 10.1113/expphysiol.2005.032854.

4 The effect of fish oil on physical aggression in schoolchildren – a randomized, double-blind, placebo-controlled trial. · Itomura M, Hamazaki K, Sawazaki S, Kobayashi M, Terasawa K, Watanabe S, Hamazaki T. · Division of Clinical Application, Dept. of Clinical Sciences, Institute of Natural Medicine, Toyama Medical and Pharmaceutical University, Toyama, Japan 9300194. · J Nutr Biochem. 2005 Mar;16(3):163–71 PubMed 15741051.

5 Omega-3 fatty acid deficiencies in neurodevelopment, aggression and autonomic dysregulation: opportunities for intervention. · Int Rev Psychiatry. 2006 Apr;18(2):107–18. Hibbeln JR, Ferguson TA, Blasbalg TL. National Institute on Alcohol Abuse and Alcoholism, Bethesda, 20892, USA PubMed 16777665.

6 High maternal intake of polyunsaturated fatty acids during pregnancy in mice alters offsprings' aggressive behavior, immobility in the swim test, locomotor activity and brain protein kinase C activity. · J Nutr. 1998 Dec;128(12):2505–11. · Raygada M, Cho E, Hilakivi-Clarke L.Lombardi · Cancer Centre, Georgetown University, Washington USA. PubMed 9868200.

7 One generation of n–3 polyunsaturated fatty acid deprivation increases depression and aggression test scores in rats. · J Lipid Res. 2006 Jan;47(1):172–80. Epub 2005 Oct 6 · DeMar JC Jr, Ma K, Bell JM, Igarashi M, Greenstein D, Rapoport SI. · Brain Physiology and Metabolism Section, National Institute on Aging, and Child Psychiatry Branch, National Institutes of Health Bethesda, MD, 20892, USA. PubMed 16210728.

8 Maternal high n–6 polyunsaturated fatty acid intake during pregnancy increases voluntary alcohol intake and hypothalamic oestrogen receptor alpha and beta levels among female offspring. · Dev Neurosci. 2000 Sep–Dec;22(5–6):488–93. · Cabanes A, de Assis S, Gustafsson JA, Hilakivi-Clarke L.Lombardi · Cancer Center, Georgetown University, Washington, DC, USA. PubMed 11111167.

9 omega–3 Fatty acid treatment of women with borderline personality disorder: a double-blind, placebo-controlled pilot study. · Am J Psychiatry. 2003 Jan;160(1):167–9. · Zanarini MC, Frankenburg FR. · Laboratory for the Study of Adult Development, McLean Hospital, Belmont, MA 02478, USA. PubMed 12505817.

10 The effect of docosahexaenoic acid on aggression in young adults. A placebo-controlled double-blind study. · T Hamazaki, S Sawazaki, M Itomura, E Asaoka, Y Nagao, N Nishimura, K Yazawa, T Kuwamori, and M Kobayashi · J Clin Invest. 1996 February 15; 97(4): 1129–1133. · The First Dept. of Internal Medicine, Toyama Medical and Pharmaceutical University, Japan. PubMed 507162.

11 Adipose tissue n–6 fatty acids and acute myocardial infarction in a population consuming a diet high in polyunsaturated fatty acids · American Jnl. of Clinical Nutrition, Vol. 77, No. 4, 796–802, April 2003 · Jeremy D Kark, Nathan A Kaufmann, Fred Binka, Nehama Goldberger and Elliot M Berry · Epidemiology Unit, Dept. of Social Medicine, Hadassah University Hospital, Jerusalem; the Dept. of Human Nutrition and Metabolism, Hebrew University-Hadassah School of Public Health, Jerusalem School of Public Health, University of Ghana.

12 The Queen of Fats Susan Allport.

13 Search across databases Fish oil OR omega–3 OR docosahexaenoic OR eicosapentaenoic.

14 Oxidative Stress and Peroxisome Proliferator–Activated Receptors Reversing the Curse? · (Circulation Research. 2004;95:1137.) · Pallavi R. Devchand, Ouliana Ziouzenkova, Jorge Plutzky · Donald W. Reynolds Cardiovascular Clinical Research Center, Cardiovascular Division, Brigham and Women's Hospital, Harvard Medical School, Boston, Mass.

15   Omega-3 fatty acids decreased irritability of patients with bipolar disorder in an add-on, open label study
        - Kemal Sagduyu, Mehmet E Dokucu, Bruce A Eddy, Gerald Craigen, Claudia F Baldassano, and Ay egül
        Yıldız, - Nutr J. 2005; 4: 6. Published online 2005 February 9. doi: 10.1186/1475-2891-4-6.

16   Leptin and adiponectin stimulate the release of proinflammatory cytokines and prostaglandins from
        human placenta and maternal adipose tissue via nuclear factor-kappaB, peroxisomal proliferator-
        activated receptor-gamma and extracellularly regulated kinase. - Lappas M, Permezel M, Rice GE. - Dept.
        of Obstetrics and Gynaecology, University of Melbourne and Mercy Perinatal Research Centre, Mercy
        Hospital for Women, Victoria, Australia Endocrinology. 2005 Aug;146(8):3334-42 PubMed 5905315.

17   Recent advances in the relationship between obesity, inflammation, and insulin resistance. - Bastard JP,
        Maachi M, Lagathu C, Kim MJ, Caron M, Vidal H, Capeau J, Feve B. - Inserm U680, Faculte de Medecine
        Pierre et Marie Curie, site Saint-Antoine, Universite Pierre et Marie Curie, Paris 6 et Service de Biochimie et
        Hormonologie, Hopital Tenon, Paris, France. - Eur Cytokine Netw. 2006 Mar;17(1):4-12. PubMed 16613757.

18   Release of interleukins and other inflammatory cytokines by human adipose tissue is enhanced in
        obesity and primarily due to the nonfat cells. - Fain JN. - Dept. of Molecular Sciences, College of Medicine,
        University of Tennessee Health Science Center, USA. - Vitam Horm. 2006;74:443-77 PubMed 17027526.

19   The inflammatory consequences of psychologic stress: relationship to insulin resistance, obesity,
        atherosclerosis and diabetes mellitus, type II. - Blac PubMed k PH.Dept. of Microbiology, Boston
        University School of Medicine, 715 Albany Street, Room L-501, Boston, MA 02118. - Med Pub Hypotheses.
        2006;67(4):879-91. PubMed 16781084.

20   The Driving Force Food Evolution and the Future - Michael Crawford & David Marsh.

21   Distribution, interconversion, and dose response of n-3 fatty acids in humans American Jnl. of Clinical
        Nutrition, - Vol. 83, No. 6, S1467-1476S, June 2006 - Linda M Arterburn, Eileen Bailey Hall and Harry Oken
        - From Martek Biosciences Corporation, Columbia, MD and the University of Maryland, Baltimore, MD

22   Omega 3 Fatty Acids, Selective Oxidation, and Human Obesity - Steven Phinney MD Ph.D. - Professor
        of Medicine University of California at DavisNewsletter Volume 2- July/Aug/Sept.

23   Omega 3 Fatty Acids, Selective Oxidation, and Human Obesity - Steven Phinney MD Ph.D. - Professor
        of Medicine University of California at Davis.

24   Dietary, but not topical, alpha-linolenic acid suppresses UVB-induced skin injury in hairless mice when
        compared with linoleic acid Photochemistry and Photobiology, Dec 2002 - by Takemura, Naoya,
        Takahashi, Kazuhiko, Tanaka, Hiroshi, Ihara, Yuka, Et al.

25   Efficiency of conversion of [alpha]-linolenic acid to long chain n-3 fatty acids in man. - Lipid metabolism and
        therapy Current Opinion in Clinical Nutrition & Metabolic Care. 5(2):127-132, March 2002.- B, J. Thomas.

26   Adipose tissue From Wikipedia, the free encyclopedia.

27   Omega 3 Fatty Acids, Selective Oxidation, and Human Obesity - Steven Phinney MD Ph.D. -University
        of California at Davis Newsletter Volume 2- July/Aug/Sept.

28   http://en.wikipedia.org/wiki/Image:Cell_membrane_detailed_diagram.svg.

29   Glyconutrients http://www.glyconutrient.biz/glycolipids.htm.

30   Polyunsaturated fatty acids and gene expression. - Curr Opin Clin Nutr Metab Care. 2004 Mar;7(2):151-6
        - Lapillonne A, Clarke SD, Heird WC. - USDA/ARS Children's Nutrition Research Center, Dept. of
        Pediatrics, Baylor College of Medicine, Houston, USA. PubMed 15075705.

31   The Driving Force - Food Evolution and the Future. - Michael Crawford and David Marsh.

32   Fatty acid content of plasma lipids and erythrocyte phospholipids are altered following burn injury. -
        Lipids. 2001 Jul;36(7):675-82 - Pratt VC, Tredget EE, Clandinin MT, Field CJ. - Dept. of Agricultural, Food
        and Nutritional Science, University of Alberta, Canada PubMed 11521965.

33   The Driving Force - Food Evolution and the Future. - Michael Crawford and David Marsh.

34   Ethanol consumption alters electroretinograms and depletes neural tissues of docosahexaenoic acid in
        rhesus monkeys: nutritional consequences of a low n-3 fatty acid diet. - Pawlosky RJ, Bacher J, Salem
        N. - Food Composition Laboratory, Beltsville Human Nutrition Research Center ARS, Maryland, USA.
        - Alcohol Clin Exp Res. 2001 Dec;25(12):1758-65. PubMed 11781509.

35   Perspectives on alcohol consumption: liver polyunsaturated fatty acids and essential fatty acid
        metabolism. - Pawlosky RJ, Salem N. - Division of Intramural Clinical and Biological Research, National
        Institutes of Health, National Institute on Alcohol Abuse and Alcoholism, National Institutes of Health,
        Rockville, USA. Alcohol. 2004 Aug;34(1):27-33 PubMed 15670662.

36   Development of alcoholic fatty liver and fibrosis in rhesus monkeys fed a low n-3 fatty acid diet. -
        Pawlosky RJ, Salem N. - Laboratory of Membrane Biochemistry and Biophysics, National Institute on
        Alcohol Abuse and Alcoholism, - Intramural Clinical and Biological Research, Maryland USA. - Alcohol.
        2004 Aug;34(1):27-33 PubMed 15597091.

37   Elevated oxidation of docosahexaenoic acid, 22:6 (n − 3), in brain regions of rats undergoing ethanol withdrawal · Ginger L. Milne, Jason D. Morrow and Matthew J. Picklo, · Sr. Division of Clinical Pharmacology, Vanderbilt University School of Medicine, Nashville, TN, United States Dept. of Pharmacology, Physiology, and Therapeutics, School of Medicine and Health Sciences, University of North Dakota, Grand Forks, · USA Volume 405, Issue 3, 25 September 2006, Pages 172–174 18061502.

38   Ethanol exposure causes a decrease in docosahexaenoic acid and an increase in docosapentaenoic acid in feline brains and retinas. · Pawlosky RJ, Salem N. · Laboratory of Membrane Biochemistry and Biophysics, National Institute on Alcoholism and Alcohol Abuse, Rockville, USA. · Am J Clin Nutr. 1995 Jun;61(6):1284–9 PubMed 7762532.

39.   Ethanol consumption alters electroretinograms and depletes neural tissues of docosahexaenoic acid in rhesus monkeys: nutritional consequences of a low n–3 fatty acid diet. · Pawlosky RJ, Bacher J, Salem N. · Food Composition Laboratory, Beltsville Human Nutrition Research Centre ARS, USDA, Beltsville, Maryland 20705, USA. · Alcohol Clin Exp Res. 2001 Dec;25(12):1758–65 PubMed 11781509.

40   Fatty acid composition, eicosanoid production and permeability in skin tissues of rainbow trout (Oncorhynchus mykiss) fed a control or an essential fatty acid deficient diet. · Ghioni C, Bell JG, Bell MV, Sargent JR. · NERC Unit of Aquatic Biochemistry, School of Natural Sciences, University of Stirling, UK. · Prostaglandins Leukot Essent Fatty Acids. 1997 Jun;56(6):479–89 PubMed 9223661.

41   Effect of randomized supplementation with high dose olive, flax or fish oil on serum phospholipid fatty acid levels in adults with attention deficit hyperactivity disorder. · Young GS, Conquer JA, Thomas R.Human · Biology and Nutritional Sciences, University of Guelph, Guelph, Ontario Canada. · Reprod Nutr Dev. 2005 Sep–Oct;45(5):549–58. PubMed 16188207.

42   Origins and evolution of the Western diet: health implications for the 21st century.· Loren Cordain, S Boyd Eaton, Anthony Sebastian, Neil Mann, Staffan Lindeberg, Bruce A Watkins, James H O'Keefe and Janette Brand·Miller · Dept. of Health and Exercise Science, Colorado State University, Fort Collins; the Dept. s of Radiology and Anthropology, Emory University, Atlanta the Dept. of Medicine and UCSF/Moffitt General Clinical Research Center, University of California, San Francisco the Dept. of Food Science, RMIT University, Melbourne, Australia the Dept. of Medicine, Lund University, Sweden the Dept. of Food Science, Lipid Chemistry and Molecular Biology Laboratory, Purdue University, West Lafayette, IN the Mid America Heart Institute, Cardiovascular Consultants, Kansas City, MO ; and the Human Nutrition Unit, Dept. of Biochemistry, University of Sydney, Australia.

43   Omega–3 fatty acid deficiencies in neurodevelopment, aggression and autonomic dysregulation: opportunities for intervention. · Hibbeln, J. R., T. A. Ferguson, et al. (2006). · Int Rev Psychiatry 18(2): 107–18.

44   Docosahexaenoic acid and neurologic development in animals. · Heinemann, K. M. and J. E. Bauer (2006). · J Am Vet Med Assoc 228(5): 700–5, 655. · Heinemann KM, Bauer JE. Comparative Nutrition Laboratory, Department of Small Animal Clinical Sciences, College of Veterinary Medicine, Texas A&M University, College Station, TX 77843, USA. Pub Med 16506930.

45   Role of omega–3 fatty acids in brain development and function: potential implications for the pathogenesis and prevention of psychopathology. · McNamara RK, Carlson SE.· Dept. of Psychiatry, University of Cincinnati College of Medicine, Cincinnati, USA. · Prostaglandins Leukot Essent Fatty Acids. 2006 Oct–Nov;75(4–5):329–49. Epub 2006 Sep. PubMed 16949263.

46   Serotonin, testosterone and alcohol in the etiology of domestic violence · David T. George, John C. Umhau, Monte J. Phillips, Devadatham Emmela Paul W. Ragan, Susan E. Shoaf and Robert R. Rawlings · Laboratory of Clinical Studies, DICBR, National Institute on Alcohol Abuse and Alcoholism, Bethesda, MD 20892, USA Dept. of Psychiatry, Vanderbilt University Medical Center, 1211 22nd Ave. S.,TN, USA. · Psychiatry Research Volume 104, Issue 1, 10 October 2001, Pages 27–37. PubMed 11600187.

47   Effect of testosterone on serotonin and noradrenaline concentrations and taste bud cell number of rat circumvallate papilla · Chemical Senses 7: 109–116 J. · Cano, A. Machado, C. Roza and E. Rodriguez-Echandia · Departamento de Morfología, Facultad de Medicina, Universidad Autónoma de Madird, y Departamento de Bioquímica y Biología Molecular, CSIC, Facultad de Ciencias, Universidad Autónoma de Madrid Spain.

48   See 47 above

49   Aggression: The Testosterone·Serotonin Link · Moshe BirgerMD, Marnina SwartzMD, David CohenMA, Ya'akov Alesh MD, Chaim GrishpanMD and Moshe KotelrMD · Forensic Psychiatric Division and Directorate, Be'er Yaakov Mental Health Center, Magen Prison, Ramleh, Israel Abarabnel Mental Health Center, Bat·Yam, Israel Both affiliated to Sackler Faculty of Medicine, Tel Aviv University, Ramat Aviv, Israel.

50   Simple Test may Detect Breast Cancers · Chris Gupta.

51 Nutritional Intervention With Omega-3 Fatty Acids in a Case of Malignant Fibrous Histiocytoma of the Lungs - Ronald S. Pardini, David Wilson, Steven Schiff, Stephen A. Bajo, and Randall Pierce - Nutr Cancer. 2005;52(2):121-9 Department of Biochemistry, College of Agriculture, Biotechnology and Natural Resources, University of Navada, Reno, NV 89557, USA Pubmed 16201843.

52 Arachidonic acid metabolism in benign and malignant prostatic tissue in vitro: effects of fatty acids and cyclooxygenase inhibitors. - Chaudry AA, Wahle KW, McClinton S, Moffat LE. - Nutr Cancer. 2005;52(2):121-9 Dept of Urology, Aberdeen Royal Infirmary, UK Pubmed 7512536.

53 Maternal and perinatal long-chain fatty acids: possible roles in preterm birth. - Reece MS, McGregor JA, Allen KG, Harris MA. - Dept. of Food Science and Human Nutrition, Colorado State University, Fort Collins 80523, USA. - Am J Obstet Gynecol. 1997 Apr;176(4):907-14 Pubmed 9125620.

54 Delay of preterm delivery in sheep by omega-3 long-chain polyunsaturates. - Baguma-Nibasheka M, Brenna JT, Nathanielsz PW. - Laboratory for Pregnancy and Newborn Research, College of Veterinary Medicine, Cornell University, Ithaca, New York, 14853, USA. - Biol Reprod. 1999 Mar;60(3):698-701 Pubmed 10026118.

55 Long-chain n-3 PUFA: plant v. marine sources. - The Institute of Food Research, University of East Anglia, Norwich, UK, 28 June-1 July 2005 - Proceedings of the Nutrition Society. 65(1):42-50, February 2006. - Williams, Christine M. I, Burdge, Graham.

56 Is Docosahexaenoic Acid (DHA) Essential? Lessons from DHA Status Regulation, Our Ancient Diet, Epidemiology and Randomized Controlled Trials - Frits A. J. Muskiet, M. Rebecca Fokkema, Anne Schaafsma, E. Rudy Boersma and Michael A. Crawford - Pathology and Laboratory Medicine, Groningen University Hospital, The Netherlands; Friesland Nutrition Research, Leeuwarden, The Netherlands; Emeritus Professor of Pediatrics, Groningen, The Netherlands; and Institute of Brain Chemistry and Human Nutrition, University of North London, London, UK - The American Society for Nutritional Sciences J. Nutr. 134:183-186, January 2004.

57 Variation in [U-13C] alpha linolenic acid absorption, beta-oxidation and conversion to docosahexaenoic acid in the pre-term infant fed a DHA-enriched formula. - Mayes C, Burdge GC, Bingham A, Murphy JL, Tubman R, Wootton SA. - Neonatal Intensive Care Unit, Royal Maternity Hospital, Belfast, - Pediatr Res. 2006 Feb;59(2):271-5 Pubmed 16439591.

58 The Biochemistry of N3 Polyunsaturated Fats - Donald B Jump - PHD Dept. of Physiology, Biochemistry and Molecular Biology Michigan State University JCB17 December 2001 - manuscript R100062200.

59 Olestra and Gastrointestinal Problems - Megan Castle.

60 Gastroenterology symptom information - VirtualMedicalCentre.com.

61 Relationship of total and abdominal adiposity with CRP and IL-6 in women. - Rexrode, K. M., Pradhan, A., Manson, J. E., Buring, J. E., Ridker, P. M.Author - Center of Cardiovascular Disease Prevention, Division of Preventive Medicine, Dept. of Medicine, Brigham and Women's Hospital and Harvard Medical School, 900 Commonwealth Avenue East, Boston, MA USA. - Annals of Epidemiology, 2003 (Vol. 13) (No. 10) 674-682.

62 Blood inflammatory markers and risk of dementia: The Conselice Study of Brain Aging. -Ravaglia G, Forti P, Maioli F, Chiappelli M, Montesi F, Tumini E, Mariani E, Licastro F, Patterson C. - Dept. of Internal Medicine, Cardioangiology, and Hepatology, University Hospital S. Orsola-Malpighi, Bologna, Italy. - Neurobiol Aging. 2006 Sep 28; PubMed 17011077.

63 The best of hypertension 2005-Chamontin B. Arch Mal Coeur Vaiss. - 2006 Jan;99 Spec No I(1):35-41Service de médecine interne-HTA, CHU Rangueil, 1, TSA 50032-31059 Toulouse. Chamontin. PubMed 16479962.

64 Decrease of interleukin 6 during the first 12 months is a prognostic marker for clinical outcome during 36 months treatment with disease-modifying anti-rheumatic drugs. - Br J Rheumatol. 1997 Dec;36(12):1298-303 - Straub RH, Müller-Ladner U, Lichtinger T, Schölmerich J, Menninger H, Lang B. - Dept. of Internal Medicine I, University Medical Centre, Regensburg, Germany. PubMed 9448591.

65 Influence of anti-tumour necrosis factor therapy on cardiovascular risk factors in patients with active rheumatoid arthritis. - Ann Rheum Dis. 2005 Feb;64(2):303-5. Epub 2004 Jul 1. - Popa C, Netea MG, Radstake T, Van der Meer JW, Stalenhoef AF, van Riel PL, Barerra P. - Rheumatology Dept., UMC St Radboud, HB Nijmegen, The Netherlands. PubMed 15231512.

66 Association of serum interleukin-6 and high-sensitivity C-reactive protein levels with insulin resistance in gestational diabetes mellitus. - Nan Fang Yi Ke Da Xue Xue Bao. 2007 Jun;27(6):799-801 - Yu F, Xue YM, Li CZ, Shen J, Gao F, Yu YH, Fu XJ. - Dept. of Endocrinology, Nangfang Hospital, Southern Medical University, Guangzhou China. PubMed 17584642.

67 Serum imbalance of cytokines in melanoma patients. - Moretti S, Chiarugi A, Semplici F, Salvi A, De Giorgi V, Fabbri P, Mazzoli S. - Second Dermatology Unit, S.M. Nuova Hospital, Azienda Sanitaria di

Firenze, Dept. of Dermatological Science, 50121 Florence, Italy. · Melanoma Res. 2001 Aug;11(4):395-9. PubMed 11479428.

68 Interleukin-6 is a potent inducer of S100P, which is up-regulated in androgen-refractory and metastatic prostate cancer. · Int J Biochem Cell Biol. 2005 Feb;37(2):442-50 · Hammacher A, Thompson EW, Williams ED. Bernard O'Brien · Institute of Microsurgery, University of Melbourne, Fitzroy, Vic. 3065, Australia. PubMed 15474988.

69 Interleukin-6 is increased in breath condensate of patients with non-small cell lung cancer. · Int J Biol Markers. 2002 Apr-Jun;17(2):141-5 · Carpagnano GE, Resta O, Foschino-Barbaro MP, Gramiccioni E, Carpagnano F. · Institute of Respiratory Diseases, University of Bari, Italy. PubMed 12113582.

70 IL6, aspirin, nonsteroidal anti-inflammatory drugs, and breast cancer risk in women living in the southwestern United States. · Cancer Epidemiol Biomarkers Prev. 2007 Apr;16(4):747-55 . · Slattery ML, Curtin K, Baumgartner R, Sweeney C, Byers T, Giuliano AR, Baumgartner KB, Wolff RR. · Health Research Center, University of Utah, Salt Lake City, UT. PubMed 17416766.

71 The IL-6/sIL-6R complex as a novel target for therapeutic approaches. · Expert Opin Ther Targets. 2007 May;11(5):613-24. · Rose-John S, Waetzig GH, Scheller J, Grötzinger J, Seegert D. · Biochemisches Institut, Christian-Albrechts-Universität zu Kiel, Kiel, Germany. PubMed 17465721.

72 Interleukin-6 trans-signalling in chronic inflammation and cancer. · Scheller J, Ohnesorge N, Rose-John S. · Biochemisches Institut, Christian-Albrechts-Universität zu Kiel, Scand J Immunol. 2006 May;63(5):321-9. PubMed 16640655.

73 Interleukin-6 biology is coordinated by membrane-bound and soluble receptors: role in inflammation and cancer. · J Leukoc Biol. 2006 Aug;80(2):227-36. Epub 2006 May 17 · Rose-John S, Scheller J, Elson G, Jones SA · Biochemisches Institut, Christian-Albrechts-Universität zu Kiel, Olshausenstr. 40, D-24098 Kiel. PubMed 16707558.

74 Depot differences in steroid receptor expression in adipose tissue: possible role of the local steroid milieu. · Am J Physiol Endocrinol Metab 288: E200-E207, 2005. · S. Rodriguez-Cuenca, M. Monjo, A. M. Proenza, and P. Roca · Grup de Metabolisme Energètic i Nutrició, Departament de Biologia Fonamental i Ciències de la Salut, Institut Universitari d'Investigació en Ciències de la Salut, Palma de Mallorca, Spain.

75 The Driving Force · Michael Crawford and David Marsh.

76 Marine microalgae as a source of w3 fatty acids · Ide Ni Fhaolain & Stephen Fitzpatrick · Galway-Mayo Institute of Technology.

77 Effects of various dietary fats on cardiolipin acyl composition during ontogeny of mice. · Berger A, Gershwin ME, German JB. · Lipids. 1992 Aug;27(8):605-12 Department of Food Science and Technology, University of California, Davis 95616. PubMed 1406071.

78 The Driving Force, Evolution and The Future · Michael Crawford and David Marsh · Harper & Row,

79 Brain-specific lipids from marine, lacustrine, or terrestrial food resources: potential impact on early African Homo sapiens. · Comp Biochem Physiol B Biochem Mol Biol. 2002 Apr;131(4):653-73 Broadhurst CL, Wang Y, Crawford MA, Cunnane SC, Parkington JE, Schmidt WF.US Department of Agriculture, Environmental Chemistry Laboratory, Agricultural Research Service, Beltsville, MD 20705, USA. PubMed 11923081.

80 Lessons from experimental disruption of estrous cycles and behaviors. · Med Sci Sports Exerc. 2003 Sep;35(9):1573-80. Wade GN, Jones JE. · Center for Neuroendocrine Studies, University of Massachusetts, Amherst. PubMed 12972879.

81 Decrease in Neuron Size in Docosahexaenoic Acid-Deficient Brain. · 218 Pediatric Neurology Vol 26. No.3 · Aneeq Ahmad, PhD, Toru Moriguchi, PhD, and Norman Salem, Jr, PhD.

82 Poxvirus-induced alteration of arachidonate metabolism. · G J Palumbo, W C Glasgow, and R M Buller · Laboratory of Viral Diseases, National Institute of Allergy and Infectious Diseases, National Institutes of Health, Bethesda, MD 20892. · Proc Natl Acad Sci U S A. 1993 March 1; 90(5): 2020-2024 PubMed 46012.

83 Egg yolk as a source of long-chain polyunsaturated fatty acids in infant feeding · Artemis P Simopoulos and Norman Salem · Jr. Am j Clin 1992;55:411-4. Center for Genetics, Nutrition and Health, Washington, DC 20009.

84 Retinal and brain accretion of long-chain polyunsaturated fatty acids in developing felines: the effects of corn oil-based maternal diets. · Pawlosky RJ, Denkins Y, Ward G, Salem N. · Laboratory of Membrane Biochemistry and Biophysics, National Institute on Alcoholism and Alcohol Abuse, Rockville, MD 20852, USA. · Am J Clin Nutr. 1997 Feb;65(2):465-72.

85 Is dietary arachidonic acid necessary for feline reproduction? · Pawlosky RJ, Salem N. · National Institute on Alcoholism and Alcohol Abuse, Division of Intramural Clinical and Biological Research, Rockville, MD 20852, USA. ·1996 Apr;126(4 Suppl):1081S-5S.

86   Egg yolk as a source of long-chain polyunsaturated fatty acids in infant feeding. · Artemis P Simopoulos and Norman Salem · Jr. Am j Clin 1992;55:411–4.

87   Composition of lipids in human serum and adipose tissue during prolonged feeding of a diet high in unsaturated fat. · Jnl. of Lipid Research, Vol. 7, 103–111, January 1966 · Seymour Dayton , Sam Hashimoto Wilfrid Dixon , and Morton Lee Pearce · Medical Services of Wadsworth Hospital and Domiciliary and Research Service, Veterans Administration Center, and Dept.s of Medicine and of Preventive Medicine, School of Medicine, University of California, Los Angeles, California

88   Essential fatty acids in health and chronic disease. · American Jnl. of Clinical Nutrition, Vol. 70, No. 3, 560S–569S, Sept 1999 · Artemis P Simopoulos. The Center for Genetics, Nutrition and Health,

89   Nutritional Intervention With Omega–3 Fatty Acids in a Case of Malignant Fibrous Histiocytoma of the Lungs · Ronald S. Pardini, David Wilson, Steven Schiff, Stephen A. Bajo, and Randall Pierce. · PubMed 16201843.

90   Different ratios of eicosapentaenoic and docosahexaenoic omega–3 fatty acids in commercial fish oils differentially alter pro-inflammatory cytokines in peritoneal macrophages from C57BL/6 female mice. · J Nutr Biochem. 2007 Jan;18(1):23–30. Epub 2006 Mar 24 · Bhattacharya A, Sun D, Rahman M, Fernandes G.Division of Clinical Immunology and Rheumatology, Dept. of Medicine, University of Texas Health Science Center at San Antonio, San Antonio, TX 78229–3900, USA. PubMed 16563716.

91   Elevated concentrations of plasma omega–3 polyunsaturated fatty acids among Alaskan Eskimos · AJ. American Jnl. of Clinical Nutrition, Vol 59, 384–388. · Parkinson, AL Cruz, WL Heyward, LR Bulkow, D Hall, L Barstaed and WE Connor · Arctic Investigations Program, National Center for Infectious Diseases, Anchorage, AK 99501.

92   (a) n–3 Fatty acids and cardiovascular disease risk factors among the Inuit of Nunavik ·American Jnl. of Clinical Nutrition, Vol. 74, No. 4, 464–473, October 2001. · Eric Dewailly, Carole Blanchet, Simone Lemieux, Louise Sauvé, Suzanne Gingras, Pierre Ayotte and Bruce John Holub · Public Health Research Unit, CHUL Research Center, Centre Hospitalier Universitaire de Quebec, Ste-Foy, Canada; the Dept.s of Social and Preventive Medicine and of Food Sciences and Nutrition, Laval University, Ste-Foy, and the Dept. of Human Biology and Nutritional Sciences, Guelph, Canada.

93   (n–3) Fatty Acids and Infectious Disease Resistance. · The American Society for Nutritional Sciences J. Nutr. 132:3566–3576, December 2002 · Michele Anderson and Kevin L. Fritsche · Dept.s of Nutritional Sciences, Animal Sciences, and Molecular Microbiology and Immunology, University of Missouri, Columbia, MO 65211.

94   Effect of diets containing n–3 fatty acids on muscle long-chain n–3 fatty acid content in lambs fed low and medium quality roughage diets · E N Ponnampalam, A J Sinclair, A R Egan, S K Blakeley, and B J Leury · Dept. of Animal Production, University of Melbourne, Victoria Australia.

95   Essential fatty acids in health and chronic disease · Artemis P Simopoulos · American Jnl. of Clinical Nutrition, Vol. 70, No. 3, 560S–569S, September 1999.

96   Smart Fats M A Schmidt.

97   The evaluations contained in this publication were prepared by the Joint FAO/WHO Expert Committee on Food Additives which met in Geneva, 25 June – 4 July 1973] World Health Organization Geneva 1974.

98   Gamma-linolenic acid dietary supplementation can reverse the aging influence on rat liver microsome delta 6–desaturase activity. · Biochim Biophys Acta. 1991 May 8;1083(2):187–92. · Biagi PL, Bordoni A, Hrelia S, Celadon M, Horrobin DF. · Centro Ricerche sulla Nutrizione, University of Bologna, Italy. 674661.

99   n–3 Fatty acids and cardiovascular disease risk factors among the Inuit of Nunavik · Eric Dewailly, Carole Blanchet, Simone Lemieux, Louise Sauvé, Suzanne Gingras, Pierre Ayotte and Bruce John Holub Public Health Research Unit, CHUL Research Center, Centre Hospitalier Universitaire de Quebec, Ste-Foy, Canada; the Dept.s of Social and Preventive Medicine and of Food Sciences and Nutrition, Laval University, Ste-Foy, Canada; and the Dept. of Human Biology and Nutritional Sciences, Guelph, Canada. · American Jnl. of Clinical Nutrition, Vol. 74, No. 4, 464–473, October 2001.

100   Elevated concentrations of plasma omega–3 polyunsaturated fatty acids among Alaskan Eskimos. · American Jnl. of Clinical Nutrition, Vol 59, 384–388 . · AJ Parkinson, AL Cruz, WL Heyward, LR Bulkow, D Hall, L Barstaed and WE Connor · Arctic Investigations Program, National Center for Infectious Diseases, Anchorage, AK 99501.

101   Symposium Highlights – Omega–3 Fatty Acids: Recommendations for Therapeutics and Prevention · CME Posted 10/19/2005 · Heather Hutchins, MS, RD.

102   A defect in the activity of Delta6 and Delta5 desaturases may be a factor predisposing to the development of insulin resistance syndrome. · Prostaglandins Leukot Essent Fatty Acids. 2005 May;72(5):343–50. · Das UN. PubMed 15850715.

103   Origins and evolution of the Western diet (See 42).

104   Origins and evolution of the Western diet: health implications for the 21st century (See 42)[2].

105   Origins and evolution of the Western diet: health implications for the 21st century (See 42).

106   Origins and evolution of the Western diet: health implications for the 21st century (See 42).

107   The Merck Manuals Online Medical Dictionary.

108   Vegan Society.

109   Variability of iodine content in common commercially available edible seaweeds. · Thyroid. 2004 Oct;14(10):836–41· Teas J, Pino S, Critchley A, Braverman LE. Department of Health Promotion Education and Behavior, Norman J. Arnold School of Public Health, University of South Carolina and the South Carolina Cancer Center, Columbia, South Carolina, USA PubMed 15588380.

110   Nutrient Requirements of Beef Cattle · http://books.nap.edu/openbook/0309069343/gifmid/26.gif

111   Long-chain conversion of [13C] linoleic acid and a-linolenic acid in response to marked changes in their dietary intake in men. · Jnl. of Lipid Research, Vol. 46, 269–280, February 2005 ·Nahed Hussein, Eric Ah-Sing, Paul Wilkinson, Clare Leach, Bruce A. Griffin and D. Joe Millward.Centre for Nutrition and Food Safety, School of Biomedical and Molecular Sciences, University of Surrey, Guildford, Surrey GU2 7XH, United Kingdom

112   Smart Fats M Schmidt.

113   The immune system and the skin Dr Victoria Lewis. · http://www.netdoctor.co.uk/skin_hair/skin_immune_system_003741.htm.

114   Cell cycle arrest and apoptosis of melanoma cells by docosahexaenoic acid: association with decreased pRb phosphorylation. · Cancer Res. 2000 Aug 1;60(15):4139–45 · Albino AP, Juan G, Traganos F, Reinhart L, Connolly J, Rose DP, Darzynkiewicz Z. · The American Health Foundation, Valhalla, New York 10595, USA. PubMed 10945621.

115   Membrane transport of long-chain fatty acids: evidence for a facilitated process · The Jnl. of Lipid Research, Vol. 39, 2309–2318, December 1998 · Nada Abumrad, Carroll Harmon, and Azeddine Ibrahimi · Dept. of Physiology and Biophysics, State University of New York, Stony Brook, NY 11794.

116   Power of a Human Brain · The Physics Factbook™.

117   High blood pressure induces low fat metabolism in heart muscle · Gwen Ericson · Washington University.

118   Comparative effects of perilla and fish oils on the activity and gene expression of fatty acid oxidation enzymes in rat liver · Biochim Biophys Acta. 2000 May 6;1485(1):23–35 Ide T, Kobayashi H, Ashakumary L, Rouyer IA, Takahashi Y, Aoyama T, Hashimoto T, Mizugaki M. · Laboratory of Nutrition Biochemistry, National Food Research Institute, Ministry of Agriculture, Forestry and Fisheries, Tsukuba Science , Japan. PubMed 10802246.

119   Cardiovascular Risk Factors Emerge After Artificial Selection for Low Aerobic Capacity · Ulrik Wisløff, Sonia M. Najjar, Øyvind Ellingsen, Per Magnus Haram, Steven Swoap, Qusai Al-Share, Mats Fernström,3 Khadijeh Rezaei, Sang Jun Lee, Lauren Gerard Koch, Steven L. Britton.

120   Essential fatty acids in health and chronic disease · Artemis P Simopoulos. · Center for Genetics, Nutrition and Health, Washington, DC. · American Jnl. of Clinical Nutrition, Vol. 70, No. 3, 560S–569S, Sept 1999

121   The Biochemistry of n-3 Polyunsaturated Fatty Acids · J. Biol. Chem., Vol. 277, Issue 11, 8755–8758, March 15, 2002 · Donald B. Jump · Dept.s of Physiology, Biochemistry, and Molecular Biology, Michigan State University, East Lansing, Michigan 48824.

122   Chronic Docosahexaenoic Acid Intake Enhances Expression of the Gene for Uncoupling Protein 3 and Affects Pleiotropic mRNA Levels in Skeletal Muscle of Aged C57BL/6NJcl Mice. · Jnl. of Nutrition. 2001;131:2636–2642. · Seung Hun Cha, Akiko Fukushima, Keiko Sakuma and Yasuo Kagawa · Dept.s of Medical Chemistry and Molecular Nutrition, Kagawa Nutrition University, 3-9-21 Chiyoda, Sakado, Saitama, Japan and Dept. of Biochemistry, Jichi Medical School, Kawachi, Tochigi, 329–0498, Japan.

123   The Effects of Diet on Inflammation Emphasis on the Metabolic Syndrome. · J Am Coll Cardiol, 2006; 48:677–685, doi:10.1016/j.jacc.2006.03.052 · Dario Giugliano, Antonio Ceriello, and Katherine Esposito, · Division of Metabolic Diseases, Center of Excellence for Cardiovascular Diseases, University of Naples, Italy. Warwick Medical School, Coventry, U.K

124   Role of omega-3 fatty acids in brain development and function: potential implications for the pathogenesis and prevention of psychopathology. · Prostaglandins Leukot Essent Fatty Acids. 2006 Oct–Nov;75(4–5):329–49 · McNamara RK, Carlson SE. · Dept. of Psychiatry, University of Cincinnati College of Medicine, Cincinnati, USA. PubMed 16949263.

125   Potential mechanisms connecting asthma, esophageal reflux, and obesity/sleep apnea complex—A hypothetical review - Aiman Kasasbeh, , Ehab Kasasbeh and Guha Krishnaswamy -Division of Allergy and Immunology, Dept. of Internal Medicine, Quillen College of Medicine, East Tennessee State University, Johnson City, TN 37614-0622, UK.

126   Impact of sleep and sleep loss on neuroendocrine and metabolic function. - Horm Res. 2007;67 Suppl l:2-9. - Van Cauter E, Holmback U, Knutson K, Leproult R, Miller A, Nedeltcheva A, Pannain S, Penev P, Tasali E, Spiegel K. - Dept. of Medicine, University of Chicago, Chicago, IL 60637, USA. PubMed 17308390.

127   Dietary docosahexaenoic acid-enriched phospholipids normalize urinary melatonin excretion in adult (n-3) polyunsaturated fatty acid-deficient rats. - Zaouali Ajina, M : Gharib, A : Durand, G : Gazzah, N : Claustrat, B : Gharib, C : Sarda, N - J-Nutr. 1999 Nov; 129(11): 2074-80.

128   Dietary docosahexaenoic acid-enriched phospholipids normalize urinary melatonin excretion in adult (n-3) polyunsaturated fatty acid-deficient rats. - J Nutr. 1999 Nov;129(11):2074-80 - Zaouali-Ajina M, Gharib A, Durand G, Gazzah N, Claustrat B, Gharib C, Sarda N. - Laboratoire de Physiologie de l'Environnement, Faculte de Medecine Lyon Grange-Blanche, Lyon France. PubMed 10539787.

129   Bidirectional communication between the pineal gland and the immune system. - Can J Physiol Pharmacol. 2003 Apr;81(4):342-9 - Skwarlo-Sonta K, Majewski P, Markowska M, Oblap R, Olszanska B. - Dept. of Vertebrate Physiology, Faculty of Biology, Warsaw University, Poland. PubMed 12769226.

130   Melatonin effect on arachidonic acid metabolism to cyclooxygenase derivatives in human platelets - Marta Martinuzzo, Maria de las M. Del Zar, Daniel P. Cardinali Luis O. Carreras and Maréa I. Departamento de Fisiologia, Facultad de Medicina, Universidad de Buenos Aires, Argentina and 2Seccion Hemostasia y Trombosis, Division Hematologia, Hospital de Clinicas "Jose de San Martin," Universidad de Buenos Aires, Argentina

131   Features of fatty acid synthesis.

132   Potential mechanisms connecting asthma, esophageal reflux, and obesity/sleep apnea complex—A hypothetical review - Aiman Kasasbeh, , Ehab Kasasbeh and Guha Krishnaswamy -Sleep Med Rev 2007;11(1):47-58. Division of Allergy and Immunology, Department of Internal Medicine, Quillen College of Medicine, East Tennessee State University, Johnson City, TN

133   Impact of sleep and sleep loss on neuroendocrine and metabolic function. - Horm Res. 2007;67 Suppl l:2-9 - Van Cauter E, Holmback U, Knutson K, Leproult R, Miller A, Nedeltcheva A, Pannain S, Penev P, Tasali E, Spiegel K. - Dept. of Medicine, University of Chicago, Chicago, IL 60637, USA. PubMed 17308390.

134   Leptin Levels Are Dependent on Sleep Duration: Relationships with Sympathovagal Balance, Carbohydrate Regulation, Cortisol, and Thyrotropin - Karine Spiegel, Rachel Leproult, Mireille L'Hermite-Balériaux, Georges Copinschi, Plamen D. Penev and Eve Van Cauter - Dept. of Medicine, University of Chicago, Chicago, Illinois 60637; and Laboratory of Physiology, Université Libre de Bruxelles, - The Jnl. of Clinical Endocrinology & Metabolism Vol. 89, No. 11 5762-5771.

135   Docosa-hexaenoic acid (DHA) accumulation is regulated by the polyunsaturated fat content of the diet: Is it synthesis or is it incorporation? - Gibson RA.

136   Effect of dietary alpha-linolenic acid intake on incorporation of docosahexaenoic and arachidonic acids into plasma phospholipids of term infants. - Lipids. 1996 Mar;31 Suppl:S131-5 - Sauerwald TU, Hachey DL, Jensen L, Chen H, Anderson RE, Heird WC. USDA, ARS, - Children's Nutrition Research Center, Dept. of Pediatrics, Baylor College of Medicine, Houston, Texas 77030, USA PubMed 8729107.

137   Eicosapentaenoic and docosapentaenoic acids are the principal products of alpha-linolenic acid metabolism in young men - Br J Nutr. 2002 Oct;88(4):355-63 - Burdge GC, Jones AE, - Wootton SA. Institute of Human Nutrition, Level C, West Wing, Southampton General Hospital, Tremona Road, Southampton PubMed 12323085.

138   Effect of altered dietary n-3 fatty acid intake upon plasma lipid fatty acid composition, conversion of [13C]alpha-linolenic acid to longer-chain fatty acids and partitioning towards beta-oxidation in older men. - Br J Nutr. 2003 Aug;90(2):311-21 - Burdge GC, Finnegan YE, Minihane AM, Williams CM, Wootton SA. - Institute of Human Nutrition, University of Southampton, UK PubMed 12908891.

139   Conversion of alpha-linolenic acid to eicosapentaenoic, docosapentaenoic and docosahexaenoic acids in young women. - Br J Nutr. 2002 Oct;88(4):411-20 Burdge GC, Wootton SA. - Institute of Human Nutrition, University of Southampton, Southampton, UK. PubMed 12323090.

140   The Driving Force - Food Evolution and the Future - Michael Crawford and David Marsh

141   The Driving Force - Food Evolution and the Future - Michael Crawford & David Mashall.

142   The Driving Force - Food Evolution and the Future - Michael Crawford and David Marsh.

143 Metabolic fuels and reproduction in female mammals. · Neurosci Biobehav Rev.1992 Summer;16(2):235–72.· Wade GN, Schneider JE · Dept. of Psychology and Neuroscience, University of Massachusetts, Amherst 01003. PubMed 1630733.

144 Neuroendocrinology of nutritional infertility · Neurosci Biobehav Rev. 1992 Summer;16(2):235–72 · Wade GN, Schneider JE. · Dept. of Psychology and Neuroscience, University of Massachusetts, Amherst 01003.

145 Nutrition and reproduction in women · The ESHRE Capri Workshop Group1 Human Reproduction Update 2006 12(3):193–207; doi:10.1093/humupd/dmk003.

146 Origins and evolution of the Western diet: (See 42).

147 MayoClinic.com Tools for healthier lives Rheumatoid arthritis.

148 Introduction to lipid peroxidation.

149 Oxidative Stress and Peroxisome Proliferator–Activated Receptors Circulation Research. 2004;95:1137 · Pallavi R. Devchand, Ouliana Ziouzenkova, Jorge Plutzky · Donald W. Reynolds Cardiovascular Clinical Research Center, Cardiovascular Division, Brigham and Women's Hospital, Harvard Medical School.

150 Telomere From Wikipedia, the free encyclopedia.

151 Mutational spectrum and genotoxicity of the major lipid peroxidation product, trans–4–hydroxy–2–nonenal, induced DNA adducts in nucleotide excision repair-proficient and · deficient human cells. · Feng Z, Hu W, Amin S, Tang MS. · Biochemistry, 42 (25), 7848–7854, 2003. 10.1021/bi034343lg S0006–2960(03)04431–3· Dept.s of Environmental Medicine, Medicine, and Pathology, New York University School of Medicine, Tuxedo, New York 10987, and Division of Carcinogenesis and Molecular Epidemiology, American Health Foundation, Valhalla, New York 10595.

152 Formation of cyclic deoxyguanosine adducts from omega–3 and omega–6 polyunsaturated fatty acids under oxidative conditions. · Pan J, Chung FL. Chem·Res·Toxicol. 2002 Mar; 15(3): 367–72. Departments of Environmental Medicine, Medicine, and Pathology, New York University School of Medicine, Tuxedo, New York 10987, and Division of Carcinogenesis and Molecular Epidemiology, American Health Foundation, Valhalla, New York 10595

153 Nanomedicine, Volume I: Basic Capabilities © 1999 Landes Bioscience, TX, 1999 · Robert A. Freitas Jr.

154 The role of docosahexaenoic acid in mediating mitochondrial membrane lipid oxidation and apoptosis in colonocytes · Carcinogenesis 2005 Nov;26(11):1914–21. Epub 2005 Jun 23. Ng Y, · Barhoumi R, Tjalkens RB, Fan YY, Kolar S, Wang N, Lupton JR, Chapkin RS · Faculty of Nutrition, Texas A&M University, College Station, TX 77843, USA. PubMed 15975958.

155 Effects of various dietary fats on cardiolipin acyl composition during ontogeny of mice · Lipids. 1992 Aug;27(8):605–12. · Berger A, Gershwin ME, German JB. · Dept. of Food Science and Technology, University of California, Davis 95616. PubMed 1406071.

156 PUFA and aging modulate cardiac mitochondrial membrane lipid composition and Ca2+ activation of PDH · Am J Physiol Heart Circ Physiol 276: H149–H158, 1999 · Salvatore Pepe, Naotaka Tsuchiya, Edward G. Lakatta, and Richard G. Hansford · Laboratory of Cardiovascular Science, Gerontology Research Center, National Institute on Aging, National Institutes of Health, Baltimore, Maryland 21224.

157 Docosahexaenoic acid accumulates in cardiolipin and enhances HT–29 cell oxidant production. · Steven M Watkins, Lynne C Carter and J Bruce · German Dept. of Food Science and Technology, University of California, Davis, CA 95616.

158 Cardiolipins from Rats Fed Different Dietary Lipids Affect Bovine Heart Cytochrome c Oxidase · Activity. Sakiyo Yamaoka-Koseki, Reiko Urade and Makoto Kito · Research Insitute for Food Science, Kyoto University, Uji, Kyoto611 Japan.

159 Brief communication: omega–3 essential fatty acid supplementation and erythrocyte oxidant/antioxidant status in rats. · Ann Clin Lab Sci. 2005 Spring;35(2):169–73 · Iraz M, Erdogan H, Ozyurt B, Ozugurlu F, Ozgocmen S, Fadillioglu E. · Dept. of Pharmacology, Inonu University Faculty of Medicine, Malatya PubMed 15943181.

160 Oxidative Stress and Peroxisome Proliferator–Activated Receptors · Circulation Research. 2004;95:1137. · Pallavi R. Devchand, Ouliana Ziouzenkova, Jorge Plutzky · Donald W. Reynolds Cardiovascular Clinical Research Center, Cardiovascular Division, Brigham and Women's Hospital, Harvard Medical School, Boston, Mass.

161 Effect of fish oil supplementation on plasma oxidant/antioxidant status in rats. · Prostaglandins Leukot Essent Fatty Acids. 2004 Sep;71(3):149–52 · Erdogan H, Fadillioglu E, Ozgocmen S, Sogut S, Ozyurt B, Akyol O, Ardicoglu O. · Dept. of Physiology, Faculty of Medicine, Gaziosmanpasa University, Tokat , Turkey. PubMed 5253883.

162   Oxidized phospholipids as modulators of inflammation in atherosclerosis. · Curr Opin Lipidol. 2003 Oct;14(5):421-30 · Leitinger N. · Dept. of Vascular Biology and Thrombosis Research, University of Vienna, Vienna, Austria. PubMed 14501580.

163   Oxidized lipids: the two faces of vascular inflammation · Curr Atheroscler Rep. 2006 May;8(3):223-31 · Birukov KG · .Dept. of Medicine, University of Chicago, 929 East 57th Street, W410, Chicago, IL 60637, USA. PubMed 16640959.

164   Menopause Modifies the Association of Leukocyte Telomere Length with Insulin resistance and Inflammation · Jnl. of Clinical Endocrinology & Metabolism, doi:10.1210/jc.2005-1814 · Abraham Aviv Ana Valdes, Jeffrey P Gardner Rami Swaminathan Masayuki Kimura Tim D Spector.

165   Functional Estrogen Receptors in the Mitochondria of Breast Cancer · MBC Vol. 17, Issue 5, 2125-2137, May 2006 · Ali Pedram, Mahnaz Razandi, Douglas C. Wallace,and Ellis R. Levin. Division of Endocrinology, Veterans Affairs Medical Center, Long Beach, Long Beach, CA 90822; Department of Medicine, University of California, Irvine, Irvine CA 92717; Department of Biochemistry, University of California, Irvine, Irvine CA 92717; Department of Pharmacology, University of California, Irvine, Irvine CA 92717; and Department of the Center for Molecular and Mitochondrial Medicine and Genetics, University of California, Irvine, Irvine CA 92717

166   Lower serum zinc in Chronic Fatigue Syndrome (CFS): relationships to immune dysfunctions and relevance for the oxidative stress status in CFS. · J Affect Disord. 2006 Feb;90(2-3):141-7 · Maes M, Mihaylova I, De Ruyter M. M · Care4U Outpatient Clinics, Olmenlaan 9, 2610 Antwerp-Wilrijk, Belgium. PubMed 16338007.

167   Anti-inflammatory properties of lipid oxidation products. · J Mol Med. 2003 Oct;81(10):613-26 · Bochkov VN, Leitinger N. · Dept. of Vascular Biology and Thrombosis Research, University of Vienna, 1090 Vienna, Austria. PubMed 13679995.

168   Dietary ratio of (n-6)/(n-3) polyunsaturated fatty acids alters the fatty acid composition of bone compartments and biomarkers of bone formation in rats · J Nutr. 2000 Sep;130(9):2274-84 · Watkins BA, Li Y, Allen KG, Hoffmann WE, Seifert MF. · Dept. of Food Science, Lipid Chemistry and Molecular Biology Laboratory, Purdue University, West Lafayette, IN 47907, USA. PubMed 10958824.

169   Correlation between arachidonic acid oxygenation and luminol-induced chemiluminescence in neutrophils: inhibition by diethyldithiocarbamate. · Chabannes B, Perraut C, El Habib R, Moliere P, Pacheco Y, Lagarde M. · INSERM U352, Laboratoire de Biochimie et Pharmacologie, Institut National des Sciences Appliquees, Villeurbanne, France. · Biochem Pharmacol. 1997 Apr 4;53(7):927-35 PubMed 9174105.

170   Blood cell redox status and fatty acids. Prostaglandins · Leukot Essent Fatty Acids. 1995 Feb-Mar;52(2-3):159-61· Lagarde M, Vericel E, Chabannes B, Prigent AF. · INSERM U352, Chimie Biologique INSA-Lyon, Villeurbanne, France PubMed 7784452.

171   Dietary omega-3 polyunsaturated fatty acids inhibit phosphoinositide formation and chemotaxis in neutrophils. · J Clin Invest. 1993 Feb;91(2):651-60 · Sperling RI, Benincaso AI, Knoell CT, Larkin JK, Austen KF, Robinson DR. · Dept. of Medicine, Harvard Medical School, Boston, MA 02115. PubMed 8381824.

172   The effects of dietary n-3 polyunsaturated fatty acids on neutrophils · Proc Nutr Soc. 1998 Nov;57(4):527-34 · Sperling RI. Dept. of Medicine, Harvard Medical School, Brigham & Women's Hospital, Boston, USA. PubMed 10096112.

173   Effect of low-to-moderate amounts of dietary fish oil on neutrophil lipid composition and function Lipids. · 2000 Jul;35(7):763-8 Healy DA, Wallace FA, Miles EA, Calder PC, Newsholm P. · Dept. of Biochemistry, The Conway Institute of Biomolecular and Biomedical Research, University College Dublin, PubMed 10941877.

174   Docosahexaenoic acid concentrations are higher in women than in men because of estrogenic effects · Am J Clin Nutr. 2004 Nov;80(5):1167-74 · Giltay EJ, Gooren LJ, Toorians AW, Katan MB, Zock PL. · Psychiatric Center GGZ Delfland, Delft, Netherlands. PubMed 15531662.

175   Hibbeln JR and Salem N Jr. Dietary polyunsaturated fatty acids and depression: when cholesterol does not satisfy. · Am J Clinical Nutr 1995; 62: 1-9; · Hibbeln JR and Salem N Jr. Risks of cholesterol-lowering therapies. · Biological Psychiatry 1996; 40: 7: 686-687. · Hibbeln JR, Umhau JC, George DT, and Salem N Jr. · Do Plasma Polyunsaturates predict Hostility and Violence? World Rev Nutr Diet 1996; 82: 175-186.

176   Changes in relative fatty acid composition of serum lecithin and cholesterol ester after treatment with two gonane progestins administered alone and in combination with ethinyl estradiol. · Arch Gynecol. 1984;236(1):35-40 · Crona N, Enk L, Samsioe G, Silfverstolpe G. PubMed 6239594.

177   Docosahexaenoic acid concentrations are higher in women than in men because of estrogenic effects · Am J Clin Nutr. 2004 Nov;80(5):1167-74 · Giltay EJ, Gooren LJ, Toorians AW, Katan MB, Zock PL. · Psychiatric Center GGZ Delfland, Netherlands. PubMed 15531662.

178   Raloxifene and hormone replacement therapy increase arachidonic acid and docosahexaenoic acid levels in postmenopausal women. · Jnl. of Endocrinology, Vol 182, Issue 3, 399-408 · Giltay EJ, Duschek EJ, Katan MB, Zock PL, Neele SJ, Netelenbos JC. · Psychiatric Center GGZ Delfland, Delft, The Netherlands.

179   Cloning, Expression, and Fatty Acid Regulation of the Human D-5 Desaturase · J Biol Chem, Vol. 274,
        Issue 52, 37335-37339, December 24, 1999 · Hyekyung P. Cho, Manabu Nakamura, and Steven D. Clarke
        · Program of Nutritional Sciences and the Institute for Cellular and Molecular Biology, The University of
        Texas-Austin, Austin, Texas 78712.

180   Metabolic fuels and reproduction in female mammals. · Neurosci Biobehav Rev. 1992 Summer;16(2):235-72
        · Wade GN, Schneider JE.· Dept. of Psychology and Neuroscience, University of Massachusetts. PubMed
        1630733.

181   Midwivesonline.com.

182   Relative fatty acid composition of serum lecithin in the second half of the normal pregnancy · Gynecol
        Obstet Invest. 1982;14(3):225-35 · Rosing U, Johnson P, Olund A, Samsioe G. PubMed 7129232.

183   Current Status of the Hypothesis That Mammleian Ovulation is comparable to an Inflamatory Reaction.
        · Biology of Reproduction 50, 233-238 (1994) · Lawrence L Espey iology Dept., Trinity Universtiy, San
        Antonio Texas 78212-7200.

184   Synthesis and biological evaluation of selective aromatase expression regulators in breast cancer cells.
        · J Med Chem. 2007 Apr 5;50(7):1635-44 · Su B, Landini S, Davis DD, Brueggemeier RW. · Division of
        Medicinal Chemistry and Pharmacognosy, College of Pharmacy, and Ohio State Biochemistry Program,
        The Ohio State University, Columbus, Ohio 43210, USA. PubMed 17315855.

185   Raloxifene and hormone replacement therapy increase arachidonic acid and docosahexaenoic acid
        levels in postmenopausal women.· J Endocrinol. 2004 Sep;182(3):399-408 · Giltay EJ, Duschek EJ, Katan
        MB, Zock PL, Neele SJ, Netelenbos JC · Psychiatric Center GGZ Delfland, Delft, The Netherlands.
        PubMed 15350182.

186   British Jnl. of Nutrition (2003), 90, 993-995.

187   Fin Nutritional paper 4 - feeding fish meal improves cow fertility.

188   Docosahexaenoic acid concentrations are higher in women than in men because of estrogenic effects.
        · Am J Clin Nutr. 2004 Nov;80(5):1167-74 Giltay EJ, Gooren LJ, Toorians AW, Katan MB, Zock PL.
        Psychiatric Center GGZ Delfland, Delft, PubMed 15531662.

189   Fatty acid compositions of serum phospholipids of postmenopausal women: a comparison between
        Greenland Inuit and Canadians before and after supplementation with fish oil. · Nutrition. 2002
        Jul-Aug;18(7-8):627-Stark KD, Mulvad G, Pedersen HS, Park EJ, Dewailly E, Holub BJ. · Dept. of Human
        Biology and Nutritional Sciences, University of Guelph, Guelph, Ontario, Canada. PubMed 12093443.

190   Milk composition in women from five different regions of China: the great diversity of milk fatty acids. · J
        Nutr. 1995 Dec;125(12):2993-8 · Ruan C, Liu X, Man H, Ma X, Lu G, Duan G, DeFrancesco CA, Connor WE.
        · Central Laboratory, Dalian Medical University, China.

191   Human milk fatty acid composition from nine countries varies most in DHA. · Lipids Vol 41 no 9 Sept
        2006 · Yuhas R, Pramuk K, Lien EL. · Dept. of Nutrition Research, Wyeth Nutrition, 500 Arcola Road,
        Collegeville, Pennsylvania 19426, USA.

192   Sperm fatty acid composition in subfertile men. · Prostaglandins Leukot Essent Fatty Acids. 2006
        Aug;75(2):75-9 · Aksoy Y, Aksoy H, Altinkaynak K, Aydin HR, Ozkan A. · Dept. of Urology, School of
        Medicine, Ataturk University, TR-25240 Erzurum, Turkey. PubMed16893631.

193   The fatty acid composition of phospholipids of spermatozoa from infertile patients. · Mol Hum Reprod.
        1998 Feb;4(2):111-8 Zalata AA, Christophe AB, Depuydt CE, Schoonjans F, Comhaire FH. · University
        Hospital Ghent, Dept. of Internal Medicine, Belgium. PubMed 9542967.

194   Combined effect of DHA and alpha-tocopherol enrichment on sperm quality and fertility in the turkey.
        · Theriogenology. 2006 Jun;65(9):1813-27 Zaniboni L, Rizzi R, Cerolini S. · Dept. of Veterinary sciences and
        Technologies for Food Safety (VSA), University of Milan, Via Trentacoste 2, 20134 Milan, Italy. PubMed
        16298425.

195   Expression and Regulation of D5-Desaturase, D6-Desaturase, Stearoyl-Coenzyme A (CoA) Desaturase
        1, and Stearoyl-CoA Desaturase 2 in Rat Testis. · Biol Reprod 2003, 10.1095/biolreprod.102.014035 · Thomas
        Sæther, Thien N. Tran, Helge Rootwelt, Bjørn O. Christophersen and Trine B. Haugen. Andrology
        Laboratory, Department of Gynecology and Obstetrics, Institute of Clinical Biochemistry and Department
        of Clinical Chemistry, Rikshospitalet University Hospital, N-0027 Oslo, Norway

196   Combined effect of DHA and alpha-tocopherol enrichment on sperm quality and fertility in the turkey.
        · Theriogenology. 2006 Jun;65(9):1813-27 · Dept. of Veterinary Sciences and Technologies for Food Safety
        (VSA), · University of Milan, Via Trentacoste 2, 20134 Milan, PubMed 16298425.

197   Effect of feeding a DHA-enriched nutriceutical on the quality of fresh, cooled and frozen stallion semen.
        · Theriogenology. 2005 Mar 15;63(5):1519-27 · Brinsko SP, Varner DD, Love CC, Blanchard TL, Day BC,
        Wilson ME. · Dept. of Large Animal Medicine and Surgery, College of Veterinary Medicine, Texas A&M
        University 77843-4475, USA. PubMed 15725455.

198   Evaluation of the ratio of omega(6: omega3 fatty acids and vitamin E levels in the diet on the reproductive performance of cockerels. - Arch Tierernahr. 2003 Dec;57(6):429–42. Zanini SF, Torres CA, Bragagnolo N, Turatti JM, Silva MG, Zanini MS. - Dept. of Rural Economics and Animal Science, Center of Agrarian Sciences, Federal University of Espírito Santo, Alegre, PubMed 14982322.

199   Effect of long-term supplementation with arachidonic or docosahexaenoic acids on sperm production in the broiler chicken - J Reprod Fertil. 2000 Nov;120(2):257–64. - Surai PF, Noble RC, Sparks NH, Speake BK. - Dept. of Biochemistry and Nutrition, Scottish Agricultural College, Auchincruive, Ayr KA6 5HW, UK. PubMed 11058441.

200   Expression and Regulation of D5–Desaturase, D6–Desaturase, Stearoyl-Coenzyme A ....See 195 above.

201   Arachidonic acid and prostaglandin E2 stimulate testosterone production by goldfish testis in vitro. - Author: Wade, M G : Van der Kraak, G - Gen-Comp-Endocrinol. 1993 Apr; 90(1): 109-18.

202   Evidence for metabolic and reproductive phenotypes in mothers of women with polycystic ovary syndrome. - Proc Natl Acad Sci U S A. 2006 May 2;103(18):7030–5 - Sam S, Legro RS, Essah PA, Apridonidze T, Dunaif A. - Division of Endocrinology, Metabolism, and Molecular Medicine, Dept. of Medicine, Feinberg School of Medicine, Northwestern University, Chicago, IL 60611, USA. PubMed 16632599.

203   Prostaglandin receptors are mediators of vascular function in endometrial pathologies. - Mol Cell Endocrinol. 2006 Jun 27;252(1–2):191–200. Epub 2006 May 15 - Jabbour HN, Sales KJ, Smith OP, Battersby S, Boddy SC. MRC - Human Reproductive Sciences Unit, Centre for Reproductive Biology, The Queen's Medical Research Institute, Edinburgh. PubMed 16701939.

204   Assessment of premenstrual dysphoric disorder symptoms: population of women in Casablanca - Encephale. 2002 Nov–Dec;28(6 Pt 1):525–30 - Tahiri SM, Moussaoui D, Kadri N. - Centre Psychiatrique Universitaire Ibn Rochd, Casablanca, Maroc. PubMed 12506265.

205   Effects of altering dietary fatty acid composition on prostaglandin synthesis and fertility. - Prostaglandins Leukot Essent Fatty Acids. 1999 Nov;61(5):275–87 - Abayasekara DR, Wathes DC. - Reproduction and Development Group, Dept. of Veterinary Basic Sciences, Royal Veterinary College, London, UK. PubMed 10670689.

206   Prostaglandin receptors are mediators of vascular function in endometrial pathologies. - Mol Cell Endocrinol. 2006 Jun 27;252(1–2):191–200. - Jabbour HN, Sales KJ, Smith OP, Battersby S, Boddy SC. MRC - Human Reproductive Sciences Unit, Centre for Reproductive Biology, The Queen's Medical Research Institute, 47 Little France Crescent, Edinburgh EH16 4TJ, United Kingdom. PubMed 16701939.

207   Effects of altering dietary fatty acid composition on prostaglandin synthesis and fertility. - Prostaglandins Leukot Essent Fatty Acids. 1999 Nov;61(5):275–87 - Abayasekara DR, Wathes DC. - Reproduction and Development Group, Dept. of Veterinary Basic Sciences, Royal Veterinary College, London, UK. PubMed 10670689.

208   Dietary fatty acid intakes and the risk of ovulatory infertility - American Jnl. of Clinical Nutrition, Vol. 85, No. 1, 231–237, January 2007 - Jorge E Chavarro, Janet W Rich-Edwards, Bernard A Rosner and Walter C Willett - Dept.s of Nutrition (JEC and WCW), Epidemiology (JEC, JWR-E, and WCW), and Biostatistics (BAR), Harvard School of Public Health, Boston, MA; and the Dept. of Ambulatory Care and Prevention (JWR-E) and the Channing Laboratory, Dept. of Medicine, Brigham and Women's Hospital (JWR-E, BAR, and WCW), Harvard Medical School, Boston, MA

209   Daily Telegraph 02/11/05 - Roger Highfield - Attractive women are more that just a pretty face.

210   A maternal diet high in n–6 polyunsaturated fats alters mammary gland development, puberty onset, and breast cancer risk among female rat offspring. - Proc Natl Acad Sci U S A. 1997 Aug 19;94(17):9372–7 - Hilakivi-Clarke L, Clarke R, Onojafe I, Raygada M, Cho E, Lippman M. - Lombardi Cancer Center, Georgetown University Medical Center, Washington, DC , USA. PubMed 9256489.

211   Essential fatty acid deficiency delays the onset of puberty in the female rat. - Endocrinology. 1989 Sep;125(3):1650–9 - Smith SS, Neuringer M, Ojeda SR. - Dept. of Anatomy, Hahnemann University, Philadelphia, Pennsylvania PubMed 2759037.

212   A maternal diet high in n–6 polyunsaturated fats alters mammary gland development. See 210 above.

213   Timing of dietary fat exposure and mammary tumorigenesis: role of estrogen receptor and protein kinase C activity. - Mol Cell Biochem. 1998 Nov;188(1–2):5–12 - Hilakivi-Clarke L, Clarke R. - Lombardi Cancer Center, Georgetown University, Washington, DC 20007–2197, USA. PubMed 9823005.

214   Neuregulins signaling via a glial erbB–2–erbB–4 receptor complex contribute to the neuroendocrine control of mammalian sexual development. - J Neurosci. 1999 Nov 15;19(22):9913–27 - Ma YJ, Hill DF, Creswick KE, Costa ME, Cornea A, Lioubin MN, Plowman GD, Ojeda SR. - Division of Neuroscience, Oregon Regional Primate Research Center, Beaverton, Oregon 97006, USA. PubMed 10559400.

215   Essential fatty acid deficiency delays the onset of puberty in the female rat. See 211 above.

216   n-3 Fatty acids and the metabolic syndrome · Yvon A Carpentier, Laurence Portois and Willy J Malaisse · L Deloyers Laboratory of Experimental Surgery, Université Libre de Bruxelles, Brussels, Belgium · American Jnl. of Clinical Nutrition, Vol. 83, No. 6, S1499–1504S, June 2006.

217   Unfavorable effect of type 1 and type 2 diabetes on maternal and fetal essential fatty acid status: a potential marker of fetal insulin resistance · American Jnl. of Clinical Nutrition, Vol. 82, No. 6, 1162–1168, December 2005 · Min Y, Lowy C, Ghebremeskel K, Thomas B, Offley-Shore B, Crawford M. · Institute of Brain Chemistry and Human Nutrition, London Metropolitan University, and the Endocrine and Diabetic Day Centre, Guy's and St Thomas' Hospital Trust, London,

218   Type 1 diabetes compromises plasma arachidonic and docosahexaenoic acids in newborn babies. · Lipids. 2004 Apr;39(4):335–42 · Ghebremeskel K, Thomas B, Lowy C, Min Y, Crawford MA. · Institute of Brain Chemistry and Human Nutrition, London Metropolitan University. PubMed 15357021.

219   Essential fatty acids in infant nutrition: lessons and limitations from animal studies in relation to studies on infant fatty acid requirements · American Jnl. of Clinical Nutrition, Vol. 71, No. 1, 238S–244S, January 2000 · Sheila M Innis · Dept. of Paediatrics, University of British Columbia, Vancouver.

220   Smart Fats A Schmidt.

221   Role of omega-3 fatty acids in brain development and function: potential implications for the pathogenesis and prevention of psychopathology. · Prostaglandins Leukot Essent Fatty Acids. 2006 Oct–Nov;75(4–5):329–49. · McNamara RK, Carlson SE. ·Dept. of Psychiatry, University of Cincinnati College of Medicine, Cincinnati, OH USA. PubMed 16949263.

222   Omega-3 fatty acid deficiencies in neurodevelopment, aggression and autonomic dysregulation: opportunities for intervention. · Int Rev Psychiatry. 2006 Apr;18(2):107–18. · Hibbeln JR, Ferguson TA, Blasbalg TL. · National Institute on Alcohol Abuse and Alcoholism, Bethesda, USA PubMed 16777665.

223   Reversal of docosahexaenoic acid deficiency in the rat brain, retina, liver, and serum · Jnl. of Lipid Research Vol. 42, 419–427, March 200 · Toru Moriguchi, James Loewke, Megan Garrison, Janice Nicklay Catalan, and Norman Salem, Jr. · Laboratory of Membrane Biochemistry & Biophysics, National Institutes on Alcohol Abuse & Alcoholism, NIH, Bethesda, MD 20892 USA.

224   Intakes of essential n-6 and n-3 polyunsaturated fatty acids among pregnant Canadian women · American Jnl. of Clinical Nutrition, Vol. 77, No. 2, 473–478, February 2003 · Sheila M Innis and Sandra L Elias · Dept. of Pediatrics, University of British Columbia, Vancouver, Canada.

225   Fatty acid composition of human colostrum in Slovenian women living in urban and rural areas · Biology of the Neonate 2001;79:15–20 (DOI: 10.1159/000047060 · Fidler Natasa ; Salobir Karl; Stibilj Vekoslava · Institute of Nutrition, Biotechnical Faculty, University of Ljubljana, Slovenie.

226   Human milk fatty acid composition from nine countries varies most in DHA. · Lipids. 2006 Sep;41(9):851–8 · Yuhas R, Pramuk K, Lien EL. · Dept. of Nutrition Research, Wyeth Nutrition, 500 Arcola Road, Collegeville, Pennsylvania PubMed 17152922.

227   Milk composition in women from five different regions of China: the great diversity of milk fatty acids. · J Nutr. 1995 Dec;125(12):2993–8 · Ruan C, Liu X, Man H, Ma X, Lu G, Duan G, DeFrancesco CA, Connor WE. · Central Laboratory, Dalian Medical University, China. PubMed 7500177.

228   Long-chain polyunsaturated fatty acids in maternal and infant nutrition. · Prostaglandins Leukot Essent Fatty Acids. 2006 Sep;75(3):135–44 · Muskiet FA, van Goor SA, Kuipers RS, Velzing-Aarts FV, Smit EN, Bouwstra H, Janneke Dijck-Brouwer DA, Rudy Boersma E, Hadders-Algra M. · Pathology and Laboratory Medicine, University Medical Center Groningen, The Netherlands PubMed 16876396.

229   Supplementing lactating women with flaxseed oil does not increase docosahexaenoic acid in their milk · American Jnl. of Clinical Nutrition, Vol. 77, No. 1, 226–233, January 2003 · Cindy A Francois, Sonja L Connor, Linda C Bolewicz and William E Connor · Division of Endocrinology, Metabolism and Clinical Nutrition, the Dept. of Medicine, Oregon Health and Science University, Portland.

230   Intakes of essential n-6 and n-3 polyunsaturated fatty acids among pregnant Canadian women · American Jnl. of Clinical Nutrition, Vol. 77, No. 2, 473–478, February 2003 · Sheila M Innis and Sandra L Elias · Dept. of Pediatrics, University of British Columbia, Vancouver, Canada.

231   Arachidonic acid and prostacyclin signaling promote adipose tissue development : a human health concern? · Florence Massiera, Perla Saint-Marc, Josiane Seydoux, Takahiko Murata, Takuya Kobayashi Shuh Narumiya, Philippe Guesnet, Ez-Zoubir Amri, Raymond Negrel and Gérard Ailhaud · Institut de Recherche Signalisation, Centre Médical Universitaire, Dept. of Pharmacology, Kyoto University, Laboratoire de Nutrition et Sécurité Alimentaire, · JLR Papers in Press, November 4, 2002. DOI 10.1194/jlr. M200346-JLR200.

232 Distribution, interconversion, and dose response of n–3 fatty acids in humans · American Jnl. of Clinical Nutrition, Vol. 83, No. 6, S1467–1476S, June 2006 · Linda M Arterburn, Eileen Bailey Hall and Harry Oken · From Martek Biosciences Corporation, Columbia, MD (LMA and EBH), and the University of Maryland, Baltimore, MD (HO).

233 Docosahexaenoic and arachidonic acid concentrations in human breast milk worldwide · American Jnl. of Clinical Nutrition, Vol. 85, No. 6, 1457–1464, June 2007 · J Thomas Brenna, Behzad Varamini, Robert G Jensen, Deborah A Diersen-Schade, Julia A Boettcher and Linda M Arterburn · Division of Nutritional Sciences, Cornell University, Ithaca, NY (JTB and BV); the Dept. of Nutritional Sciences, University of Connecticut, Storrs, CT (RGJ); Mead Johnson & Company, Evansville, IN (DAD and JAB); and Martek Biosciences Corporation, Columbia, MD (LMA).

234 Supplementing lactating women with flaxseed oil does not increase docosahexaenoic acid in their milk · American Jnl. of Clinical Nutrition, Vol. 77, No. 1, 226–233, January 2003 · Cindy A Francois, Sonja L Connor, Linda C Bolewicz and William E Connor · Division of Endocrinology, Metabolism and Clinical Nutrition, the Dept. of Medicine, Oregon Health and Science University, Portland.

235 Essential fatty acids in infant nutrition: lessons and limitations from animal studies in relation to studies on infant fatty acid requirements See 219.

236 Trans, n–3, and n–6 fatty acids in Canadian human milk. · Lipids. 1996 Mar;31 Suppl:S279–82. · Ratnayake WM, Chen ZY. · Nutrition Research Division, Health Canada, Ottawa, Canada. PubMed 8729134.

237 Trans Fatty Acids in Subcutaneous Fat of Pregnant Women and in Human Milk in the Czech Republic · Annals of the New York Academy of Sciences 967:544–547 (2002) · Pavel Dlouhya, Eva Tvrzicka, Barbora Stankova. Marta Buchtikova, Rajmund Pokornya. Olga Wiereova,Diana Bilkova, Jolana Rambouskova and Michal Andel.

238 Infant plasma trans, n–6, and n–3 fatty acids and conjugated linoleic acids are related to maternal plasma fatty acids, length of gestation, and birth weight and length · American Jnl. of Clinical Nutrition, Vol. 73, No. 4, 807–814, April 2001 · Sandra L Elias and Sheila M Innis · Dept. of Paediatrics, University of British Columbia, Vancouver, Canada.

239 Trans fatty intakes during pregnancy, infancy and early childhood. · Atheroscler Suppl. 2006 May;7(2):17–20 · Innis SM. · Nutrition Research Program, Child and Family Research Institute, Dept. of Pediatrics, University of British Columbia, Vancouver, Canada. PubMed 16713384.

240 Inverse association between trans isomeric and long-chain polyunsaturated fatty acids in cord blood lipids of full-term infants · American Jnl. of Clinical Nutrition, Vol. 74, No. 3, 364–368, September 2001 · Tamás Decsi, István Burus, Szilárd Molnár, Hajnalka Minda and Volker Veitl · Dept. of Paediatrics, University of Pécs, Pécs, Hungary, and the Research Dept., Milupa GmbH, Salzburg, Austria.

241 Trans fatty intakes during pregnancy, infancy and early childhood. (seeabove).

242 Planet Ark.

243 Incorporation of trans long-chain n–3 polyunsaturated fatty acids in rat brain structures and retina. · Grandgirard A, Bourre JM, Julliard F, Homayoun P, Dumont O, Piciotti M, Sebedio JL. · INRA, Station de Recherches sur la Qualité des Aliments de l'Homme, Unité de Nutrition Lipidique, Dijon, France.

244 Breastfeeding mom's diet and baby's brain development · http://www.007b.com/breastfeeding_intelligence_diet.php.

245 Supplementing lactating women with flaxseed oil does not increase docosahexaenoic acid in their milk (See above).

246 Synthesis of long-chain polyunsaturated fatty acids in lactating mammary gland role of {Delta}5 and {Delta}6 desaturases, SREBP-1, PPAR{alpha}, and PGC-1 · Maricela Rodriguez-Cruz Originally published In Press as doi:10.1194/jlr.M500407–JLR200 on December 6, 2005 · Armando R. Tovar§, Berenice Palacios-González, Martha del Prado and Nimbe Torresl · Unidad de Investigación Médica en Nutrición, Coordinación de Investigación en Salud, Centro Médico Nacional Siglo XXI, Instituto Mexico City Posgrado en Ciéncias Biológicas, Mexico City Departamento de Fisiología de la Nutrición, Mexico City,

247 Trans fatty acids may impair biosynthesis of long-chain polyunsaturates and growth in man · Acta Paediatr. 1992 Apr;81(4):302–6 · Koletzko B. · Kinderklinik Heinrich-Heine-Universität, Düsseldorf, Germany. PubMed 1606388.

248 Effects of n–3 polyunsaturated fatty acid supplementation in pregnancy on maternal and fetal erythrocyte fatty acid composition. · Acta Paediatr. 1992 Apr;81(4):302–6 Eur J Clin Nutr. 2004 Mar;58(3):429–37 · Dunstan JA, Mori TA, Barden A, Beilin LJ, Holt PG, Calder C, Taylor AL, Prescott SL. · School of Paediatrics and Child Health, University of Western Australia, Perth, Australia. PubMed 14985680.

249   n–6 and n–3 Long-chain polyunsaturated fatty acids in the erythrocyte membrane of Brazilian preterm and term neonates and their mothers at delivery · Prostaglandins Leukot Essent Fatty Acids. 2006 Feb;74(2) · Pontes PV, Torres AG, Trugo NM, Fonseca VM, Sichieri R. · Laboratório de Bioquímica Nutricional e de Alimentos, Instituto de Química, Universidade Federal do Rio de Janeiro, RJ, Brazil PubMed 16364619.

250   Blood fatty acid composition of pregnant and nonpregnant Korean women: red cells may act as a reservoir of arachidonic acid and docosahexaenoic acid for utilization by the developing fetus. · Lipids. 2000 May;35(5):567–74 · Ghebremeskel K, Min Y, Crawford MA, Nam JH, Kim A, Koo JN, Suzuki H. · Institute of Brain Chemistry and Human Nutrition, The University of North London, PubMed 10907792.

251   The influence of a vegetarian diet on the fatty acid composition of human milk and the essential fatty acid status of the infant. · J Pediatr. 1992 Apr;120(4 Pt 2):S71–7. · Sanders TA, Reddy S. · Dept. of Nutrition and Dietetics, King's College, University of London. PubMed 1560329.

252   Arachidonic and docosahexaenoic acids are biosynthesized ir 18–carbon precursors in human infants · Proc Natl Acad Sci U S A. 1996 Jan 9;93(1):49–54 · Salem N Jr, Wegher B, Mena P, Uauy R. · Laboratory of Membrane Biochemistry and Biophysics, National Institute of Alcohol Abuse and Alcoholism, National Institutes of Health, Rockville, MD 20852, USA. PubMed 8552667.

253   Essential fatty acids in infant nutrition: lessons and limitations from animal studies in relation to studies on infant fatty acid requirements See 219.

254   Plausible explanations for effects of long chain polyunsaturated fatty acids (LCPUFA) on neonates.

255   Arachidonic and Docosahexaenoic Acids are Biosynthesized ir 18–Carbon Precursors in Human Infants (see above).

256   Benefits and risks of modifying maternal fat intake in pregnancy and lactation. David L Hachey – Am J Clin Nutr 1994;59 (suppl):545s–64s.

257   Emerging drug therapies for preventing spontaneous preterm labor and preterm birth · Lamont, Ronald F; Jaggat, Anilla N · Expert Opinion on Investigational Drugs, Volume 16, Number 3, March 2007, pp. 337–345(9).

258   Raised dietary n–6 polyunsaturated fatty acid intake increases 2–series prostaglandin production during labour in the ewe. · J Physiol. 2005 Jan 15;562(Pt 2):583–92. · Elmes M, Green LR, Poore K, Newman J, Burrage D, Abayasekara DR, Cheng Z, Hanson MA, Wathes DC. · Reproduction and Development Group, Royal Veterinary College, Hawkshead Lane, North Mymms, Hatfield, Herts AL9 7TA, UK. PubMed 15513945.

259   The effect of a diet supplemented with the n–6 polyunsaturated fatty acid linoleic acid on prostaglandin production in early- and late-pregnant ewes. · J Endocrinol. 2005 Jan;184(1):165–78 · Cheng Z, Elmes M, Kirkup SE, Chin EC, Abayasekara DR, Wathes DC. · Reproduction and Development Group, Royal Veterinary College, Hawkshead Lane, North Mymms, Hatfield, Herts AL9 7TA, PubMed UK. 15642793.

260   Delay of preterm delivery in sheep by omega–3 long-chain polyunsaturates · Biol Reprod. 1999 Mar;60(3):698–701 · Baguma-Nibasheka M, Brenna JT, Nathanielsz PW. · Laboratory for Pregnancy and Newborn Research, College of Veterinary Medicine, Cornell University, Ithaca, New York, 14853, USA. PubMed 10026118.

261   Delay of preterm delivery in sheep by omega–3 long-chain polyunsaturates (Above).

262   Aspirin inhibits both lipid peroxides and thromboxane in preeclamptic placentas. · Free Radic Biol Med. 1995 Mar;18(3):585–91 · Wang Y, Walsh SW. · Dept. of Obstetrics and Gynecology, Medical College of Virginia, Virginia Commonwealth University, Richmond, USA. PubMed 9101251.

263   Neutrophils from pregnant women produce thromboxane and tumor necrosis factor-alpha in response to linoleic acid and oxidative stress. · Am J Obstet Gynecol. 2005 Sep;193(3 Pt 1):830–5 · Vaughan JE, Walsh SW. · Dept.s of Obstetrics and Gynecology, Virginia Commonwealth University Medical Center, Richmond, VA, USA. PubMed 16150282.

264   Maternal and perinatal long-chain fatty acids: possible roles in preterm birth. · Am J Obstet Gynecol. 1997 Apr;176(4):907–14 · Reece MS, McGregor JA, Allen KG, Harris MA. · Dept. of Food Science and Human Nutrition, Colorado State University, Fort Collins 80523, USA. PubMed 9125620.

265   Essential fatty acid content of maternal erythrocyte phospholipids. A study in preterm and full-term human newborns · Rev Med Chil. 1998 Apr;126(4):391–6. · Araya J, Rojas M, Fernández P, Mateluna A. · Departamentos de Nutrición y de Ginecología y Obstetricia, Facultad de Medicina, Santiago, Chile. PubMed 9699369.

266   Erythrocyte omega–3 and omega–6 polyunsaturated fatty acids and preeclampsia risk in Peruvian women. · Arch Gynecol Obstet. 2006 May;274(2):97–103. Epub 2006 Mar 7 · Qiu C, Sanchez SE, Larrabure G, David R, Bralley JA, Williams MA. · Center for Perinatal Studies, Swedish Medical Center, 747 Broadway (Suite 4 North), Seattle, WA 98122, USA. 16520922.

267   Seafood consumption, the DHA content of mothers' milk and prevalence rates of postpartum depression: a cross-national, ecological analysis - Arch Gynecol Obstet. 2006 May;274(2):97-103. - Qiu C, Sanchez SE, Larrabure G, David R, Bralley JA, Williams MA. - Center for Perinatal Studies, Swedish Medical Center, Seattle, USA. PubMed 12103448.

268   Seafood consumption, the DHA content of mothers' milk and prevalence rates of postpartum depression: a cross-national, ecological analysis.- Hibbeln JR.- Laboratory of Membrane Biophysics and Biochemistry, National Institute on Alcohol Abuse and Alcoholism, Rockville, MD 20892, USA. PubMed 12103448.

269   Increased risk of postpartum depressive symptoms is associated with slower normalization after pregnancy of the functional docosahexaenoic acid status. - Otto SJ, de Groot RH, Hornstra G.- Dept. of Public Health, Erasmus MC, University Medical Center Rotterdam, P.O. Box 1738, DR Rotterdam 3000, The Netherlands. PubMed 12907133.

270   Reduced Brain DHA Content After a Single Reproductive Cycle in Female Rats Fed a Diet Deficient in N-3 Polyunsaturated Fatty Acids - Beth Levant, Jeffery D. Radel and Susan E. Carlson A - Dept.s of Pharmacology, Toxicology, and Therapeutics, Kansas Occupational Therapy Education, Dietetics and Nutrition, Smith Mental Retardation Research Center, University of Kansas Medical Center, Kansas, USA.

271   Visual maturation of term infants fed long-chain polyunsaturated fatty acid-supplemented or control formula for 12 mo. - Birch, EE; Castaneda, YS; Wheaton, DH; Birch, DG; Uauy, RD; Hoffman, DR. Retina Foundation of the Southwest, Dallas, TX, USA.

272   n-3 Fatty acids and cognitive and visual acuity development: methodologic and conceptual considerations American Jnl. of Clinical Nutrition, - Vol. 83, No. 6, S1458-1466S, June 2006 - Carol L Cheatham, John Colombo and Susan E Carlson - Dept. of Dietetics and Nutrition, The Schiefelbusch Institute for Life Span Studies and the Dept. of Psychology Lawrence, and the RL Smith Mental Retardation and Developmental Disabilities Research Center, University of Kansas Medical Center, Kansas City, USA.

273   Plausible explanations for effects of long chain polyunsaturated fatty acids (LCPUFA) on neonates - Arch Dis Child Fetal Neonatal Ed 1999;80:F148-F154 - L O Kurlak, T J Stephenson - Division of Child Health School of Human Development University Hospital Queens Medical Centre Nottingham NG7 2UH.

274   Essential fatty acids in infant nutrition: lessons and limitations from animal studies in relation to studies on infant fatty acid requirements See 219.

275   Lysosomal Enzyme Activities Are Decreased in the Retina and Their Circadian Rhythms Are Different from Those in the Pineal Gland of Rats Fed an -Linolenic Acid-Restricted Diet - (Jnl. of Nutrition. 2000;130:3059-3062.) - Atsushi Ikemoto, Akiko Fukuma, Yoichi Fujii and Harumi Okuyama - Dept. of Biological Chemistry, Faculty of Pharmaceutical Sciences, Nagoya City University, Nagoya, Japan.

276   Plausible explanations for effects of long chain polyunsaturated fatty acids (LCPUFA) on neonates (See Above).

277   Is docosahexaenoic acid, an n-3 long-chain polyunsaturated fatty acid, required for development of normal brain function? - American Jnl. of Clinical Nutrition, Vol. 82, No. 2, 281-295, August 2005 - An overview of evidence from cognitive and behavioral tests in humans and animals Joyce - C McCann and Bruce N Ames - Nutrition, Metabolism and Genomics Center, Children's Hospital Oakland Research Institute, Oakland, CA

278   Reversal of docosahexaenoic acid deficiency in the rat brain, retina, liver, and serum - Jnl. of Lipid Research, see 223.

279   Role of omega-3 fatty acids in brain development and function: potential implications for the pathogenesis and prevention of psychopathology - Prostaglandins Leukot Essent Fatty Acids. 2006 Oct-Nov;75(4-5) - McNamara RK, Carlson SE. - Dept. of Psychiatry, University of Cincinnati College of Medicine, Cincinnati, USA. PubMed 16949263.

280   Maternal Dietary (n-3) Fatty Acid Deficiency Alters Neurogenesis in the Embryonic Rat Brain - American Society for Nutrition J. Nutr. 136:1570-1575, June 2006 - Pauline Coti Bertrand, John R. O'Kusky and Sheila M. Innis3 - The Nutrition Research Program, Child and Family Research Institute, University of British Columbia, Vancouver, British Columbia V5Z 4H4, Canada.

281   Polyunsaturated fatty acids in maternal diet, breast milk, and serum lipid fatty acids of infants in relation to atopy. - Allergy. 2001 Jul;56(7):633-8. - Kankaanpää P, Nurmela K, Erkkilä A, Kalliomäki M, Holmberg-Marttila D, Salminen S, Isolauri E. - Dept.s of Biochemistry and Food Chemistry, and Pediatrics, University of Turku, Turku, Finland. PubMed 11421921.

282   Serum levels of phospholipid fatty acids in mothers and their babies in relation to allergic disease European Jnl. of Pediatrics - Vol 157 no 4 March 1998 - Dept. of Paediatrics, University Hospital, S-Linköping, Sweden G. Yu and B. Björkstén.

283 Atopic sensitization during the first year of life in relation to long chain polyunsaturated fatty acid levels in human milk. · Pediatr Res. 1998 Oct;44(4):478-84 · Duchen K, Yu G, Bjorksten B. · Dept. of Paediatrics, Linköping University, Sweden. PubMed 9773834.

284 Breast milk from mothers of children with newly developed atopic eczema has low levels of long chain polyunsaturated fatty acids. · J Allergy Clin Immunol. 1993 Jun; 91(6) :1134-9 · Businco L, Ioppi M, Morse NL, Nisini R, Wright S. · Dept. of Paediatrics, Università La Sapienza, Rome, Italy. PubMed 8509576.

285 Polyunsaturated fatty acids in school children in relation to allergy and serum IgE levels. · Pediatr Allergy Immunol. 1998 Aug;9(3):133-8. · Yu G, Bjorksten B. · Dept. of Health and Environment, Linköping University, Sweden. PubMed 9814727.

286 Reversal of docosahexaenoic acid deficiency in the rat brain, retina, liver, and serum · See 223.

287 Dietary n-6:n-3 fatty acid ratio in the perinatal period affects bone parameters in adult female rats · Br J Nutr. 2004 Oct;92(4):643-8 · Korotkova M, Ohlsson C, Hanson LA, Strandvik B. · Dept. of Pediatrics, Göteborg University, Sweden. PubMed 15522133.

288 Can prenatal N-3 fatty acid deficiency be completely reversed after birth? Effects on retinal and brain biochemistry and visual function in rhesus monkeys. · Pediatr Res. 2005 Nov;58(5):865-72 · Anderson GJ, Neuringer M, Lin DS, Connor WE. · Division of Endocrinology, Diabetes and Clinical Nutrition, Dept. of Medicine, Oregon National Primate Research Center, Oregon Health and Science University, Portland, Oregon, USA. PubMed 16257925.

289 Reversibility of n-3 fatty acid deficiency-induced changes in dopaminergic neurotransmission in rats : critical role of developmental stage · Jnl. of Lipid Research, Vol. 43, 1209-1219, August 2002 · Ercem Kodas, Sylvie Vancassel, Bernard Lejeune, Denis Guilloteau and Sylvie Chalon · INSERM U316, UFR des Sciences Pharmaceutiques, Laboratoire de Biophysique Médicale et Pharmaceutique, Université François Rabelais, and Laboratoire de Biophysique et Mathématiques, UFR des Sciences Pharmaceutiques, Tours, INRA, Laboratoire de Nutrition et Sécurité Alimentaire, Jouy-en-Josas, France.

290 Reversibility of n-3 fatty acid deficiency-induced alterations of learning behavior in the rat: level of n-6 fatty acids as another critical factor · Jnl. of Lipid Research, Vol. 42, 1655-1663, October 2001 · Atsushi Ikemoto, Masayo Ohishi, Yosuke Sato, Noriaki Hata, Yoshihisa Misawa, Yoichi Fujii, and Harumi Okuyama · Dept. of Biological Chemistry, Faculty of Pharmaceutical Sciences, Nagoya City University, 3-1 Tanabedori, Mizuhoku, Nagoya 467-8603, Japan Applied Research Dept., Harima Chemicals, Tsukuba, Ibaraki 300-26, Japan.

291 Can prenatal N-3 fatty acid deficiency be completely reversed after birth? Effects on retinal and brain biochemistry and visual function in rhesus monkeys Jnl. of Lipid Research · Vol. 42, 1655-1663, October 2001 · Anderson GJ, Neuringer M, Lin DS, Connor WE. · Division of Endocrinology, Diabetes and Clinical Nutrition, Dept. of Medicine, Oregon National Primate Research Center, Oregon Health and Science University, Portland, Oregon 97239-3098, USA. PubMed 16257925.

292 Testosterone and aggressiveness · Marco Giammanco, Garden Tabacchi, Santo Giammanco, Danila Di Majo and Maurizio La Guardia · Endocrinology (2005) Entrez PubMed 16210377.

293 Induction of PGE2 by estradiol mediates developmental masculinization of sex behavior · Nature Neuroscience 7, 643 - 650 (2004) Published online: 23 May 2004; | doi:10.1038/nn1254 ·Stuart K Amateau & Margaret M McCarthy. · Program in Neuroscience and Dept. of Physiology, University of Maryland at Baltimore School of Medicine, Baltimore, Maryland 21201, USA.

294 A maternal diet high in n-6 polyunsaturated fats alters mammary gland development, See 210 above.

295 Timing of dietary fat exposure and mammary tumorigenesis: role of estrogen receptor and protein kinase C activity · Mol Cell Biochem. 1998 Nov;188(1-2):5-12 · Hilakivi-Clarke L, Clarke R, Onojafe I, Raygada M, Cho E, Lippman M.· Lombardi Cancer Center, Georgetown University Medical Center, Washington, DC USA. PubMed 9823005.

296 A maternal diet high in n-6 polyunsaturated fats alters mammary gland development, · See 210 above.

297 Essential fatty acid deficiency delays the onset of puberty in the female rat. (See 211 above).

298 Plausible mechanisms for effects of long-chain polyunsaturated fatty acids on growth. · J Pediatr. 2003 Oct;143(4 Suppl):S9-16 · Lapillonne A, Clarke SD, Heird WC. · Dept. of Pediatrics, Baylor College of Medicine, Houston, Texas, USA. PubMed 14597909.

299 Omega-3 fatty acids and decidual cell prostaglandin production in response to the inflammatory cytokine IL-1beta. · Am J Obstet Gynecol. 2006 Dec;195(6) · Roman AS, Schreher J, Mackenzie AP, Nathanielsz PW · Obstetrics and Gynecology, NYU School of Medicine, New York, USA. PubMed 16792994.

300 Today's CPE - Polycystic Ovary Syndrome Today's Dietitian · Carol Brannon, Vol. 6, No. 10, p. 14.

301   Involvement of arachidonic acid and the lipoxygenase pathway in mediating luteinizing hormone-induced testosterone synthesis in rat Leydig cells · Endocr Res. 1997 Feb-May;23(1-2):15-26. · Mele PG, Dada LA, Paz C, Neuman I, Cymeryng CB, Mendez CF, Finkielstein CV, Cornejo Maciel F, Podestá EJ. ·Dept. of Biochemistry, School of Medicine, University of Buenos Aires, Argentina. PubMed 9187535.

302   A Healthy Menstrual Cycle · Joseph L. Mayo , CNI509 Rev. 7/98 Clinical Nutrition Insights Vol5 No 9.

303   Mifepristone-Induced Vaginal Bleeding Is Associated with Increased Immunostaining for Cyclooxygenase-2 and Decrease in Prostaglandin Dehydrogenase in Luteal Phase Endometrium · The Jnl. of Clinical Endocrinology & Metabolism Vol. 87, No. 11 5229-5234 · Dharani K. Hapangama, Hilary O. D. Critchley, Teresa A. Henderson and David T. Baird · Contraceptive Development Network, Centre for Reproductive Biology, University of Edinburgh, Edinburgh, U.K.

304   Womens Health Abnormal Vaginal Bleeding: Premenopausal Vaginal Bleeding.
       From ACP Medicine Online Alan H. DeCherney, M.D. 06/07/2006.

305   Supplementation with omega-3 polyunsaturated fatty acids in the management of dysmenorrhea in adolescents. · Am J Obstet Gynecol. 1996 Apr;174(4):1335-8 · Harel Z, Biro FM, Kottenhahn RK, Rosenthal SL. · Division of Adolescent Medicine, Children's Hospital Medical Center, Cincinnati, OH 45229, USA.

306   Dysmenorrhea (Menstrual Cramps) · Health-cares.net http://womens-health.health-cares.net/ dysmenorrhea.php.

307   Painful menstruation. · Pediatr Endocrinol Rev. 2006 Jan;3 Suppl 1:160-3 · Tzafettas J. · 2nd Dept. of Obstetrics and Gynecology, Aristotle University, Thessaloniki, Greece. PubMed 16641851.

308   Prostaglandin E2 Increases Cyp19 Expression in Rat Granulosa Cells: Implication of GATA-4 2006 November 13. doi: 10.1016/j.mce.2006.09.012. · Zailong Cai, Jakub Kwintkiewicz, Mary Elizabeth Young, and Carlos Stocco · Dept. of Obstetrics, Gynecology and Reproductive Science, Yale School of Medicine, USA. PubMed 1779458.

309   Inhibition of gonadotropin-stimulated ovarian steroid production by polyunsaturated fatty acids in teleost fish. · Lipids. 1995 Jun;30(6):547-54 · Mercure F, Van Der Kraak G. Dept. of Zoology, University of Guelph, Ontario, Canada PubMed 7651083.

310   Managing endometriosis pain with NSAIDs · Ros Wood and Ellen T Johnson.

311   Ratio of n-6 to n-3 fatty acids and bone mineral density in older adults: the Rancho Bernardo Study. · Am J Clin Nutr. 2005 Apr;81(4):934-8 · Weiss LA, Barrett-Connor E, von Muhlen D. PubMed 15817874.

312   Modulatory effect of omega-3 polyunsaturated fatty acids on osteoblast function and bone metabolism. · Prostaglandins Leukot Essent Fatty Acids. 2003 Jun;68(6):387-98 · Watkins BA, Li Y, Lippman HE, Feng S. · Center for Enhancing Foods to Protect Health, Lipid Chemistry and Molecular Biology Laboratory, Dept. of Food Science, Purdue University, West Lafayette, IN 47907, USA. PubMed 12798659.

313   Conjugated linoleic acid and bone biology. ·J Am Coll Nutr. 2000 Aug;19(4):478S-486S Purdue University, Dept. of Food Science, Lipid Chemistry and Molecular Biology Laboratory, West Lafayette, Indiana PubMed 10963468.

314   Inhibition of osteoporosis due to restricted food intake by the fish oils DHA and EPA and perilla oil in the rat. · Biosci Biotechnol Biochem. 2004 Dec;68(12):2613-5 · Sun L, Tamaki H, Ishimaru T, Teruya T, Ohta Y, Katsuyama N, Chinen I.· Laboratories of Applied Biochemistry, Faculty of Agriculture, University of the Ryukyus, Okinawa 903-0213, Japan. PubMed 15618634.

315   Melatonin inhibits fatty acid-induced triglyceride accumulation in ROS17/2.8 cells: implications for osteoblast differentiation and osteoporosis · Am J Physiol Regul Integr Comp Physiol 292: R2208-R2215, 2007 · M. Sanchez-Hidalgo, Z. Lu, D.-X. Tan, M. D. Maldonado, R. J. Reiter, and R. I. Gregerman · Dept. of Cellular and Structural Biology, Geriatric Research Education and Clinical Center, Audie L. Murphy Division, and Division of Geriatrics and Gerontology, University of Texas Health Science.

316   Tayside University Hospitals Trust Hirsutism.

317   Androgen status in women with late onset or persistent acne vulgaris · C.R. Darley, J.W. Moore, G.M. Besser, D.D. Munro, C.R.W. Edwards, L.H. Rees, J.D. Kirby (1984) · Clinical and Experimental Dermatology 9 (1), 28-35. doi:10.1111/j.1365-2230.1984.tb00751.x.

318   ACTH stimulation tests and plasma dehydroepiandrosterone sulfate levels in women with hirsutism · N Engl J Med. 1990 Sep 27;323(13):849-54 .Siegel SF, Finegold DN, Lanes R, Lee PA. · Dept. of Pediatrics, University of Pittsburgh School of Medicine, PA. PubMed 2168515.

319   Source localization of androgen excess in adolescent girls. · J Clin Endocrinol Metab. 1994 Dec;79(6) :1778-84 · Ibanez L, Potau N, Zampolli M, Prat N, Gussinye M, Saenger P, Vicens-Calvet E, Carrascosa A. · Endocrinology Unit, Hospital Materno-Infantil Vall d'Hebron, Autonomous University, Barcelona, Spain. PubMed 7989484.

320 Fish oil constituent docosahexa-enoic acid selectively inhibits growth of human papillomavirus immortalized keratinocytes Carcinogenesis, · Vol. 20, No. 2, 249–254, February 1999 · DaZhi Chen and Karen Auborn · Long Island Jewish Medical Center, The Long Island Campus for Albert Einstein College of Medicine, Otolaryngology, NY USA.

321 Effects of selenium deficiency on fatty acid metabolism in rats fed fish oil-enriched diets. · J Trace Elem Med Biol. 2004;18(1):89–97 · Institute of Animal Nutrition, Freie Universität Berlin, Germany. PubMed 15487769.

322 Cloning, Expression, and Nutritional Regulation of the Mammalian D–6 Desaturase · J Biol Chem, Vol. 274, Issue 1, 471–477, January 1, 1999 · Program of Nutritional Sciences and the Institute for Cellular and Molecular Biology, The University of Texas-Austin, Austin, Texas 78712.

323 Dietary Polyunsaturated Fat that Is Low in (n–3) and High in (n–6) Fatty Acids Alters the SNARE Protein Complex and Nitrosylation in Rat Hippocampus. · J Nutr. 2007 Aug;137(8):1852–6 · Pongrac JL, Slack PJ, Innis SM. · The Nutrition Research Program, Child and Family Research Institute, University of British Columbia, Vancouver, Canada PubMed 17634254.

324 Roles of unsaturated fatty acids (especially omega–3 fatty acids) in the brain at various ages · See 336.

325 Dietary polyunsaturated fatty acids and depression: when cholesterol does not satisfy. · Am J Clinical Nutr 1995; 62: 1–9; ·Hibbeln JR and Salem N Jr. · Risks of cholesterol-lowering therapies. Biological Psychiatry 1996; 40: 7: 686-687. · Hibbeln JR, Umhau JC, George DT, and Salem N Jr. · Do Plasma Polyunsaturates predict Hostility and Violence? World Rev Nutr Diet 1996; 82: 175-186.

326 Depressive Symptoms, omega–6:omega–3 Fatty Acids, and Inflammation in Older Adults · Psychosomatic Medicine 69:217–224 (2007) · Janice K. Kiecolt-Glaser, PhD, Martha A. Belury, PhD, Kyle Porter, MAS, David Q. Beversdorf, MD, Stanley Lemeshow, PhD and Ronald Glaser, PhD · Dept.s of Psychiatry, Human Nutrition, Neurology, Molecular Virology, Immunology, and Medical Genetics, Ohio State Institute for Behavioral Medicine Research; Ohio State University, Ohio.

327 Suicide attempters and PUFAS: lower plasma eicosapentaenoic acid alone predicts greater psychopathology. · Hibbeln JR, Enstrom G, Majchrzak S, Salem Jr. N, Traskman-Benz L. · 4th Congress of the International Society for the Study of Lipids and Fatty Acids 2000; P–5–28:

328 Omega–3 fatty acids in the treatment of psychiatric disorders. · Drugs. 2005;65(8):1051–9 · Peet M, Stokes C. · Swallownest Court Hospital, Doncaster and South Humber Healthcare NHS Trust, Sheffield, UK PubMed 15907142.

329 Improvements in hostility and depression in relation to dietary change and cholesterol lowering. · Ann Int Med 1992; 117: 820–823. · Weidner G, Connor SL, Hollis JF, Connor WE

330 A replication study of violent and nonviolent subjects: Cerebrospinal fluid metabolites of serotonin and dopamine are predicted by plasma essential fatty acids.· Hibbeln JR; Umhau JC; Linnoila M; George DT; Ragan PW; Shoaf SE; Vaughan MR; Rawlings R; Salem · N. Biological Psychiatry 1998; 44: 243 249.

331 Individual Differences in Alcohol-Induced Aggression Alcohol Research & Health, · Wntr, 2001 by J. Dee Higley A Nonhuman-Primate.

332 CSF 5–HIAA, testosterone, and sociosexual behaviors in free-ranging male rhesus macaques in the mating season. · Psychiatry Res. 1997 Sep 19;72(2):89–102 · Mehlman PT, Higley JD, Fernald BJ, Sallee FR, Suomi SJ, Linnoila M. · LABS of Virginia, Inc., Yemassee, SC PubMed 9335200.

333 DHA May Benefit Heart Disease Related Depression Lithium and Fish Oils Can Boost DHA Levels · A.S. Gissen ttp://intelegen.com/nutrients/dha_may_benefit_heart_disease_re.htm.

334 Self Destructive Behavior and Role of the I function · Karen Taverna · Bryn Mawr College Neurobiology and Behavior Professor Grobstein 7 April 1998.

335 Sex differences in adult ADHD: a double dissociation in brain activity and autonomic arousal. · Hermens DF, Williams LM, Lazzaro I, Whitmont S, Melkonian D, Gordon E. · The Brain Dynamics Centre, Acacia House, Westmead Hospital, Hawkesbury Road, Westmead, Australia. PubMed 15099695.

336 Omega–3 fatty acids in ADHD and related neurodevelopmental disorders. · Int Rev Psychiatry. 2006 Apr;18(2):155–72 Richardson AJ. · Dept of Physiology, Human Anatomy and Genetics, University of Oxford. PubMed 16777670.

337 National Insitute on Alcohol Abuse and Alcoholism No. 63 2004.

338 Roles of unsaturated fatty acids (especially omega–3 fatty acids) in the brain at various ages and during ageing · J Nutr Health Aging. 2004;8(3):163–74. · Bourre JM. INSERM Research Director. Unit U26 Neuropharmaco-nutrition. Hopital Fernand Widal, 200 rue du Faubourg Saint Denis. 75745 Paris cedex 10. PubMed 15129302.

339   The role of nutritional factors on the structure and function of the brain: an update on dietary requirements - Rev Neurol (Paris). 2004 Sep;160(8-9):767-92 - Bourre JM. - Unité de recherches en Neuro-Pharmaco-Nutrition, INSERM U26, Hôpital Fernand Widal, Paris. 15454864.

340   Reversal of docosahexaenoic acid deficiency in the rat brain, retina, liver, and serum Jnl. of Lipid Research, - Vol. 42, 419-427, March 2001 - Toru Moriguchi, James Loewke, Megan Garrison, Janice Nicklay Catalan, and Norman Salem, Jr. - Laboratory of Membrane Biochemistry & Biophysics, National Institutes on Alcohol Abuse & Alcoholism, NIH, Bethesda, MD 20892.

341   Astrocytes in culture require docosahexaenoic acid to restore the n-3/n-6 polyunsaturated fatty acid balance in their membrane phospholipids. - J Neurosci Res. 2004 Jan 1;75(1):96-106 Champeil-Potokar G, Denis I, Goustard-Langelier B, Alessandri JM, Guesnet P, Lavialle M. - Laboratoire de Nutrition et Sécurité Alimentaire, Institut National de la Recherche Agronomique, Jouy-en-Josas, France. PubMed 14689452.

342   The effects of dietary alpha-linolenic acid on the composition of nerve membranes, enzymatic activity, amplitude of electrophysiological parameters, resistance to poisons and performance of learning tasks in rats. - J Nutr. 1989 Dec;119(12):1880-92 - Bourre JM, Francois M, Youyou A, Dumont O, Piciotti M, Pascal G, Durand G. - Institut National de la Santé et de la Recherche Médicale, INSERM Unité 26, Hôpital Fernand Widal, Paris. PubMed 2576038.

343   Effects of docosapentaenoic acid on neuronal apoptosis. - Lipids. 2003 Apr;38(4):453-7 - Kim HY, Akbar M, Lau A. - Section of Mass Spectrometry, Laboratory of Membrane Biochemistry and Biophysics, National Institute on Alcohol Abuse and Alcoholism, NIH Rockville, MA USA. PubMed 12848293.

344   Omega-3 Fatty Acids in Inflammation and Autoimmune Diseases - Artemis P. Simopoulos - Jnl. of the American College of Nutrition, Vol. 21, No. 6, 495-505 (2002) , MD, FACN The Center for Genetics, Nutrition and Health, Washington, D.C.

345   Docosahexaenoic Acid and Eicosapentaenoic Acid Antagonize the Proinflammatory Interactions of Pneumolysin with Human Neutrophils. - Infection and Immunity, July 2004, p. 4327-4329, Vol. 72, No. 7 - Riana Cockeran, Annette J. Theron, Charles Feldman, Timothy J. Mitchell, and Ronald Anderson - Medical Research Council for Inflammation and Immunity, Dept. of Immunology, Faculty of Health Sciences, University of Pretoria, and Tshwane Academic Division of the National Health Laboratory Services, Pretoria,1 Division of Pulmonology, University of the Witwatersrand, Johannesburg, South Africa,2 Division of Infection and Immunity, , University of Glasgow, Glasgow, Scotland.

346   Smart Fats A Scmidt.

347   Polyunsaturated fatty acid synthesis and release by brain-derived cells in vitro. - J Mol Neurosci. 2001 Apr-Jun;16(2-3):195-200; discussion 215-21 - Moore SA. - Dept. of Pathology, The University of Iowa, Iowa City 52242, USA. PubMed 11478374.

348   Cloning, Expression, and Nutritional Regulation of the Mammalian D-6 Desaturase - J Biol Chem, Vol. 274, Issue 1, 471-477, January 1, 1999 - Hyekyung P. Cho, Manabu T. Nakamura, and Steven D. Clarke Program of Nutritional Sciences and the Institute for Cellular and Molecular Biology, The University of Texas-Austin, Austin, Texas 78712.

349   Essential fatty acids in infant nutrition: lessons and limitations from animal studies in relation to studies on infant fatty acid requirements See 219.

350   Reversal of docosahexaenoic acid deficiency in the rat brain, retina, liver, and serum See 223.

351   Roles of unsaturated fatty acids (especially omega-3 fatty acids) in the brain at various . . . See 336.

352   Can Prenatal N-3 Fatty Acid Deficiency Be Completely Reversed after Birth? Effects on Retinal and Brain Biochemistry and Visual Function in Rhesus Monkeys.

353   Half-lives of docosahexaenoic acid in rat brain phospholipids are prolonged by 15 weeks of nutritional deprivation of n-3 polyunsaturated fatty acids - J Neurochem. 2004 Dec;91(5):1125-37 - DeMar JC Jr, Ma K, Bell JM, Rapoport SI. - Brain Physiology and Metabolism Section, National Institute on Aging, NIH, Bethesda, Maryland USA. PubMed 15569256.

354   The effect of dietary docosahexaenoic acid on plasma lipoproteins and tissue fatty acid composition in humans. - Lipids. 1997 Nov;32(11):1137-46 Nelson GJ, Schmidt PC, Bartolini GL, Kelley DS, Kyle D. - Western Human Nutrition Research Center, San Francisco, California USA PubMed 9397398.

355   Gene expression and molecular composition of phospholipids in rat brain in relation to dietary n-6 to n-3 fatty acid ratio. - Biochim Biophys Acta. 2003 Jun 10;1632(1-3):72-9 - Barcelo-Coblijn G, Kitajka K, Puskas LG, Hogyes E, Zvara A, Hackler L Jr, Farkas T. - Biological Research Center, Institute of Biochemistry, Hungarian Academy of SciencesSzeged, Hungary. PubMed 12782153.

356   Differential effects of eicosapentaenoic and docosahexaenoic acids upon oxidant-stimulated release and uptake of arachidonic acid in human lymphoma U937 cells. - Pharmacol Res. 2005 Aug;52(2):183-91 - Obajimi O, Black KD, MacDonald DJ, Boyle RM, Glen I, Ross BM. - Scottish Association for Marine Science, Dunstaffnage Marine Laboratory, Oban, Scotland. PubMed 15967385.

357 Roles of unsaturated fatty acids (especially omega–3 fatty acids) in the brain at various ... See 336.

358 Docosahexaenoic acid-rich phospholipid supplementation: effect on behavior, learning ability, and retinal function in control and n–3 polyunsaturated fatty acid deficient old mice. - Nutr Neurosci. 2002 Feb;5(1):43–52. - Carrie I, Smirnova M, Clement M, DE JD, Frances H, Bourre JM. - INSERM U26, Unité de Neuro-Pharmaco-Nutrition, Paris, France. PubMed 11929197.

359 Malignant Melanoma and Other Types of Cancer Preceding Parkinson Disease. - Epidemiology. 2006 Sep;17(5):582–7. - Olsen JH, Friis S, Frederiksen K. - Institute of Cancer Epidemiology, Danish Cancer Society, Strandboulevarden 49, DK–2100 Copenhagen, Denmark. PubMed 16837822.

360 Reversal of docosahexaenoic acid deficiency in the rat brain, retina, liver, and serum See 223.

361 Retinal light damage in rats with altered levels of rod outer segment docosahexaenoate. - Invest Ophthalmol Vis Sci. 1996 Oct;37(11):2243–57. - Organisciak DT, Darrow RM, Jiang YL, Blanks JC. - Petticrew Research Laboratory, Wright State University, Daylon, Ohio 45435, USA. PubMed 8843911.

362 Reversal of docosahexaenoic acid deficiency in the rat brain, retina, liver, and serum See 223.

363 Omega–3 Treatment of Childhood Depression: A Controlled, Double–Blind Pilot Study - Am J Psychiatry 163:1098–1100, June 2006 - Hanah Nemets, M.D., Boris Nemets, M.D., Alan Apter, M.D., Ziva Bracha, M.D. and R.H. Belmaker, M.D.

364 Docosahexaenoic acid promotes neurite growth in hippocampal neurons. - J Neurochem. 2004 Aug;90(4):979–88 - Calderon F, Kim HY - Section of Mass Spectrometry, Laboratory of Membrane Biochemistry and Biophysics, National Institute on Alcohol Abuse and Alcoholism, NIH, Bethesda, Maryland, USA. PubMed 15287904.

365 Effects of supplementation with omega 3 long-chain polyunsaturated fatty acids on retinal and cortical development in premature infants. - Hoffman DR, Birch EE, Birch DG, Uauy RD. - Dept. of Pediatrics, University of Texas Southwestern Medical Center, Dallas. PubMed 8475899.

366 Astrocytes in culture require docosahexaenoic acid to restore the n–3/n–6 polyunsaturated fatty acid balance in their membrane phospholipids. - Am J Clin Nutr. 1993 May;57(5 Suppl):807S–812S - Hoffman DR, Birch EE, Birch DG, Uauy RD. - Dept. of Pediatrics, University of Texas Southwestern Medical Center, Dallas. PubMed 14689452.

367 One generation of n–3 polyunsaturated fatty acid deprivation increases depression and aggression test scores in rats - Jnl. of Lipid Research, Vol. 47, 172–180, January 2006 - James C. DeMar, Jr., Kiazong Ma, Jane M. Bell, Miki Igarashi, Deanna Greenstein and Stanley I. Rapoport - National Institute of Mental Health, NIH, Bethesda, MD 20892.

368 Influence of a dietary n–3 fatty acid deficiency on the cerebral catecholamine contents, EEG and learning ability in rat. - Behav Brain Res. 2002 Apr 1;131(1–2):193–203 - Takeuchi T, Fukumoto Y, Harada E. - Dept. of Veterinary Physiology, Faculty of Agriculture, Tottori University, 680–0945, Tottori, Japan. PubMed 11844586.

369 Reduced G protein-coupled signaling efficiency in retinal rod outer segments in response to n–3 fatty acid deficiency - J Biol Chem. 2004 Jul 23;279(30):31098–104. Epub 2004 May 15 - Niu SL, Mitchell DC, Lim SY, Wen ZM, Kim HY, Salem N Jr, Litman BJ. - Laboratory of Membrane Biochemistry and Biophysics, National Institute on Alcohol Abuse and Alcoholism, Rockville, Maryland 20852, USA. PubMed 15145938.

370 An extraordinary degree of structural specificity is required in neural phospholipids for optimal brain function: n–6 docosapentaenoic acid substitution for docosahexaenoic acid leads to a loss in spatial task performance. - Lim SY, Hoshiba J, Salem N Jr. - J Neurochem. 2005 Nov;95(3):848–57. Epub 2005 Aug 31 - Division of Marine Environment and Bioscience, Korea Maritime University, Busan PubMed 16135079.

371 Essential fatty acids in infant nutrition: lessons and limitations from animal studies in relation to studies on infant fatty acid requirements See 219.

372 Visual membranes: specificity of fatty acid precursors for the electrical response to illumination. - Science. 1975 Jun 27;188(4195):1312–4 - Wheeler TG, Benolken RM, Anderson RE PubMed 1145197.

373 One generation of n–3 polyunsaturated fatty acid deprivation increases depression and aggression test scores in rats - Jnl. of Lipid Research, Vol. 47, 172–180, January 2006 - James C. DeMar, Jr, Kiazong Ma, Jane M. Bell, Miki Igarashi, Deanna Greenstein and Stanley I. Rapoport - Brain Physiology and Metabolism Section, National Institute on Aging, and Child Psychiatry Branch, National Institute of Mental Health, MD USA.

374 Omega–3 fatty acids decreased irritability of patients with bipolar See 15.

375 The effect of docosahexaenoic acid on aggression in young adults. A placebo-controlled double-blind study. - J Clin Invest. 1996 February 15; 97(4): 1129–1133 T - Hamazaki, S Sawazaki, M Itomura, E Asaoka, Y Nagao, N Nishimura, K Yazawa, T Kuwamori, and M Kobayashi - The First Dept. of Internal Medicine, Toyama Medical and Pharmaceutical University, Toyama, Japan. PubMed 507162.

376   Serum omega–3 fatty acids are associated with variation in mood, personality and behavior in hypercholesterolemic community volunteers. · Psychiatry Res. 2007 Jul 30;152(1):1–10. Epub 2007 Mar 23 · Conklin SM, Harris JI, Manuck SB, Yao JK, Hibbeln JR, Muldoon MF. · Cardiovascular Behavioral Medicine Postdoctoral Training Program, Dept. of Psychiatry, University of Pittsburgh, PA, PubMed 17383013.

377   Lower omega–3 polyunsaturated fatty acids and lower docosahexaenoic acid in men with paedophila. · Neuro Endocrinol Lett. 2006 Dec;27(6):719–23 Mincke E, Cosyns P, Christophe AB, De Vriese S, Maes M. · Dept. of Psychiatry, Antwerp Forensic Center, University of Antwerp, Edegem, and Dept. of Internal Medicine, Ghent University Hospital, Belgium. PubMed 17187003.

378   Induction of PGE2 by estradiol mediates developmental masculinization of sex behavior · Nature Neuroscience 7, 643 – 650 (2004) · Published online: 23 May 2004; | doi:10.1038/nn1254 ·Stuart K Amateau & Margaret M McCarthy · Program in Neuroscience and Dept. of Physiology, University of Maryland at Baltimore School of Medicine, Baltimore, Maryland.

379   Gene Environment Effects: Stress and Memory Dysfunctions Caused by Stress and Gonadal Factor Irregularities during Puberty in Control And TGF· Hypomorphic Mice · Neuropsychopharmacology 2 May 2007; doi: 10.1038/sj.npp.1301436 · Kyoko Koshibul and Pat Levitt · Dept. of Neurobiology and Center for Neural Basis of Cognition, University of Pittsburgh, PA,. Dept. of Pharmacology and Vanderbilt Kennedy Center for Research on Human Development, Vanderbilt University, Nashville, TN, USA.

380   Arachidonic acid and prostaglandin E2 stimulate testosterone production by goldfish testis in vitro. · Author: Wade, M G : Van der Kraak, G Citation: Gen·Comp·Endocrinol. 1993 Apr; 90(1): 109–18 PubMed 126399.

381   Suicide attempt and n–3 fatty acid levels in red blood cells: A case control study in China · Mingming Huan, Kei Hamazaki, Yueji Sun, Miho Itomura, Hongyan Liu, Wei Kang, Shiro Watanabe, Katsutoshi Terasawa and Tomohito Hamazaki · Division of Clinical Application, Dept. of Clinical Sciences, Institute of Natural Medicine, Toyama Medical and Pharmaceutical University, Sugitani, Toyama-City, Japan University Hospital, Toyama Medical and Pharmaceutical University, Toyama-City, JapanDept. of Neuropsychology, Dalian Medical University Psychiatry Dept. (HL), Dalian Friendship Hospital Dalian Blood Component Analysis Center (WK), Dalian-City, Liaoning-Province, China.

382   Omega–3 Polyunsaturated Essential Fatty Acid Status as a Predictor of Future Suicide Risk · M. Elizabeth Sublette, M.D., Ph.D., Joseph R. Hibbeln, M.D., Hanga Galfalvy, Ph.D., Maria A. Oquendo, M.D. and J. John Mann, Ph.D.

383   Omega–3 fatty acids decreased irritability of patients with bipolar disorder See 15.

384   Omega–3 fatty acids in the treatment of psychiatric disorders. See 328.

385   Selective deficits in the omega–3 Fatty Acid docosahexaenoic Acid in the postmortem orbitofrontal cortex of patients with major depressive disorder. · Biol Psychiatry. 2007 Jul 1;62(1):17–24 · McNamara RK, Hahn CG, Jandacek R, Rider T, Tso P, Stanford KE, Richtand NM. · Dept. of Psychiatry, University of Cincinnati College of Medicine, Ohio. PubMed 17188654.

386   Abnormalities in the fatty acid composition of the postmortem orbitofrontal cortex of schizophrenic patients: gender differences and partial normalization with antipsychotic medications. · Schizophr Res. 2007 Mar;91(1–3):37–50 · McNamara RK, Jandacek R, Rider T, Tso P, Hahn CG, Richtand NM, Stanford KE. · Dept. of Psychiatry, University of Cincinnati College of Medicine, Cincinnati, OH PubMed 17236749.

387   Essential fatty acids, lipid membrane abnormalities, and the diagnosis and treatment of schizophrenia. · Biol Psychiatry. 2000 Jan 1;47(1):8–21 · Fenton WS, Hibbeln J, Knable M. Stanley Treatment Programs at Chestnut Lodge,. Maryland, USA. PubMed 10650444.

388   Membrane phospholipids and cytokine interaction in schizophrenia.· Int Rev Neurobiol. 2004;59:297–326. · Yao JK, van Kammen DP. VA Pittsburgh Healthcare System, Pittsburgh, Pennsylvania 15206, USA. PubMed 15006493.

389   Significantly reduced docosahexaenoic and docosapentaenoic acid concentrations in erythrocyte membranes from schizophrenic patients compared with a carefully matched control group · Biol Psychiatry. 2001 Mar 15;49(6):510–22. · Assies J, Lieverse R, Vreken P, Wanders RJ, Dingemans PM, Linszen DH. · Dept. of Adolescent Psychiatry, Academic Medical Center, University of Amsterdam. PubMed 11257236.

390   Effects of dietary n–3 or n–6 fatty acids on interleukin-1ß–induced anxiety, stress, and inflammatory responses in rats · Jnl. of Lipid Research, Vol. 44, 1984–1991, October 2003 · Cai Song, Xuwen Li, Brian E. Leonard and David F. Horrobin · Dept. of Psychiatry, University of British Columbia, Canada Brain and Behaviour Research Institute, Academic Hospital Maastricht, University of Maastricht, The Netherlands Laxdale Research, Stirling, Scotland, UK.

391 Anti-stress effects of DHA. - Biofactors. 2000;13(1-4):41-5 - Hamazaki T, Itomura M, Sawazaki S, Nagao Y. - Dept. of Clinical Application, Institute of Natural Medicine, Toyama Medical and Pharmaceutical University, Japan. PubMed 11237197.

392 Plasma phospholipid essential fatty acids and prostaglandins in alcoholic, habitually violent and impulsive offenders. - Biol Psychiatry 1987; 22: 1087-1096. - Virkkunen ME, Horroboin DF, Jenkins DK, Manku MS

393 The fatty acid composition of human gliomas differs from that found in nonmalignant brain tissue. - Lipids. 1996 Dec;31(12):1283-8. Martin DD, Robbins ME, Spector AA, Wen BC, Hussey DH. - Dept. of Radiology, University of Iowa Hospitals and Clinics, Iowa City, USA.

394 Phospholipids and fatty acids in human brain tumors. - Acta Physiol Hung. 1992;79(4):381-7. - Ledwozyw A, Lutnicki K. - Dept. of Pathophysiology, Veterinary Faculty of Agricultural Academy, Lublin, Poland. PubMed 1343190.

395 Role of -3 polyunsaturated fatty acids on cyclooxygenase-2 metabolism in brain-metastatic melanoma - Yvonne Denkins, Doty Kempf, Melissa Ferniz, Shilpa Nileshwar and Dario Marchetti - Jnl. of Lipid Research, Vol. 46, 1278-1284, June 2005 - Dept. of Comparative Biomedical Sciences, School of Veterinary Medicine, Louisiana State University, Baton Rouge, LA 70803.

396 Neurodegeneration from mitochondrial insufficiency: nutrients, stem cells, growth factors, and prospects for brain rebuilding using integrative management. - Altern Med Rev. 2005 Dec;10(4):268-93. - Kidd PM. - University of California, Berkeley, USA. PubMed 16366737.

397 Mediators of injury in neurotrauma: intracellular signal transduction and gene expression. - J Neurotrauma. 1995 Oct;12(5):791-814. - Bazan NG, Rodriguez de Turco EB, Allan G. - LSU Neuroscience Center, Louisiana State University Medical Center, New Orleans, USA. PubMed 8594208.

398 Lipid signaling in neural plasticity, brain repair, and neuroprotection. - Mol Neurobiol. 2005 Aug;32(1):89-103. - Bazan NG. - LSU Neuroscience Center of Excellence and Dept. of Ophthalmology, Louisiana State University Health Sciences Center, New Orleans, LA, USA. PubMed 16077186.

399 Neuroprotectin D1: a docosahexaenoic acid-derived docosatriene protects human retinal pigment epithelial cells from oxidative stress - Proc Natl Acad Sci U S A. 2004 Jun 1;101(22):8491-6. - Mukherjee PK, Marcheselli VL, Serhan CN, Bazan NG. - Neuroscience Center of Excellence and Dept. of Ophthalmology, Louisiana State University Health Sciences Center of Medicine, New Orleans, USA. PubMed 15152078.

400 Brain response to injury and neurodegeneration: endogenous neuroprotective signaling. - Ann N Y Acad Sci. 2005 Aug;1053:137-47 Bazan NG, Marcheselli VL, Cole-Edwards K. - LSU Neuroscience Center and Dept. of Ophthalmology, Louisiana State University Health Sciences Center School of Medicine, 2020 Gravier Street, Suite D, New Orleans, Louisiana PubMed 16179516.

401 Estimates of direct medical costs for microvascular and macrovascular complications resulting from type 2 diabetes mellitus in the United States in 2000. - Clin Ther. 2003 Mar;25(3):1017-38. - O'Brien JA, Patrick AR, Caro J. Caro - Research Institute, Concord, Massachusetts 01742, USA. PubMed 12852716.

402 Wrong Diagnosis - Statistics on Heart Attacks.

403 Origins and evolution of the Western diet: (See 42).

404 Fructose, insulin resistance, and metabolic dyslipidemia - Nutr Metab (Lond). 2005; 2: 5 - Heather Basciano, Lisa Federico, and Khosrow Adeli - Clinical Biochemistry Division, Dept. of Laboratory Medicine and Pathobiology, Hospital for Sick Children, University of Toronto, Toronto, Ontario, Canada. PubMed 15723702.

405 See 406.

406 Origins and evolution of the Western diet: (See 42).

407 Serum phospholipid fatty acids, adipose tissue, and metabolic markers in obese adolescents. - Obesity 14:1931-1939 (2006) - Karlsson M, Mårild S, Brandberg J, Lönn L, Friberg P, Strandvik B. - Dept. of Pediatrics, Göteborg University, Queen Silvia Children's Hospital, SE 41685 Göteborg, Sweden.

408 Serum phospholipid fatty acids, adipose tissue, and metabolic markers in obese adolescents. See 407.

409 Arachidonic acid and prostacyclin signaling promote adipose tissue development ... See 231 Above.

410 Genotype and diet effects in lean and obese Zucker rats fed either safflower or coconut oil diets - Society for Experimental Biology and Medicine, Vol 220, 153-161 - MP Cleary, FC Phillips and RA Morton - Hormel Institute, University of Minnesota, Austin 55912, USA.

411 Turnover of plasma-free arachidonic and oleic acids in resting and exercising human subjects. Metabolism. - 1975 Jul;24(7):799-806 - Hagenfeldt L, Wahren J. PubMed 1138155.

412 Dietary n-3 fatty acids affect mRNA level of brown adipose tissue uncoupling protein 1, and white adipose tissue leptin and glucose transporter 4 in the rat. - Br J Nutr. 2000 Aug;84(2):175-84. - Takahashi Y, Ide T. Laboratory of Nutrition Biochemistry, National Food Research Institute, Ministry of Agriculture, Forestry and Fisheries, Ibaraki, Japan.

413 Dietary fatty acid composition influences energy accretion in rats. · Jnl. of Nutrition Vol. 123 No. 12 December 1993, pp. 2109–2114 · Su W, Jones PJ. Division of Human Nutrition, University of British Columbia, Vancouver, Canada.

414 Dietary n–3 fatty acids affect mRNA level of brown adipose tissue uncoupling protein 1, and white adipose tissue leptin and glucose transporter 4 See 413.

415 Polyunsaturated fatty acids of marine origin upregulate mitochondrial biogenesis and induce beta-oxidation in white fat. · Flachs P, Horakova O, Brauner P, Rossmeisl M, Pecina P, Franssen-van Hal N, Ruzickova J, Sponarova J, Drahota Z, Vlcek C, Keijer J, Houstek J, Kopecky J. · Dept. of Adipose Tissue Biology, Institute of Physiology, Academy of Sciences of the Czech Republic, Prague. PubMed 16205884.

416 Brown fat thermogenesis in rats fed high-fat diets enriched with n–3 polyunsaturated fatty acids· Diabetologia. 2005 Nov;48(11):2365–75 · Oudart H, Groscolas R, Calgari C, Nibbelink M, Leray C, Le Maho Y, Malan A. · Centre d'Ecologie et Physiologie Energetiques, associe a l'Universite Louis Pasteur, Strasbourg. PubMed 9368817.

417 Comparative effects of perilla and fish oils on the activity and gene expression of fatty acid oxidation enzymes in rat liver. · Biochim Biophys Acta. 2000 May 6;1485(1):23–35. · Ide T, Kobayashi H, Ashakumary L, Rouyer IA, Takahashi Y, Aoyama T, Hashimoto T, Mizugaki M. · Laboratory of Nutrition Biochemistry, National Food Research Institute, Ministry of Agriculture, Forestry and Fisheries, Tsukuba Science City, Japan. PubMed 10802246.

418 Developmental programming of obesity in mammals · Experimental Physiology 92.2 pp 287–298 · P. D. Taylor and L. Poston · Division of Reproduction & Endocrinology, King's College London.

419 Randomized trial of weight-loss-diets for young adults varying in fish and fish oil content. · International Jnl. of Obesity 15 May 2007 · Thorsdottir I, Tomasson H, Gunnarsdottir I, Gisladottir E, Kiely M, Parra MD, Bandarra NM, Schaafsma G, Martinéz JA. · Unit for Nutrition Research, Dept. of Food Science and Human Nutrition, Landspitali University Hospital, University of Iceland, Reykjavik.

420 Perilla oil prevents the excessive growth of visceral adipose tissue in rats by down-regulating adipocyte differentiation · The Jnl. of Nutrition Vol. 127 No. 9 September 1997, pp. 1752–1757 · Okuno M, Kajiwara K, Imai S, Kobayashi T, Honma N, Maki T, Suruga K, Goda T, Takase S, Muto Y, Moriwaki H.First · Dept. of Internal Medicine, Gifu University School of Medicine, Gifu 500, Japan.

421 Docosahexaenoic Acid Inhibits Adipocyte Differentiation and Induces Apoptosis in 3T3-L1 Preadipocytes · American Society for Nutrition J. Nutr. 136:2965–2969, December 2006 · Hye-Kyeong Kim, MaryAnne Della-Fera, Ji Lin and Clifton A. Baile · Dept. of Animal and Dairy Science, and Dept. of Foods and Nutrition, University of Georgia, Athens, GA 30602.

422 Dietary fish oils limit adipose tissue hypertrophy in rats · C. Metabolism. 1990 Mar;39(3):217–9. · C. Parrish, D. A. Pathy and A. Angel · Dept. of Medicine, University of Toronto, Ontario, Canada. PubMed 2308514.

423 Dietary fish oils modify adipocyte structure and function. · J Cell Physiol. 1991 Sep;148(3):493–502. · Parrish CC, Pathy DA, Parkes JG, Angel A. · Dept. of Medicine, University of Toronto, Canada. PubMed 1655818.

424 Perilla Oil Prevents the Excessive Growth of Visceral Adipose Tissue in Rats by Down-Regulating Differentiation See 415.

425 Docosahexaenoic Acid Inhibits Adipocyte Differentiation and Induces Apoptosis in 3T3–See 416.

426 Omega–3 PUFA of marine origin limit diet-induced obesity in mice by reducing cellularity of adipose tissue.· Ruzickova J, Rossmeisl M, Prazak T, Flachs P, Sponarova J, Veck M, Tvrzicka E, Bryhn M, Kopecky J. · Dept. of Adipose Tissue Biology and Centre for Integrated Genomics, Institute of Physiology, Academy of Sciences of the Czech Republic, 142 20 Prague, Czech Republic. PubMed 15736913.

427 Perilla Oil Prevents the Excessive Growth of Visceral Adipose Tissue in Rats by Down-Regulating Differentiation See 415.

428 Suppression of hepatic fatty acid oxidation and food intake in men. Nutrition.·1999 Nov–Dec;15(11–12):819–28 · Kahler A, Zimmermann M, Langhans W. · Institute of Animal Sciences, Swiss Federal Institute of Technology, Zurich, Switzerland. PubMed 10575655.

429 The influence of the type of dietary fat on postprandial fat oxidation rates: monounsaturated (olive oil) vs saturated fat (cream). · Jnl. of Obesity Vol 26 no6 p 814–821 June 2002 · Piers LS, Walker KZ, Stoney RM, Soares MJ, O'Dea K. · Menzies School of Health Research, Casuarina, Australia.

430 Food intake in dieters and nondieters after a liquid meal containing medium-chain triglycerides · American Jnl. of Clinical Nutrition, Vol 48, 66–71 · BJ Rolls, N Gnizak, A Summerfelt and LJ Laster · Dept. of Psychiatry and Behavioral Sciences, Johns Hopkins University School of Medicine, Baltimore, MD 21205.

431 Increased uncoupling protein2 mRNA in white adipose tissue, and decrease in leptin, visceral fat, blood glucose, and cholesterol in KK-Ay mice fed with eicosapentaenoic and docosahexaenoic acids in addition to linolenic acid. · Biochem Biophys Res Commun. 1999 May 27;259(1):85-90. · Hun CS, Hasegawa K, Kawabata T, Kato M, Shimokawa T, Kagawa Y. · Dept. of Biochemistry, Jichi Medical School, Tochigi-ken, 329-0498, Japan. PubMed 10334920.

432 Interactions of saturated, n-6 and n-3 polyunsaturated fatty acids to modulate arachidonic acid metabolism. · J Lipid Res. 1990 Feb;31(2):271-7. Garg ML, Thomson AB, Clandinin MT. · Nutrition and Metabolism Research Group, University of Alberta, Edmonton, Canada. PubMed 2109031.

433 Fish oil reduces cholesterol and arachidonic acid content more efficiently in rats fed diets containing low linoleic acid to saturated fatty acid ratios · Biochim Biophys Acta. 1988 Oct 14;962(3):337-44. · Garg ML, Wierzbicki AA, Thomson AB, Clandinin MT. · Dept. of Foods and Nutrition, Faculty of Home Economics, University of Alberta, Edmonton, Canada. PubMed 2844278.

434 Relationship between Adipocyte Size and Adipokine Expression and Secretion · The Jnl. of Clinical Endocrinology & Metabolism Vol. 92, No. 3 1023-1033 · Thomas Skurk, Catherine Alberti-Huber, Christian Herder and Hans Hauner · Else Kröner-Fresenius-Center for Nutritional Medicine of the Technical University Munich D-85350 Freising; and the German Diabetes Clinic, German Diabetes Center, Leibniz Center at Heinrich-Heine-University Düsseldorf, Germany.

435 Dietary Factors That Promote or Retard Inflammation · Arteriosclerosis, Thrombosis, and Vascular Biology. 2006;26:995. · Arpita Basu; Sridevi Devaraj; Ishwarlal Jialal · Laboratory for Atherosclerosis and Metabolic Research, University of California Davis Medical Center, Sacramento, Calif.

436 See 406.

437 Effects of an Ad Libitum Low-Fat, High-Carbohydrate Diet on Body Weight, Body Composition, and Fat Distribution in Older Men and Women A Randomized Controlled Trial · Arch Intern Med. 2004;164:210-217. · Nicholas P. Hays, PhD; Raymond D. Starling, PhD; Xiaolan Liu, MD; Dennis H. Sullivan, MD; Todd A. Trappe, PhD; James D. Fluckey, PhD; William J. Evans, PhD Arch.

438 Dietary Factors That Promote or Retard Inflammation Arteriosclerosis, Thrombosis, and Vascular Biology. (See 435).

439 Site-specific differences in the fatty acid composition of abdominal adipose tissue in an obese population from a Mediterranean area: relation with dietary fatty acids, plasma lipid profile, serum insulin, and central obesity · Marta Garaulet, Francisca Pérez-Llamas, Millán Pérez-Ayala, Pedro Martínez, Fermín Sánchez de Medina, Francisco J Tebar and Salvador Zamora · Dept. of Physiology and Pharmacology, University of Murcia, Murcia, Spain; Dept. of Biochemistry, University of Granada, Granada, Spain; Dept. s of Biochemistry and Endocrinology, Arrixaca Hospital, Murcia, Spain.

440 Distribution, interconversion, and dose response of n-3 fatty acids in humans. · American Jnl. of Clinical Nutrition, Vol. 83, No. 6, S1467-1476S, June 2006 · Arterburn LM, Hall EB, Oken H. · Martek Biosciences Corporation, Columbia, MD.

441 Site-specific differences in the fatty acid composition (See above 442).

442 Incorporation of dietary n-3 fatty acids into the fatty acids of human adipose tissue and plasma lipid classes · American Jnl. of Clinical Nutrition, Vol 62, 68-73 · DA Leaf, WE Connor, L Barstad and G Sexton · Dept. of Medicine, West Los Angeles Veterans Administration Medical Center, CA 90073, USA.

443 The effect of different dietary fats on fat cell size and number in rat epididmyal fat pad. · Janet Kirtland M I Gurr.

444 Arachidonic acid and prostacyclin signaling promote adipose tissue development : a human health concern? (See 231).

445 See 406 above.

446 Consuming Fructose-sweetened Beverages Increases Body Adiposity in Mice · Obesity Research 13:1146-1156 (2005) · Hella Jürgens, Wiltrud Haass, Tamara R. Castañeda, Annette Schürmann, Corinna Koebnick, Frank Dombrowski, Bärbel Otto Andrea R. Nawrocki, Philipp E. Scherer, Jochen Spranger, Michael Ristow, Hans-Georg Joost, Peter J. Havel and Matthias H. Tschöp.

447 See 406 above.

448 Long-term effects of diet on leptin, energy intake, and activity in a model of diet-induced obesity · J Appl Physiol 93: 887-893, 2002 · Christian K. Roberts, Joshua J. Berger, and R. James Barnard · Dept. of Physiological Science, University of California, Los Angeles, California.

449 Polyunsaturated fatty acids of marine origin upregulate mitochondrial biogenesis and induce beta-oxidation in white fat.· Diabetologia. 2005 Nov;48(11):2365-75 · Flachs P, Horakova O, Brauner P, Rossmeisl M, Pecina P, Franssen-van Hal N, Ruzickova J, Sponarova J, Drahota Z, Vlcek C, Keijer J, Houstek J, Kopecky J. · Dept. of Adipose Tissue Biology, Institute of Physiology, Academy of Sciences of the Czech Republic, Prague, Czech Republic. PubMed 16205884.

450   Polyunsaturated fatty acids of marine origin induce adiponectin in mice fed a high-fat diet. · Diabetologia. 2006 Feb;49(2):394-7 · Flachs P, Mohamed-Ali V, Horakova O, Rossmeisl M, Hosseinzadeh-Attar MJ, Hensler M, Ruzickov J, Kopecky J. · Dept. of Adipose Tissue Biology, Institute of Physiology, Academy of Sciences, Videnska 1083, 142 20 Prague, Czech Republic. PubMed 16397791.

451   See 406 above.

452   Recent advances in the relationship between obesity, inflammation, and insulin resistance · Eur Cytokine Netw. 2006 Mar;17(1):4-12 · Bastard JP, Maachi M, Lagathu C, Kim MJ, Caron M, Vidal H, Capeau J, Feve B. · Inserm U680, Faculte de Medecine Pierre et Marie Curie, site Saint-Antoine, Universite Pierre et Marie Curie, Paris 6 et Service de Biochimie et Hormonologie, Hopital Tenon, AP-HP, 75970 Paris France. PubMed 16613757.

453   Release of interleukins and other inflammatory cytokines by human adipose tissue is enhanced in obesity and primarily due to the nonfat cells. · Vitam Horm. 2006;74:443-77 Fain JN. · Dept. of Molecular Sciences, College of Medicine, University of Tennessee Health Science Center, Memphis, Tennessee, USA. PubMed 17027526.

454   The pathophysiologic roles of interleukin-6 in human disease · Ann Intern Med. 1998 Jan 15;128(2):127-37. · Papanicolaou DA, Wilder RL, Manolagas SC, Chrousos GP. PubMed 9441573.

455   Comparison of the Release of Adipokines by Adipose Tissue, Adipose Tissue Matrix, and Adipocytes from Visceral and Subcutaneous Abdominal Adipose Tissues of Obese Humans Endocrinology · Vol. 145, No. 5 2273-2282 · John N. Fain, Atul K. Madan, M. Lloyd Hiler, Paramjeet Cheema and Suleiman W. Bahouth · Dept.s of Molecular Sciences (J.N.F., P.C.), Surgery (A.K.M., M.L.H.), and Pharmacology (S.W.B.), College of Medicine, University of Tennessee Health Science Center,

456   Arachidonic acid content in adipose tissue is associated with insulin resistance in healthy children. · Jnl. of Pediatric Gastroenterology & Nutrition. 44(1):77-83, January 2007. · Aldámiz-Echevarría L, Prieto JA, Andrade F, Elorz J, Sanjurjo P, Rodríguez Soriano J. · Division of Metabolism, Dept. of Pediatrics, Cruces Hospital and Basque University School of Medicine, Bilbao, Spain. PubMed 17204958.

457   Selective release of human adipocyte fatty acids according to molecular structure. · Biochem J. 1997 June 15; 324(Pt 3): 911-915.· T Raclot, D Langin, M Lafontan, and R Groscolas · INSERM Unité 317, Institut Louis Bugnard, Faculté de médecine, Université Paul Sabatier, Hôpital Rangueil Toulouse PubMed 1218508.

458   Dietary Factors That Promote or Retard Inflammation · Arteriosclerosis, Thrombosis, and Vascular Biology. 2006;26:995 · Arpita Basu, Sridevi Devaraj and Ishwarlal Jialal · Laboratory for Atherosclerosis and Metabolic Research, University of California Davis Medical Center, Sacramento, Calif.

459   Beneficial effects of cytokine induced hyperlipidemia. · Z Ernahrungswiss. 1998;37 Suppl 1:66-74. · Feingold KR, Hardardottir I, Grunfeld C. Metabolism Section (111F). · Dept. of Veterans Affairs Medical Center, San Francisco, USA. PubMed 9558731.

460   The inflammatory consequences of psychologic stress: relationship to insulin resistance, obesity, atherosclerosis and diabetes mellitus, type II. · Med Hypotheses. 2006;67(4):879-91. Black PH. Dept. of Microbiology, Boston University School of Medicine, 715 Albany Street, Room L-501, Boston, MA 02118, United States. PubMed 16781084.

461   The effect of docosahexaenoic acid on the loss of appetite in pediatric patients with pneumonia · Lopez-Alarcon M, Furuya-Meguro MM, Garcia-Zuniga PA, Tadeo-Pulido I. · Unidad de Investigacion Medica en Nutricion, Hospital de Pediatria, Centro Medico Nacional Siglo XXI, Insituto Mexicano del Seguro Social. PubMed 16497254.

462   Delta 6-desaturase activity in liver microsomes of rats fed diets enriched with cholesterol and/ or omega 3 fatty acids. · Biochem J. 1988 Jan 15;249(2):351-6. · Garg ML, Sebokova E, Thomson AB, Clandinin MT. · Nutrition and Metabolism Research Group, University of Alberta, Edmonton, Canada. PubMed 3342019.

463   Effects of N-3 PUFAs supplementation on insulin resistance and inflammatory biomarkers in hemodialysis patients. · Ren Fail. 2007;29(3):321-9 Rasic-Milutinovic Z, Perunicic G, Pljesa S, Gluvic Z, Sobajic S, Djuric I, Ristic D. · Dept. of Endocrinology, University Hospital Zemun/Belgrade 17497447 Pubmed.

464   n-3 Fatty acids and the metabolic syndrome See 216 above.

465   Dietary long-chain n-3 fatty acids of marine origin and serum C-reactive protein concentrations are associated in a population with a diet rich in marine products · American Jnl. of Clinical Nutrition, Vol. 84, No. 1, 223-229, July 2006 · Kaijun Niu, Atsushi Hozawa, Shinichi Kuriyama, Kaori Ohmori-Matsuda, Taichi Shimazu, Naoki Nakaya, Kazuki Fujita, Ichiro Tsuji and Ryoichi Nagatomi · Dept.s of Medicine and Science in Sports and Exercise and Public Health and Forensic Medicine, Tohoku University Graduate School of Medicine, Sendai, Japan; the Division of Epidemiology and Community Health School of Public Health, University of Minnesota, Minneapolis,and the Center for Preventive Medicine and Salutogenesis, Tohoku Fukushi University, Sendai, Japan.

466 Relationship of Plasma Polyunsaturated Fatty Acids to Circulating Inflammatory Markers · The Jnl. of Clinical Endocrinology & Metabolism Vol. 91, No. 2 439–446 · Luigi Ferrucci, Antonio Cherubini, Stefania Bandinelli, Benedetta Bartali, Annamaria Corsi, Fulvio Lauretani, Antonio Martin, Cristina Andres-Lacueva, Umberto Senin and Jack M. Guralnik · Longitudinal Studies, Clinical Research Branch, National Institute on Aging, Baltimore, Maryland; Dept. of Clinical and Experimental Medicine, Institute of Gerontology and Geriatrics, Perugia University Medical School, Perugia, Italy; Dept. of Geriatric Rehabilitation, Tuscany Regional Health Agency Florence, Italy; Division of Nutritional Sciences, Cornell University, Ithaca, New York; Human Nutrition Research Center on Aging Tufts University, Boston, Massachusetts 02111; Dept. of Nutrition and Food Science , University of Barcelona, Barcelona, Spain; and Laboratory of Epidemiology, Demography, and Biometry National Institute on Aging, Bethesda, Maryland 20892.

467 Fish Consumption Among Healthy Adults Is Associated With Decreased Levels of Inflammatory Markers Related to Cardiovascular Disease · J Am Coll Cardiol, 2005; 46:120–124 The ATTICA Study · Antonis Zampelas, PhD, Demosthenes B. Panagiotakos, PhD, Christos Pitsavos, MD, PhD, FACC, Undurti N. Das, MD, FAMA, Christina Chrysohoou, MD, PhD, Yannis Skoumas, MD and Christodoulos Stefanadis, MD, PhD, FACC · Dept. of Nutrition and Dietetics, Harokopio University, Athens, Greece First Cardiology Clinic, School of Medicine, University of Athens, Athens, Greece UND Life Sciences, Walpole, Massachusetts, USA.

468 Depressive Symptoms, omega–6:omega–3 Fatty Acids, and Inflammation in Older Adults See 326 Above.

469 Lack of effect of dietary n–6:n–3 PUFA ratio on plasma lipids and markers of insulin responses in Indian Asians living in the UK. · European Jnl. of Nutrition Vol44 No1 jan 2005 · Minihane AM, Brady LM, Lovegrove SS, Lesauvage SV, Williams CM, Lovegrove JA. Hugh Sinclair Unit of Human Nutrition, School of Food Biosciences, University of Reading, Reading RG6 6AP, UK.

470 Moderate fish-oil supplementation reverses low-platelet, long-chain n–3 polyunsaturated fatty acid status and reduces plasma triacylglycerol concentrations in British Indo-Asians. · Lovegrove JA, Lovegrove SS, Lesauvage SV, Brady LM, Saini N, Minihane AM, Williams CM. · Hugh Sinclair Unit of Human Nutrition, School of Food Biosciences, The University of Reading, PubMed 15159226.

471 Dietary PUFA and the metabolic syndrome in Indian Asians living in the UK.· Am J Clin Nutr. 2004 Jun;79(6):974–82 · Brady LM, Williams CM, Lovegrove JA. · Hugh Sinclair Human Nutrition Unit, School of Food Biosciences, PO Box 226, University of Reading, UK. PubMed 15159226.

472 Milk Composition in Women from Five Different Regions of China: The Great Diversity of Milk Fatty Acids · Jnl. of Nutrition Vol. 125 No. 12 December 1995, pp. 2993–2998 · Ruan Chulei, Liu Xiaofang, Man Hongsheng, Ma Xiulan, Lin Guizheng, Duan Gianhong, Carol A. DeFrancesco and William E. Connor · Central Laboratory Dept. of Hygiene, Dalian Medical University, Dalian, China Dept. of Medicine, Oregon Health Sciences University, Portland, OR.

473 Site-specific differences in the fatty acid composition (See 442).

474 The relation between dietary intake and adipose tissue composition of selected fatty acids in US women · American Jnl. of Clinical Nutrition, Vol 67, 25–30 · M Garland, FM Sacks, GA Colditz, EB Rimm, LA Sampson, WC Willett and DJ Hunter · Dept. of Epidemiology, Harvard School of Public Health, Boston, USA.

475 Adipose tissue n–6 fatty acids and acute myocardial infarction in a population consuming a diet high in polyunsaturated fatty acids · American Jnl. of Clinical Nutrition, Vol. 77, No. 4, 796–802, April 2003 · Jeremy D Kark, Nathan A Kaufmann, Fred Binka, Nehama Goldberger and Elliot M Berry · Epidemiology Unit, Dept. of Social Medicine, Hadassah University Hospital, Jerusalem; the Dept. of Human Nutrition and Metabolism, Hebrew University-Hadassah School of Public Health, Jerusalem; and the School of Public Health, University of Ghana, Legon, Accra, Ghana.

476 Human milk fatty acid composition from nine countries varies most in DHA · Lipids Vol 41 No9 Sept 2006 · Rebecca Yuhas Kathryn Pramuk Eric L Lien · Dept. of Nutrition Research, Wyeth Nutrition, Pennsylvania.

477 Leptin secretion from subcutaneous and visceral adipose tissue in women.· Van Harmelen V. Reynisdottir S. Eriksson P. Thorne A. Hoffstedt J. Lonnqvist F. Arner P. · Dept. of Medicine and Research Center, Huddinge University Hospital, Karolinska Institute, Arteriosclerosis Research Unit, King Gustaf V Research Institute, Karolinska Institute, Dept. of Surgery, Huddinge University Hospital, Karolinska Institute, Stockholm, Suede.

478 Surgical removal of visceral fat reverses hepatic insulin resistance. · Diabetes. 1999 Jan;48(1):94–8 · Barzilai N, She L, Liu BQ, Vuguin P, Cohen P, Wang J, Rossetti L. · Dept. of Medicine, and Diabetes Research and Training Center, Albert Einstein College of Medicine, Bronx, New York USA. PubMed 9892227.

479   Effects of antidepressants on the production of cytokines · Gunter Kenis Michael Maes · Cambridge University Press 28 Nov 2002 · Dept. of Psychiatry and Neuropsychology, University of Maastricht, The Netherlands.

480   The inflammatory response system and the availability of plasma tryptophan in patients with primary sleep disorders and major depression · J Affect Disord. 1998 Jun;49(3):211–9. · Song C, Lin A, Bonaccorso S, Heide C, Verkerk R, Kenis G, Bosmans E, Scharpe S, Whelan A, Cosyns P, de Jongh R, Maes M. · Clinical Research Center for Mental Health, University Dept. of Psychiatry, Antwerp, Belgium. PubMed 9629951.

481   Site-specific differences in the fatty acid composition (see 442).

482   Thin people may be fat on the inside, doctors warn. · CBCnews. Associated Press.

483   Perilla Oil Prevents the Excessive Growth of Visceral Adipose Tissue in Rats by Down-Regulating Adipocyte Differentiation See 415.

484   Novel treatments for obesity and osteoporosis: targeting apoptotic pathways in adipocytes. · Curr Med Chem. 2005;12(19):2215–25 · Nelson-Dooley C, Della-Fera MA, Hamrick M, Baile CA. · Dept.s of Animal and Dairy Sciences, University of Georgia, USA. PubMed 16178781.

485   See 406.

486   Desaturation function does not decline after menopause in human females. · Horm-Metab-Res. 2000 Jan; 32(1): 26–32 · Liu YW, Medeiros LC, Revesz E, O'Dorisio TM. · The Ohio State University, Dept. of Human Nutrition and Food Management, USA.

487   Fatty acid composition and estimated desaturase activities are associated with obesity and lifestyle variables in men and women. · Nutr Metab Cardiovasc Dis. 2006 Mar;16(2):128–36. · Warensjö E, Ohrvall M, Vessby B · Unit for Clinical Nutrition Research, Dept. of Public health and Caring sciences, Uppsala University. PubMed 16487913.

488   Improvements in glucose tolerance and insulin sensitivity after lifestyle intervention are related to changes in serum fatty acid profile and desaturase activities: the SLIM study. · Diabetologia. 2006 Oct;49(10):2392–401. · Corpeleijn E, Feskens EJ, Jansen EH, Mensink M, Saris WH, de Bruin TW, Blaak EE. · Dept. of Human Biology, The Nutrition and Toxicology Research Institute NUTRIM, Maastricht University. PubMed 16896932.

489   Expression and Regulation of D5-Desaturase, D6- Desaturase, Stearoyl-Coenzyme A... See 195 above.

490   See 406.

491   Persistent elevation of plasma insulin levels is associated with increased cardiovascular risk in children and young adults. · The Bogalusa Heart Study · Circulation. 1996 Jan 1;93(1):54–9. · Bao W, Srinivasan SR, Berenson GS.Tulane · National Center for Cardiovascular Health, Tulane School of Public Health and Tropical Medicine, New Orleans, La. 70112–2824, USA. PubMed 8616941.

492   Is metabolic syndrome X a disorder of the brain with the initiation of low-grade systemic inflammatory events during the perinatal period? · J Nutr Biochem. 2007 Apr 30 · Das UN. · Dept. of Molecular and Clinical Medicine, Care Hospital, The Institute of Medical Sciences, Banjara Hills, Hyderabad–500 034, India; UND Life Sciences, Shaker Heights, OH, USA PubMed 17475465.

493   Long-chain polyunsaturated fatty acids in plasma lipids of obese childrenLipids. · 1996 Mar;31(3):305–11. · Decsi T, Molnar D, Koletzko B. · Dept. of Paediatrics, University Medical School of Pecs, Hungary. PubMed 8900460.

494   Leptin levels in rat offspring are modified by the ratio of linoleic to -linolenic acid in the maternal diet. · Jnl. of Lipid Research, Vol. 43, 1743–1749, October 2002 · Marina Korotkova, Britt Gabrielsson, Malin Lönn, Lars-Åke Hanson and Brigitta Strandvik · Dept.s of Pediatrics, Clinical Immunology, Research Centre for Endocrinology and Metabolism, Dept. of Internal Medicine, Göteborg University, Sweden.

495   Temporal changes in dietary fats: role of n–6 polyunsaturated fatty acids in excessive adipose tissue development and relationship to obesity. · Prog Lipid Res. 2006 May;45(3):203–36 · Ailhaud G, Massiera F, Weill P, Legrand P, Alessandri JM, Guesnet P. · ISDBC Centre de Biochimie UMR 6543 CNRS, Faculté des Sciences, Parc Valrose, 06108 Nice cedex 2, France. PubMed 16516300.

496   Gender-related long-term effects in adult rats by perinatal dietary ratio of n–6/n–3 fatty acids · Am J Physiol Regul Integr Comp Physiol 288: R575–R579, 2005 · Marina Korotkova, Britt G. Gabrielsson, Agneta Holmäng, Britt-Marie Larsson, Lars Å. Hanson, and Birgitta Strandvik · Dept. of Pediatrics, Research Centre for Endocrinology and Metabolism, Dept. of Internal Medicine, Cardiovascular Institute and the Wallenberg Laboratory,Dept. of Clinical Immunology, Göteborg University, Göteborg, Sweden.

497   Fatty acid composition of fats is an early determinant of childhood obesity: a short review and an opinion.
      · Obesity Reviews 5 (1), 21–26. Ailhaud G, Guesnet P. · Institut de Recherche Signalisation, Biologie du
      Développement et Cancer, Nice, France.

498   Arachidonic acid and prostacyclin signaling promote adipose tissue development, . . See 231.

499   Developmental programming of obesity in mammals · P. D. Taylor and L. Poston · Division of Reproduction
      & Endocrinology, King's College London, UK.

500   Afferent signals regulating food intake. · Proc Nutr Soc. 2000 Aug;59(3):373–84 · Bray GA · Pennington
      Biomedical Research Center, Louisiana State University, 70808, USA. PubMed 10997653.

501   Effects of hypocaloric diet low in essential fatty acids on in vitro human adipose tissue prostaglandin
      production and essential fatty acid status. · Nutrition. 1991 Jul–Aug;7(4):256–9. · Katz DP, Knittle JL. ·
      Dept. of Anesthesiology, Montefiore Medical Center, Bronx, New York. PubMed 1802215.

502   The biology of obesity. · Trayhurn P. · Neuroendocrine & Obesity Biology Unit, Liverpool Centre for
      Nutritional Genomics, School of Clinical Sciences, University of Liverpool, U.K. PubMed 15877920.

503   Long-chain polyunsaturated fatty acids in plasma lipids of obese children. · Lipids. 1996 Mar;31(3):305–11 · Decsi
      T, Molnár D, Koletzko B. · Dept. of Paediatrics, University School of Pécs, Hungary. PubMed 8900460.

504   Short-term diabetic ketosis alters n–6 polyunsaturated fatty acid content in plasma phospholipids. · J Clin
      Endocrinol Metab Bassi et al. 81 (4): 1650. A Bassi, A Avogaro, C Crepaldi, P Pavan, S Zambon, R Marin, I
      Macdonald and E Manzato · University of Padova, Italy.

505   Metabolic control of sexual function and growth: role of neuropeptide Y and leptin. · Mol Cell
      Endocrinol. 1998 May 25;140(1–2):107–13 · Aubert ML, Pierroz DD, Gruaz NM, d'Alleves V, Vuagnat BA,
      Pralong FP, Blum WF, Sizonenko PC. · Dept. of Pediatrics, School of Medicine, Geneva, Switzerland.
      PubMed 9722177.

506   Leptin directly acts within the hypothalamus to stimulate gonadotropin-releasing hormone secretion
      in vivo in rats. · J Physiol. 2002 Nov 15;545(Pt 1):255–68 · Watanobe H. Division of Internal Medicine,
      International University of Health and Welfare, Tochigi, Japan. PubMed 12433965.

507   Leptin and adiponectin stimulate the release of proinflammatory cytokines and prostaglandins from
      human placenta and maternal adipose tissue via nuclear · factor-kappaB, peroxisomal proliferator-
      activated receptor-gamma and extracellularly regulated kinase · Endocrinology. 2005 Aug;146(8):3334–42.
      Epub 2005 May 19 · Lappas M, Permezel M, Rice GE. · Dept. of Obstetrics and Gynaecology, University of
      Melbourne and Mercy Perinatal Research Centre, Mercy Hospital for Women, East Melbourne, Victoria,
      Australia. PubMed 15905315.

508   Long-term effects of diet on leptin, energy intake, and activity in a model of diet-induced obesity · J
      Appl Physiol 93: 887–893, 2002. · Christian K. Roberts, Joshua J. Berger, and R. James Barnard Dept. of
      Physiological Science, University of California, Los Angeles, California USA.

509   Analysis of paradoxical observations on the association between leptin and insulin resistance · The FASEB
      Jnl. 2002;16:1163–1176 · Rolando B. Ceddia, Heikki A. Konistinen, Juleen R. Zierath and Gary Sweeney · Dept.
      of Biology, York University, Toronto, Canada Integrative Physiology, Karolinska Institute, Stockholm,
      Sweden; and Dept. of Medicine, Division of Cardiology, Helsinki University Central Hospital, Finland.

510   Serum immunoreactive-leptin concentrations in normal-weight and obese humans. · N Engl J Med.
      1996 Feb 1;334(5):292–5 · Considine RV, Sinha MK, Heiman ML, Kriauciunas A, Stephens TW, Nyce
      MR, Ohannesian JP, Marco CC, McKee LJ, Bauer TL, et al.Division of Endocrinology, · Jefferson Medical
      College of Thomas Jefferson University, Philadelphia, USA. PubMed 8532024.

511   Leptin levels in rat offspring are modified by the ratio of linoleic to -linolenic acid in the maternal diet
      · Jnl. of Lipid Research, Vol. 43, 1743–1749, October 2002 · Marina Korotkova, Britt Gabrielsson, Malin
      Lönn, Lars-Åke Hanson and Brigitta Strandvik · Dept.s of Pediatrics, Dept. of Internal Medicine, Clinical
      Immunology, Dept. of Internal Medicine, Research Centre for Endocrinology and Metabolism, Dept. of
      Internal Medicine, Göteborg University,

512   Eicosapentaenoic fatty acid increases leptin secretion from primary cultured rat adipocytes: role of glucose
      metabolism · Am J Physiol Regul Integr Comp Physiol 288: R1682–R1688, 2005 · Patricia Pérez-Matute,
      Amelia Marti, J. Alfredo Martínez, M. P. Fernández-Otero, Kimber L. Stanhope, Peter J. Havel, and María
      J. Moreno-Aliaga · Dept. of Physiology and Nutrition, University of Navarra, Pamplona, Spain; and Dept.
      of Nutrition, University of California, USA.

513   Effect of dietary lipids on plasma fatty acid profiles and prostaglandin and leptin production in gilthead
      seabream (Sparus aurata). · Comp Biochem Physiol B Biochem Mol Biol. 2005 Dec;142(4): · Ganga R, Bell
      JG, Montero D, Robaina L, Caballero MJ, Izquierdo MS. · Grupo de Investigacion en Acuicultura. ULPGC
      & ICCM. Telde, Las Palmas, Canary Islands, PubMed 16257554.

514   Regulation of leptin release and lipolysis by PGE2 in rat adipose tissue. - Fain JN, Leffler CW, Bahouth SW, Rice AM, Rivkees - SA. Prostaglandins Other Lipid Mediat. 2000 Oct;62(4):343-50 - Dept. of Biochemistry, College of Medicine, University of Tennessee, Memphis, USA. PubMed 11060898.

515   Arachidonic acid inhibits lipogenic gene expression in 3T3-L1 adipocytes through a prostanoid pathway - The Jnl. of Lipid Research, Vol. 39, 1327-1334, July 1998 - Michelle K. Mater, David Pan, W. G. Bergen, and Donald B. Jump - Dept.s of Physiology, Animal Science, Dept.s of Physiology, Botany and Plant Pathology, Dept.s of Physiology, Michigan State University, East Lansing, Michigan 48824 Dept. of Animal and Dairy Science, Auburn University, Auburn, AL 36849.

516   Effects of Linoleic Acid (LA) and Conjugated Linoleic Acid (CLA) on Leptin - Patti Plett, H. Weiler, A. Angel - Dept. of Medicine and Nutritional Sciences, University of Manitoba, Winnipeg, MB.

517   Regulation of leptin release and lipolysis by PGE2 in rat adipose tissue. See 514.

518   Stimulation of leptin release by arachidonic acid and prostaglandin E(2) in adipose tissue from obese humans Metabolism. - 2001 Aug;50(8):921-8. - Fain JN, Leffler CW, Cowan GS, Buffington C, Pouncey L, Bahouth - SW. Dept. of Biochemistry, College of Medicine, University of Tennessee, Memphis, USA. PubMed 11474480.

519   Effects of supplemental rumen-protected conjugated linoleic acid or linoleic acid on feedlot performance, carcass quality, and leptin concentrations in beef cattle - J Anim Sci. 2004 Mar;82(3):851-9. - Gillis MH, Duckett SK, Sackmann JR, Realini CE, Keisler DH, Pringle TD. Dept. of Animal and Dairy Science, University of Georgia, USA. PubMed 15032443.

520   Team Discovers a Chemical Pathway that Causes Mice to Overeat and Gain Weight. By Mark Schrope.

521   Dietary n-3 fatty acids affect mRNA level of brown adipose tissue uncoupling protein 1, and white adipose tissue leptin and glucose transporter See 413.

522   Regulation of leptin secretion from white adipocytes by free fatty acids - Am J Physiol Endocrinol Metab 285: E521-E526, 2003 - Philippe G. Cammisotto, Yves Gélinas, Yves Deshaies, and Ludwik J. Bukowiecki - Dept. of Anatomy and Physiology, Faculty of Medicine, Laval University, Quebec, Canada.

523   Dietary n-3 fatty acids affect mRNA level of brown adipose tissue uncoupling protein 1, and white adipose tissue leptin and glucose transporter 4 (See 413).

524   Reduction of leptin gene expression by dietary polyunsaturated fatty acids. - J Lipid Res. 2001 May;42(5):743-50 - Reseland JE, Haugen F, Hollung K, Solvoll K, Halvorsen B, Brude IR, Nenseter MS, Christiansen EN, Drevon CA. - Institute for Nutrition Research, University of Oslo, P. O. Box 1046, Blindern, N-0316 Oslo, Norway. PubMed 11352981.

525   Increased uncoupling protein2 mRNA in white adipose tissue, See 431 above.

526   Chronic effects of different fatty acids and leptin in INS-1 cells. - Diabetes Res Clin Pract. 2001 Jan;51(1):1-8 - Kawai T, Hirose H, Seto Y, Fujita H, Saruta T. - Dept. of Internal Medicine, School of Medicine, Keio University, Shinjuku-ku, Tokyo 160-8582, Japan. PubMed 11137176.

527   Regulation of leptin secretion from white adipocytes by free fatty acids. - Cammisotto PG, Gelinas Y, Deshaies Y, Bukowiecki LJ. - Dept. of Anatomy and Physiology, Faculty of Medicine, Laval University, Quebec, Canada.

528   Eicosapentaenoic fatty acid increases leptin secretion from primary See 512 above.

529   Consumption of high-fructose corn syrup in beverages may play a role in the epidemic of obesity - George A Bray, Samara Joy Nielsen and Barry M Popkin - Pennington Biomedical Research Center, Louisiana State University, Baton Rouge, LA (GAB), and the Dept. of Nutrition, University of North Carolina, Chapel Hill (SJN and BMP).

530   Consuming Fructose-sweetened Beverages Increases Body Adiposity in Mice Obesity - Research 13:1146-1156 (2005) - Hella Jürgens, Wiltrud Haass, Tamara R. Castañeda, Annette Schürmann, Corinna Koebnick, Frank Dombrowski, Bärbel Otto Andrea R. Nawrocki, Philipp E. Scherer, Jochen Spranger, Michael Ristow, Hans-Georg Joost, Peter J. Havel and Matthias H. Tschöp - German Institute of Human Nutrition, Dept. of Psychiatry, University of Cincinnati Otto-von-Guericke-University, Innenstadt University Hospital, Albert Einstein College of Medicine, Bronx, New Charité University Medicine, University of California Berlin,YorkMunich,Magdeburg.

531   Consumption of high-fructose corn syrup in beverages may play a role in the epidemic of obesity - American Jnl. of Clinical Nutrition, Vol. 79, No. 4, 537-543, April 2004 - George A Bray, Samara Joy Nielsen and Barry M Popkin - Pennington Biomedical Research Center, Louisiana State University, Baton Rouge, LA (GAB), and the Dept. of Nutrition, University of North Carolina, Chapel Hill.

532   See 406.

533   The Weston A Price Foundation for Wise Traditions How To Restore Digestive Health By Jordan S. Rubin.

534   Medium-Chain Triglycerides Increase Energy Expenditure and Decrease Adiposity in Overweight Men
       · Obesity Research 11:395–402 (2003) · Marie-Pierre St-Onge, Robert Ross, William D. Parsons and Peter
       J.H. Jones School of Dietetics and Human Nutrition, McGill University, Ste-Anne-de-Bellevue, Quebec,
       Canada and School of Physical and Health Education, Queen's University, Kingston, Ontario, Canada.
535   Medium-Chain Oil Reduces Fat Mass and Down-regulates Expression of Adipogenic Genes in Rats ·
       Jianrong Han, James A. Hamilton, James L. Kirkland, Barbara E. Corkey and Wen Guo Dept. of Medicine,
       650 Albany St., Boston, MA.
536   Medium-Chain Triglycerides Increase Energy Expenditure and Decrease Adiposity in Overweight Men
       (See 534 above).
537   Increasing dietary palmitic acid decreases fat oxidation and daily energy expenditure · American Jnl. of
       Clinical Nutrition, Vol. 82, No. 2, 320–326, August 2005 · C Lawrence Kien, Janice Y Bunn and Figen
       Ugrasbul · Dept. of Pediatrics, University of Texas Medical Branch and Shriners Hospital for Children,
       Galveston, TX, and the Dept. of Medical Biostatistics, University of Vermont, USA.
538   Plasma palmitoleic acid content and obesity in children. · Am J Clin Nutr. 2005 Oct;82(4):747–50. Okada
       T, Furuhashi N, Kuromori Y, Miyashita M, Iwata F, Harada K. · Dept. of Pediatrics, Nihon University
       School of Medicine, Tokyo, Japan. Jianrong Han, James A. Hamilton, James L. Kirkland, Barbara E. Corkey
       and Wen Guo, · Dept. of Medicine, Room 805, 650 Albany St., Boston, MA PubMed 16210702.
539   Modifications induced by dietary lipid source in adipose tissue phospholipid fatty acids and their
       consequences in lipid mobilization · Brtiish Jnl. of Nutrition82: 319–327 Maria P. · Portillo, Ana I. Tueros,
       Javier S. Perona, Valentina Ruiz-Guti?rrez, Isabel Torres and M. Teresa Macarulla· Dept. of Nutrition and
       Food Science University of Pais Vasco, Spain Instituto de la Grasa (C.S.I.C.), Sevilla, Spain.
540   Production of eicosapentaenoic and docosahexaenoic acid-containing oils in transgenic land plants for
       human and aquaculture nutrition see 2 above.
541   Fish Farming May Soon Overtake Cattle Ranching As a Food Source Lester R. Brown.
542   Lipid composition and contaminants in farmed and wild salmon. · Environ. Sci. Technol., 39 (22),
       8622 –8629, 2005 · M. Coreen Hamilton, Ronald A. Hites, Steven J. Schwager, Jeffery A. Foran Barbara
       A. Knuth and David O. Carpenter · AXYS Analytical Services, Sidney, British Columbia, Canada, School
       of Public and Environmental Affairs, Indiana University, Dept. of Biological Statistics and Computational
       Biology, Cornell University, Ithaca, New York Midwest Center for Environmental Science and Public
       Policy, Milwaukee, Wisconsin Dept. of Natural Resources, Cornell University, Ithaca, New York and
       Institute for Health and the Environment, University at Albany, New York.
543   INTENSIVE MARINE FISH AQUACULTURE WWF.
544   Antarctic Krill: a case study on the ecosystem implications of fishing Lighthouse Foundation By Virginia
       Gascón & Rodolfo Werner.
545   Net loss of wild fish to produce farmed salmon.
546   Fish Farming May Soon Overtake Cattle Ranching As a Food Source · Lester R. · October 3, 2000 –92001
       Earth Policy Institute Brown.
547   *Small Farms *New Family Farms *Agricultural Alternatives Vol. 8, No. 2 Sept–Oct 1997.
548   http://www.nutritiondata.com/facts–B00001–01c2134.html.
549   Antarctic Krill: a case study on the ecosystem implications of fishing See 544.
550   Where to find omega-3 fatty acids and how feeding animals with diet enriched in omega-3 fatty acids
       to increase nutritional value of derived products for human: what is actually useful? · J Nutr Health Aging.
       2005 Jul–Aug;9(4):232–42 · Bourre JM. · INSERM Neuro-pharmaco-nutrition, Hopital Fernand Widal,
       Paris. Pubmed 15980924.
551   Comparing the Fatty Acid Composition of Organic and Conventional Milk · J. Dairy Sci. 89:1938–1950K. A.
       Ellis, G. Innocent, D. Grove-White, P. Cripps, W. G. McLean, C. V. Howard and M. Mihm · University of
       Glasgow Veterinary School University of Liverpool, Faculty of Veterinary Medicine Dept. of Pharmacology
       & Therapeutics School of Biomedical Sciences, Liverpool, Molecular Biosciences, University of Ulster
       University of Glasgow Veterinary School.
552   High omega 3 Fatty Acid Content in Alpine Cheese The Basis for an Alpine Paradox · American Heart
       Association, Inc 2004;109:103–107 · Christa B. Hauswirth, MD; Martin R.L. Scheeder, Dr sg agr; Jürg H. Beer, MD
       · Dept. of Medicine, Kantonsspital Baden, and the Federal Institute of Technology, Zürich, Switzerland.
553   Flax: New Uses and Demands Berglund, D.R. p. 358–360. In: J. Janick and A. Whipkey.
554   An integrated production system of highly purified eicosapentaenoic acid from microalgae. improvement
       of photobioreactors and downstream processing. · Cordis.

555   I. Enhancement of EPA and DHA biosynthesis by over-expression of masu salmon delta6-desaturase-like gene in zebrafish · Transgenic Res. 2005 Apr;14(2):159-65 · Alimuddin, Yoshizaki G, Kiron V, Satoh S, Takeuchi T. · Dept. of Marine Biosciences, Tokyo University of Marine Science and Technology, Japan. PubMed 16022387.

556   June 2006 ISB News Report Yifan Dai and Randall S. Prather http://www.isb.vt.edu/news/2006/news06. jun.htm.

557   Production of eicosapentaenoic and docosahexaenoic acid-containing oils in transgenic land plants for human and aquaculture nutrition. See 2 above.

558   Sleep and metabolic control: Waking to a problem? Clinical and Experimental Pharmacology and Physiology, Volume 34, Numbers 1-2, January 2007 , pp. 1-9 · Michael I Trenell, Sleep and Circadian Research Group, Woolcock Institute of Medical Research and , Nathaniel S Marshall Sleep and Circadian Research Group, Woolcock Institute of Medical Research and Central Clinical School, Faculty of Medicine, University of Sydney, Sydney, New South Wales, Australia and Naomi L Rogers Sleep and Circadian Research Group, Woolcock Institute of Medical Research and Central Clinical School, Faculty of Medicine, University of Sydney, Sydney, New South Wales, Australia. Sleep and Circadian Research Group, Woolcock Institute of Medical Research and Central Clinical School, Faculty of Medicine, University of Sydney, Australia.

559   Melatonin (with the help of Wikipedia) http://en.wikipedia.org/wiki/Melatonin.

560   Permeability of pure lipid bilayers to melatonin · J Pineal Res. 1995 Oct;19(3):123-6. · Costa EJ, Lopes RH, Lamy-Freund MT · Instituto de Física, Universidade de São Paulo, Brazil. PubMed 8750345.

561   Melatonin inhibits fatty acid transport in inguinal fat pads of hepatoma 7288CTC-bearing and normal Buffalo rats via receptor-mediated signal transduction. · Life Sci. 2001 May 11;68(25):2835-44 · Sauer LA, Dauchy RT, Blask DE. · Laboratory of Experimental Neuroendocrinology/Oncology, Bassett Research Institute, Cooperstown, NY 13326-1394, USA. PubMed 11432449.

562   Effect of an n-3 fatty acid-deficient diet on the adenosine-dependent melatonin release in cultured rat pineal. · J Neurochem. 1993 Sep;61(3):1057-63 Gazzah N, Gharib A, Delton I, Moliere P, Durand G, Christon R, Lagarde M, Sarda N. · INSERM U. 352, Laboratoire de Chimie Biologique, INSAL, Villeurbanne, France. PubMed 8360673.

563   N-3 fatty acid deficiency in the rat pineal gland: effects on phospholipid molecular species composition and endogenous levels of melatonin and lipoxygenase products. · J Lipid Res. 1998 Jul;39(7):1397-403. Zhang H, Hamilton H, Salem N Jr, Kim HY. · Section of Mass Spectrometry, National Institute on Alcohol Abuse and Alcoholism. PubMed 9684742.

564   Dietary Docosahexaenoic Acid-Enriched Phospholipids Normalize Urinary Melatonin Excretion in Adult (n-3) Polyunsaturated Fatty Acid-Deficient Rats · Jnl. of Nutrition. 1999;129:2074-2080. · Monia Zaouali-Ajina, Abdallah Gharib, Georges Durand, Noureddine Gazzah, Bruno Claustrat, Claude Gharib and Nicole Sarda · Laboratoire de Physiologie de l'Environnement, Faculté de Médecine Lyon Grange-Blanche, Laboratoire de Neuropharmacologie Moléculaire UFR Laënnec,Lyon INRA Laboratoire de Nutrition et Sécurité Alimentaire, Jouy en Josas, Laboratoire de Radiopharmacie Radioanalyse, Hôpital Neuro-Cardiologique, Lyon, France, Ecole des Cadres et Techniciens de la Santé, Monastir.

565   Long-term melatonin administration reduces hyperinsulinemia and improves the altered fatty-acid compositions in type 2 diabetic rats via the restoration of Delta-5 desaturase activity. · J Pineal Res. 2002 Jan;32(1):26-33 · Nishida S, Segawa T, Murai I, Nakagawa S. · Dept. of Biochemistry, Dept. of the Third Internal Medicine, Nihon University School of Medicine, Itabashi, Tokyo, Japan. PubMed 11841597.

566   Effect of pinealectomy on plasma levels of insulin and leptin and on hepatic lipids in type 2 diabetic rats. · J Pineal Res. 2003 Nov;35(4):251-6 · Nishida S, Sato R, Murai I, Nakagawa S. Dept. of Biochemistry, Nihon University School of Medicine, Japan. PubMed 14521630.

567   Anti-inflammatory actions of melatonin and its metabolites, N1-acetyl-N2-formyl-5-methoxykynuramine and N1-acetyl-5-methoxykynuramine, in macrophages. · J Neuroimmunol. 2005 Aug;165(1-2):139-49 · Mayo JC, Sainz RM, Tan DX, Hardeland R, Leon J, Rodriguez C, Reiter RJ. · Dept. de Morfología y Biología Celular, Universidad de Oviedo, Asturias, España PubMed 15975667.

568   Melatonin: an endogenous negative modulator of 12-lipoxygenation in the rat pineal gland · Biochem. J. (1999) 344, 487-493 · Hongjian Zhang , Mohammed Akbar and Hee-Yong Kim · Section of Mass Spectrometry, Laboratory of Membrane Biochemistry and Biophysics, NIAAA, NIH, 12501 Washington Avenue, Rockville, MD 20852, U.S.A.

569   Melatonin as a Pharmacological Agent against Neuronal Loss in Experimental Models of Huntington's Disease, Alzheimer's Disease and Parkinsonism · Annals of the New York Academy of Sciences 890:471-485 (1999) · Russel J. Reiter, Javier Cabrera, Rosma M. Sainz, Juan Carlos Mayo Lucien C.

Manchester and Dun-Xian Tan · Dept. of Cellular and Structural Biology, The University of Texas Health Science Center, San Antonio Texas.

570　Melatonin and its kynurenin-like oxidation products affect the microbicidal activity of neutrophils. · Silva SO, Carvalho SR, Ximenes VF, Okada SS, Campa A. · Departamento de Análises Clínicas e Toxicológicas, Faculdade de Ciências Farmacêuticas, Universidade de São Paulo, CEP 05508-900, São Paulo, SP, Brazil.- PubMed 16242372.

571　Melatonin and its kynurenin-like oxidation products affect the microbicidal activity of neutrophils. · Microbes Infect. 2006 Feb;8(2):420–5 Silva SO, Carvalho SR, Ximenes VF, Okada SS, Campa A. · Dept. de Análises Clínicas e Toxicológicas, Faculdade de Ciências Farmacêuticas, Universidade de São Paulo, CEP 05508-900, São Paulo, SP, Brazil. PubMed 16242372.

572　Melatonin inhibits the growth of DMBA-induced mammary tumors by decreasing the local biosynthesis of estrogens through the modulation of aromatase activity. · Cos S, Gonzalez A, Guezmes A, Mediavilla MD, Martinez-Campa C, Alonso-Gonzalez C, Sanchez-Barcelo EJ. · Dept. of Physiology and Pharmacology, School of Medicine, University of Cantabria, Santander, Spain Pathological Anatomy Service, Sierrallana Hospital, Torrelavega, Cantabria, Spain.

573　Melatonin modulates aromatase activity in MCF–7 human breast cancer cells · Int J Cancer. 2006 Jan 15;118(2):274–8 · Cos S, Martinez-Campa C, Mediavilla MD, Sanchez-Barcelo EJ. ·Dept. of Physiology and Pharmacology, School of Medicine, University of Cantabria, Santander, Spain. PubMed 15683469I:

574　Estrogen-signaling pathway: a link between breast cancer and melatonin oncostatic actions. · Cancer Detect Prev. 2006;30(2):118–28 · Cos S, Gonzalez A, Martinez-Campa C, Mediavilla MD, Alonso-Gonzalez C, Sanchez-Barcelo EJ. · Dept. of Physiology and Pharmacology, School of Medicine, University of Cantabria, 39011 Santander, Spain. PubMed 16647824.

575　Melatonin-estrogen interactions in breast cancer. · J Pineal Res. 2005 May;38(4):217–22 · Sanchez-Barcelo EJ, Cos S, Mediavilla D, Martinez-Campa C, Gonzalez A, Alonso-Gonzalez C. · Dept. of Physiology and Pharmacology, School of Medicine, University of Cantabria, Spain. PubMed 15813897.

576　Impact of fish oil and melatonin on cachexia in patients with advanced gastrointestinal cancer: a randomized pilot study. · Persson,-C; Glimelius,-B; Ronnelid,-J; Nygren,-P. Department of Oncology, Radiology and Clinical Immunology, University Hospital, Uppsala University, Sweden PubMed 15723745

577　Melatonin Attenuates Estradiol-Induced Oxidative Damage to DNA: Relevance for Cancer Prevention · Experimental Biology and Medicine 226:707–712 (2001) · Malgorzata Karbownik, Russel J. Reiter, Susanne Burkhardt, Eloisa Gitto, Dun-Xian Tan and Andrzej Lewiński · Dept. of Cellular and Structural Biology, University of Texas Health Science Center, Texas; Dept. of Thyroidology, Institute of Endocrinology, Medical University of Lódz, 5 Poland.

578　http://en.wikipedia.org/wiki/Pineal_gland.

579　Infants to Adolescents: Research Update, vol. I no. 6 Brain Watching Beverly J. Roder, Ph.D. and Mabel L. Sgan, Ph.D.

580　J Pineal Res. 2005 Sep;39(2):164–9.Protective effect of melatonin on ascorbate-Fe2+ lipid peroxidation of polyunsaturated fatty acids in rat liver, kidney and brain microsomes: a chemiluminescence study. · Leaden PJ, Catalá A. · Cátedra de Bioquímica, Facultad de Ciencias Veterinarias, Universidad Nacional de La Plata, Argentina. PubMed 16098094.

581　A maternal diet high in n6 polyunsaturated fats alters mammary gland development... See210 above.

582　Early sexual maturation, central adiposity and subsequent overweight in late adolescence. A four-year follow-up of 1605 adolescent Norwegian boys and girls: the Young HUNT study · BMC Public Health. 2007; 7: 54. · Grete H Bratberg,Tom IL Nilsen,Turid L Holmen,and Lars J Vatten · HUNT Research Centre, Norwegian University of Science and Technology, Verdal, Dept. of Public Health and General Practice, Norwegian University of Science and Technology, Trondheim, Nord-Trøndelag University College, Levanger, Norway. PubMed 18553I9.

583　Nutritional and developmental regulation of plasma leptin in dairy cattle. · J Dairy Sci. 2003 Oct;86(10):3206–14. · Block SS, Smith JM, Ehrhardt RA, Diaz MC, Rhoads RP, Van Amburgh ME, Boisclair YR. Dept. of Animal Science, Cornell University NY. USA. PubMed 14594240.

584　Age impairments in sleep, metabolic and immune functions.-ExpGerontol.2004Nov–Dec;39(11–12):1739–43 · Prinz PN. · Dept. of Biobehavioral Nursing and Health Systems, University of Washington, Box 357–266, Seattle, WA 98195, USA. PubMed 15582290.

585　Effect of pinealectomy on plasma levels of insulin and leptin and on hepatic lipids in type 2 diabetic rats. · J Pineal Res. 2003 Nov;35(4):251–6 · Nishida S, Sato R, Murai I, Nakagawa S. · Dept. of Biochemistry, Nihon University School of Medicine, Tokyo, Japan PubMed 14521630.

586   Effect of exogenous melatonin on sexual behaviours in West African Dwarf goat · J O Daramola, A A Adeloye and A O Soladoye · Dept. of Animal Production, Nigeria Dept. of Human Physiology, University of Ilorin, Nigeria.

587   Title: Effect of melatonin on photoperiod responses, ovarian secretion of oestrogen, and coital responses in the domestic cat. · Leyva, H : Madley, T : Stabenfeldt, G H · J-Reprod-Fertil-Suppl. 1989; 39135–42.

588   Effects of melatonin on progesterone production by human granulosa lutein cells in culture.· Fertil Steril. 1992 Sep;58(3):526–9. Brzezinski A, Fibich T, Cohen M, Schenker JG, Laufer N. · Dept. of Obstetrics and Gynecology, Hadassah Medical Center, Jerusalem, Israel. PubMed 1521647.

589   Development of the Cerebral Cortex:XV. Sexual Differentiation of the Central Nervous System · J Am Acad Child Adolesc Psychiatry, 37(12): 1337–1339, 1998 · Roger A. Gorski, Ph.D.

590   Testostrone and aggressiveness · Marco Giammanco, Garden Tabacchi, Santo Giammanco, Danila Di Majo and Maurizio La Guardia · Endocrinology (2005).

591   Omega–3 fatty acid deficiencies in neurodevelopment, aggression and autonomic dysregulation: opportunities for intervention · Int Rev Psychiatry. 2006 Apr;18(2):107–18. · Hibbeln JR, Ferguson TA, Blasbalg TL. National Institute on Alcohol Abuse and Alcoholism, Bethesda,USA. PubMed 16777665.

592   Relationships Between Types of Fat Consumed and Serum Estrogen and Androgen Concentrations in Japanese Men · Nutrition and Cancer 2000, Vol. 38, No. 2, Pages 163–167 · Chisato Nagata, Naoyoshi Takatsuka, Norito Kawakami, Hiroyuki Shimizu.

593   Region-Specific Regulation of Cytochrome P450 Aromatase Messenger Ribonucleic Acid by Androgen in Brains of Male Rhesus Monkeys · Biology of Reproduction 62, 1818–1822 (2000) · J.A. Resko A.C. Pereyra-Martinez, H.L. Stadelman, and C.E. Roselli · Dept. of Physiology and Pharmacology, School of Medicine, Oregon Health Sciences University, Oregon.

594   Docosahexaenoic acid concentrations are higher in women than in men because of estrogenic effects · Giltay Erik J. Gooren Louis J. G. Toorians Arno W. F. T. Katan Martijn B. Zock Peter L. · Psychiatric Center GGZ Delfland, Delft, Dept. of Endocrinology, Andrology Unit, VU University Medical Center, Amsterdam, Wageningen Center for Food Sciences, Wageningen University.

595   Docosahexaenoic acid concentrations are higher in women than ....See 594 Above.

596   Free Fatty Acids Increase Androgen Precursors in Vivo · The Jnl. of Clinical Endocrinology & Metabolism Vol. 91, No. 4 1501–1507 · K. Mai, T. Bobbert, V. Kullmann, J. Andres, H. Rochlitz, M. Osterhoff, M. O. Weickert, V. Bähr, M. Möhlig, A. F. H. Pfeiffer, S. Diederich and J. Spranger Dept. of Endocrinology, Diabetes and Nutrition Charite–University Medicine Berlin, Campus Benjamin Franklin, Berlin, Dept. of Clinical Nutrition German Institute of Human Nutrition Potsdam-Rehbrücke, Nuthetal, Germany; and Endokrinologikum (S.D.), 10117 Berlin, Germany.

597   Inhibition of gonadotropin-stimulated ovarian steroid production ...See 309 above.

598   Free fatty acids increase androgen precursors in vivo. · J Clin Endocrinol Metab. 2006 Apr;91(4):1501–7 Mai K, Bobbert T, Kullmann V, Andres J, Rochlitz H, Osterhoff M, Weickert MO, Bahr V, Mohlig M, Pfeiffer AF, Diederich S, Spranger J. · Dept. of Endocrinology, Diabetes and Nutrition, Charite-University Medicine Berlin. PubMed 16434463.

599   Prostaglandin receptors are mediators of vascular function in endometrial pathologies. · Mol Cell Endocrinol. 2006 Jun 27;252(1–2):191–200. · Jabbour HN, Sales KJ, Smith OP, Battersby S, Boddy SC. · MRC Human Reproductive Sciences Unit, Centre for Reproductive Biology, The Queen's Medical Research Institute, Edinburgh. PubMed 16701939.

600   Hormonal-induced changes on the lipid composition and DPH fluorescence anisotropy of erythrocyte ghost from pre- and postmenopausal women. · Acta Physiol Pharmacol Ther Latinoam. 1998;48(1):8–17. · Marra CA, Mangionil JO, Tavella M, del Alaniz MJ, Ortiz D, Sala C. · INIBIOLP Cátedra de Bioquimica, Facultad de Ciencias Médicas de la UNLP, La Plata, Argentina. PubMed 9504188.

601   Effect of various steroids on the biosynthesis of arachidonic acid in isolated hepatocytes and HTC cells. · Lipids. 1988 Nov;23(11):1053–8 · Marra CA, de Alaniz MJ, Brenner RR. · Instituto de Investigaciones Bioquimicas de La Plata Facultad de Ciencias Médicas, La Plata, Argentina. PubMed 3148796.

602   Effects of estradiol and environmental temperature changes on rat liver delta 6 microsomal desaturase activity. · Lipids. 1986 Jul;21(7):440–3. · Gonzalez S, Nervi AM, Peluffo RO. PubMed 3747736.

603   Deficiency of essential fatty acids and membrane fluidity during pregnancy and lactation · Proc Natl Acad Sci U S A. 1991 June 1; 88(11): 4835–4839 · R T Holman, S B Johnson, and P L Ogburn · Hormel Institute, University of Minnesota, Austin. PubMed 51761.

604   Menopause-induced changes in lipid fractions and total fatty acids in plasma. · Endocr Res. 2001 Aug;27(3):357–65 · Maynar M, Mahedero G, Maynar I, Maynar JI, Tuya IR, Caballero MJ. Dept. of Physiology, Sports Sciences School, University of Extremadura, Spain. PubMed 11678583.

605   The dietary regulation of acyltransferase and desaturase activities in microsomal membranes of rat liver.
        · Lipids. 1984 Jan;19(1):48–55 · Pugh EL, Kates M. PubMed 6708745.

606   Cloning, Expression, and the Fatty Acid Regulation of the Human D-5 Deaturase · The Jnl. of Biological
        Chemistry Vol274 No52 Dec 1999 · Hyekyung p.Cho, Manabu Nakamura, and Steven D. Clarke National
        Sciences and the Institute for Cellular and Molecular Biology, The University of Texas Austin, Texas.

607   Aromatase Inhibitors in the Treatment of Breast Cancer · Endocrine Reviews 26 (3): 331–345 · Robert
        W. Brueggemeier, John C. Hackett and Edgar S. Diaz-Cruz · Medicinal Chemistry and Pharmacognosy,
        College of Pharmacy, and Hormones and Cancer Program, Ohio State University Comprehensive Cancer
        Center, The Ohio State University, Columbus, Ohio 43210.

608   Alteration of prostaglandin production and agonist responsiveness by n-6 polyunsaturated fatty acids
        in endometrial cells from late-gestation ewes · J Endocrinol. 2004 Aug;182(2):249–56 · Cheng Z, Elmes
        M, Kirkup SE, Abayasekara DR, Wathes DC. · Reproduction and Development Group, Royal Veterinary
        College, North Mymms, Hatfield, Herts. PubMed 15283685.

609   Docosahexaenoic acid concentrations are higher in women than in men because of estrogenic effects.
        · Am J Clin Nutr. 2004 Nov;80(5):1167–74. · Giltay EJ, Gooren LJ, Toorians AW, Katan MB, Zock PL.
        · Psychiatric Center GGZ Delfland, Delft. PubMed 15531662.

610   Metabolism of alpha-linolenic acid in humans. · Prostaglandins Leukot Essent Fatty Acids. 2006
        Sep;75(3):161–8. · Burdge, G. C. · Institute of Human Nutrition, University of Southampton, Bassett
        Crescent East, Southampton SO16 7PX, UK PubMed 16828546.

611   Raloxifene and hormone replacement therapy increase arachidonic acid and docosahexaenoic acid
        levels in postmenopausal women. · Giltay EJ, Duschek EJ, Katan MB, Zock PL, Neele SJ, Netelenbos JC.
        Psychiatric Center GGZ Delfland, Delft, The Netherlands. PubMed 15350182.

612   Effects of hormone replacement therapy on circulating docosahexaenoic acid and eicosapentaenoic acid
        levels in postmenopausal women. · Endocr J. 2003 Feb;50(1):51–9. · Sumino H, Ichikawa S, Murakami M,
        Nakamura T, Kanda T, Sakamaki T, Mizunuma H, Kurabayashi M. · Second Dept. of Internal Medicine,
        Gunma University School of Medicine, Maebashi 371–8511, Japan. PubMed12733709.

613   Effects induced by two different estrogens on serum individual phospholipids and serum lecithin fatty
        acid composition. · Horm Metab Res. 1981 Mar;13(3):141–5 · Silfverstolpe G, Johnson P, Samsice G, Svanborg
        A, Gustafson A. PubMed 7239424.

614   Relative fatty acid composition of lecithin during postmenopausal replacement therapy--a comparison
        between ethinyl estradiol and estradiol valerate. · Gynecol Obstet Invest. 1984;18(6):296–302 · Ottosson
        UB, Lagrelius A, Rosing U, von Schoultz B. PubMed 6519560.

615   Inhibition of gonadotropin-stimulated ovarian steroid production See 309 above.

616   Inhibition of gonadotropin-stimulated ovarian See 309 Above.

617   Association of maternal fat and alcohol intake with maternal and umbilical hormone levels and birth
        weight · Cancer Science Volume 98 Issue 6 Page 869–873, June 2007 · Chisato Nagata Shinichi Iwasa
        Makoto Shiraki Yukari Sahashi Hiroyuki Shimizu Gifu · University Graduate School of Medicine, 1–1
        Yanagido Gifu,Iwasa Maternity 161–1 Nagara Gifu 7 Sakihai Institute, 8–1 Kogane-machi, Gifu Japan.

618   Effects of polyunsaturated fatty acids and prostaglandins on oocyte maturation in a marine teleost,
        the European sea bass (Dicentrarchus labrax). · Biology of Reproduction 64, 382–389 (2001) · Sorbera
        LA, Asturiano JF, Carrillo M, Zanuy S. · Instituto de Acuicultura (Consejo Superior de Investigaciones
        Científicas), Torre de la Sal, 12595 Castellón, Spain.

619   Potential role for arachidonic acid and eicosanoids in modulating progesterone secretion by ovine
        chorionic cells. · Acta Endocrinol (Copenh). 1993 May;128(5):478–84 · de la Llosa-Hermier MP,
        Fernandez C, Martal J, Hermier C. · Laboratoire de Biochimie des Hormones, CNRS, Gif-sur-Yvette,
        France. PubMed 8317196.

620   The effect of progesterone on the release of arachidonic acid from human endometrial cells stimulated by
        histamine. · Wilson T, Liggins GC, Aimer GP, Watkins EJ. · PubMed 3083483.

621   Influence of testosterone on polyunsaturated fatty acid biosynthesis in Sertoli cells in culture Cell
        · Biochem Funct. 2005 May–Jun;23(3):175–80. · Hurtado de Catalfo GE, de Gomez Dumm IN. · Inst.
        (INIBIOLP), Facultad de Ciencias Médicas, La Plata, Argentina PubMed 15376235.

622   Prevention of Infertility Abnormal Body Weight: A Preventable Cause of Infertility · G. William Bates,

623   Estriol sensitizes rat Kupffer cells via gut-derived endotoxin · Am J Physiol Gastrointest Liver Physiol 277:
        G671–G677, 1999 · Nobuyuki Enomoto, Shunhei Yamashina, Peter Schemmer, Chantal A. Rivera, Blair U.
        Bradford, Ayako Enomoto, David A. Brenner, and Ronald G. Thurman · Laboratory of Hepatobiology and
        Toxicology and Dept. of Pharmacology, and Division of Digestive Diseases and Nutrition and Dept. of
        Medicine, University of North Carolina.

624   Omega-3 fatty acids in inflammation and autoimmune diseases. See Above 344.
625   Oxidized omega-3 fatty acids in fish oil inhibit leukocyte-endothelial interactions through activation
       of PPAR - Blood, 15 August 2002, Vol. 100, No. 4, pp. 1340-1346 - Sanjeev Sethi, Ouliana Ziouzenkova,
       Heyu Ni, Denisa D. Wagner, Jorge Plutzky, and Tanya N. Mayadas Vascular Research Division, - Dept.
       of Medicine, Brigham and Women's Hospital and Center for Blood Research and Dept. of Pathology,
       Harvard Medical School.
626   Origins and evolution of the Western diet: (See 42).
627   Teaching nutrition to medical doctors: the potential role of the State Registered Dietitian - Jnl. of Human
       Nutrition and Dietetics Volume 9 Issue 5 Page 349-356, October 1996 - Carolyn Summerbell -Rank Dept.
       of Human Nutrition, St Bartholomew's and the Royal London Hospital School of Medicine and Dentistry,
       Whitchapel, London, UK.
628   Relationship of Plasma Polyunsaturated Fatty Acids to Circulating Inflammatory Markers See 466 above.
629   Omega-3 fatty acids in inflammation and autoimmune diseases. See Above 344.
630   Increased lipogenesis in cancer cells: new players, novel targets. - Curr Opin Clin Nutr Metab Care.
       2006 Jul;9(4):358-65 - Swinnen JV, Brusselmans K, Verhoeven G. - Laboratory for Experimental
       Medicine and Endocrinology, Katholieke Universiteit Leuven, Campus Gasthuisberg, Leuven,
       Belgium. PubMed 16778563.
631   Health benefits of docosahexaenoic acid (DHA) - Pharmacol Res. 1999 Sep;40(3):211-25 - Horrocks LA,
       Yeo YK. - Docosa Foods Ltd, Columbus, OH USA, PubMed 10479465.
632   Oxidized Omega-3 Fatty Acids Inhibit NF- B Activation Via a PPAR -Dependent Pathway -
       Arteriosclerosis, Thrombosis, and Vascular Biology. 2004;24:1621 - Archana Mishra; Ashok Chaudhary;
       Sanjeev Sethi Dept. of Pathology, University of Iowa Hospitals and Clinics, Iowa City, Iowa.
633   Oxidized omega-3 fatty acids in fish oil inhibit leukocyte-endothelial interactions through activation
       of PPAR - Blood 15 August 2002, Vol. 100, No. 4, pp. 1340-1346 - Sanjeev Sethi, Ouliana Ziouzenkova,
       Heyu Ni, Denisa D. Wagner, Jorge Plutzky, and Tanya N. Mayadas - Vascular Research Division, Dept.
       of Pathology, Cardiovascular Division, Dept. of Medicine, Brigham and Women's Hospital and Center for
       Blood Research and Dept. of Pathology, Harvard Medical School, Boston, MA.
634   Docosahexaenoic acid ingestion inhibits natural killer cell activity and production of inflammatory
       mediators in young healthy men. - Lipids. 1999 Apr;34(4):317-24. - Kelley DS, Taylor PC, Nelson GJ, Schmidt
       PC, Ferretti A, Erickson KL, Yu R, Chandra RK, Mackey BE. - Western Human Nutrition Research Center,
       Presidio of San Francisco. PubMed 10443964.
635   Acne Vulgaris A Disease of Western Civilization - Arch Dermatol. 2002; 138: 1584 -1590 - Loren Cordain,
       PhD; Staffan Lindeberg, MD,PhD; Magdalena Hurtado, PhD; Kim Hill, PhD; S. Boyd Eaton, MD; Jennie
       Brand-Miller, PhD - Dept. of Health and Exercise Science, Colorado State University, Fort Collins, Dept.
       of Community Medicine, University of Lund, Lund, Sweden; Dept. of Anthropology, University of New
       Mexico, Albuquerque, Dept. of Radiology and Anthropology, Emory University, Atlanta, Ga; and Dept.
       of Biochemistry, Human Nutrition Unit, University of Sydney, Sydney, Australia.
636   Acne vulgaris: Nutritional factors may be influencing psychological sequelae. - Med Hypotheses. 2007
       Apr 18 - Katzman M, Logan AC. - START Clinic for Mood and Anxiety Disorders, University of Toronto,
       790 Bay St., Suite 900, Toronto, Canada. Pubmed 17448607.
637   Management of acne in adolescent. - Arch Pediatr. 2007 Jul 9 - Faure M. - Service de dermatologie, hôpital
       Édouard-Herriot, pavillon R, 5, place d'Arsonval, Lyon, France. Pubmed 17624743.
638   Dietary patterns and blood fatty acid composition in children with attention-deficit hyperactivity disorder
       in Taiwan. - J Nutr Biochem. 2004 Aug;15(8):467-72 - Chen JR, Hsu SF, Hsu CD, Hwang LH, Yang SC.-
       Dept. of Nutrition and Health Sciences, Taipei Medical University. Pubmed 15302081.
639   Reversal of docosahexaenoic acid deficiency in the rat brain, retina, liver, and serum - Jnl. of Lipid Research,
       Vol. 42, 419-427, March 2001 - Toru Moriguchi, James Loewke, Megan Garrison, Janice Nicklay Catalan,
       and Norman Salem, Jr. - Laboratory of Membrane Biochemistry & Biophysics, National Institutes on
       Alcohol Abuse & Alcoholism, National Institutes of Health, Bethesda, MD 20892.
640   Cognitive and physiological effects of Omega-3 polyunsaturated fatty acid supplementation in healthy
       subjects. - Eur J Clin Invest. 2005 Nov;35(11):691-9. - Fontani G, Corradeschi F, Felici A, Alfatti F, Migliorini
       S, Lodi L. - University of Siena, Siena, Italy. Pubmed 16269019.
641   Dietary enrichment with omega-3 polyunsaturated fatty acids reverses age-related decreases in the
       GluR2 and NR2B glutamate receptor subunits in rat forebrain. - Neurobiol Aging. 2007 Mar;28(3):424-39
       - Dyall SC, Michael GJ, Whelpton R, Scott AG, Michael-Titus AT. - Neuroscience Centre, Institute of
       Cell and Molecular Sciences, St. Bartholomew's and the Royal London School of Medicine and Dentistry,
       Queen Mary, University of London. Pubmed 16500747.

642 Atopic sensitization during the first year of life in relation to long chain polyunsaturated fatty acid levels in human milk. See 283 above.

643 Human milk polyunsaturated long-chain fatty acids and secretory immunoglobulin A antibodies and early childhood allergy · Pediatr Allergy Immunol. 2000 Feb;11(1):29-39. · Duchén K, Casas R, Fagerås-Böttcher M, Yu G, Björkstén B. · Dept. of Health and Environment, Linköping University Hospital, Sweden. Pubmed 10768733.

644 Diet of lactating women and allergic reactions in their infants. · Curr Opin Clin Nutr Metab Care. 2006 May;9(3):284-8. · Palmer DJ, Makrides M.Child · Health Research Institute, and Dept. of Paediatrics, The University of Adelaide, Women's and Children's Hospital, North Adelaide, South Australia, Australia. Pubmed 16607130.

645 Short-term administration of omega 3 fatty acids from fish oil results in increased transthyretin transcription in old rat hippocampus · PNAS | February 18, 2003 | vol. 100 | no. 4 | 1580-1585.

646 Polyunsaturated fatty acids in the central nervous system: evolution of concepts and nutritional implications throughout life. · Alessandri JM, Guesnet P, Vancassel S, Astorg P, Denis I, Langelier B, Aid S, Poumes-Ballihaut C, Champeil-Potokar G, Lavialle M. · Laboratory of Functional Genomics, Biological Research Center, and Institute of Biochemistry, Biological Research Center, Hungarian Academy of Sciences, Hungary; and Dept. of Clinical and Experimental Laboratory Medicine, Semmelweis University, Budapest, Hungary. Pubmed 15762297.

647 A Diet Enriched with the Omega-3 Fatty Acid Docosahexaenoic Acid Reduces Amyloid Burden in an Aged Alzheimer Mouse Model · The Jnl. of Neuroscience, March 23, 2005, 25(12):3032-3040; · Giselle P. Lim, Frédéric Calon, Takashi Morihara, Fusheng Yang, Bruce Teter, Oliver Ubeda, Norman Salem, Jr, Sally A. Frautschy,and Greg M. Cole Dept.s of Medicine and Neurology, University of California Los Angeles, Veterans Affairs Greater Los Angeles Healthcare System and Geriatric Research Educational Clinical Center, California, Section of Nutritional Neuroscience, Laboratory of Membrane Biochemistry and Biophysics, National Institute on Alcohol Abuse and Alcoholism, National Institutes of Health, Maryland 20852.

648 Docosahexaenoic acid-rich phospholipid supplementation: effect on behavior, learning ability, and retinal function in control and n-3 polyunsaturated fatty acid deficient old mice. · Nutr Neurosci. 2002 Feb;5(1):43-52 · Carrié I, Smirnova M, Clément M, DE JD, Francès H, Bourre JM. · INSERM U26, Unité de Neuro-Pharmaco-Nutrition, Paris. Pubmed 11929197.

649 Short-term administration of omega 3 fatty acids from fish oil results in increased transthyretin transcription in old rat hippocampus · PNAS , February 18, 2003, vol. 100, no. 4, 1580-1585· László G. Puskás, Klára Kitajka, Csaba Nyakas, Gwendolyn Barcelo-Coblijn, and Tibor Farkas · Laboratory of Functional Genomics, Biological Research Center, and Institute of Biochemistry, Biological Research Center, Hungarian Academy of Sciences, Szeged, Hungary; and Dept. of Clinical and Experimental Laboratory Medicine, Semmelweis University, Budapest, Hungary.

650 Consumption of Fish and n-3 Fatty Acids and Risk of Incident Alzheimer Disease · Arch Neurol. 2003;60:940-946. · Martha Clare Morris, ScD; Denis A. Evans, MD; Julia L. Bienias ScD; Christine C. Tangney PhD, David A. Bennett, MD; Robert S. Wilson, PhD; Neelum Aggarwal, MD; Julie Schneider, MD · Rush Institute for Healthy Aging Dept.s of Internal Medicine and Preventive Medicine, Rush Alzheimer's Disease Center, and Dept.s of Clinical Nutrition Neurological Sciences, and Psychology, Rush-Presbyterian-St Luke's Medical Center, Chicago, Ill.

651 Efficacy of fish oil concentrate in the treatment of rheumatoid arthritis. · J Rheumatol. 2000 Oct;27(10):2343-6 · Volker D, Fitzgerald P, Major G, Garg M. · Discipline of Nutrition and Dietetics, Faculty of Medicine and Health Sciences, and the Centre for Clinical Epidemiology and Biostatistics, University of Newcastle, Callaghan, NSW, Australia. Rush Institute for Healthy Aging , Dept.s of Internal Medicine and Preventive Medicine , Rush Alzheimer's Disease Center, and Dept.s of Clinical Nutrition, Neurological Sciences, and Psychology, Rush-Presbyterian-St Luke's Medical Center, Chicago, Ill. PubMed 11036827.

652 An introduction to dietary/supplemental omega-3 fatty acids for general health and prevention: part II. · Urol Oncol. 2005 Jan-Feb;23(1):36-48. · Moyad MA. Phil F. Jenkins Director of Complementary & Alternative Medicine, Dept. of Urology, University of Michigan Medical Center, Ann Arbor, USA. PubMed 15885582.

653 Omega-3 fatty acids and inflammation · Curr Atheroscler Rep. 2004 Nov;6(6):461-7 · Mori TA, Beilin LJ. · School of Medicine and Pharmacology-Royal Perth Hospital Unit, The University of Western Australia, Medical Research Foundation Building, Perth. PubMed 15485592.

654   Inhibition of Osteoporosis in Autoimmune Disease Prone MRL/Mpj-Faslpr Mice by N-3 Fatty Acids • Arunabh Bhattacharya, PhD, Md, Mizanur Rahman, PhD, Jameela Banu, PhD, Richard A. Lawrence, PhD, Howard S. McGuff, DDS, I.R. Garrett, PhD, Michael Fischbach, MD and Gabriel Fernandes, PhD, • CNS Dept. of Medicine, Division of Clinical Immunology, Dept. of Pathology, University of Texas Health Science Center, OsteoScreen, Inc. (I.R.G.), San Antonio, Texas.

655   Fatty acid modulation of endothelial activation • Raffaele De Caterina, James K Liao and Peter Libby • American Jnl. of Clinical Nutrition, Vol. 71, No. 1, 213S-223S, January 2000 • CNR Institute of Clinical Physiology and the Scuola Superiore S Anna, Pisa, Italy, and the Vascular Medicine and Atherosclerosis Unit, Brigham and Women's Hospital, Boston.

656   n-3 Fatty acids and the prevention of coronary atherosclerosis • American Jnl. of Clinical Nutrition, Vol. 71, No. 1, 224S-227s, January 2000 • Clemens von Schacky • Medizinische Klinik, Klinikum Innenstadt, University of Munich, Germany.

657   n-3 fatty acids and cardiovascular disease.• Am J Clin Nutr. 2006 Jun;83(6 Suppl):1477S-1482S. • Breslow JL.• Rockefeller University, New York, NY 10021, USA PubMed 16841857.

658   Relative effects of dietary saturated, monounsaturated, and polyunsaturated fatty acids on cardiac arrhythmias in rats • American Jnl. of Clinical Nutrition, Vol 57, 207-212, • PL McLennan • Cardiac Research Unit, Commonwealth Scientific and Industrial Research Organization, Adelaide, Australia.

659   Dietary modulation of lipid metabolism and mechanical performance of the heart • Molecular and Cellular Biology Vol 116 no1-2 Oct 1992 • John S. Charnock, Peter L. McLennan and Mahinda Y Abeywardena CSIRO, • Division of Human Nutrition, Glenthorne Laboratories, South Australia.

660   Antiarrhythmic and electrophysiological effects of long-chain omega-3 polyunsaturated fatty acids. • Naunyn Schmiedebergs • Arch Pharmacol. 2005 Mar;371(3):202-11. • Dhein S, Michaelis B, Mohr FW.• Clinic for Cardiac Surgery, University of Leipzig, Heart Center, Leipzig, Germany. PubMed 15900514.

661   Induction of mitochondrial nitrative damage and cardiac dysfunction by chronic provision of dietary omega-6 polyunsaturated fatty acids. • Free Radic Biol Med. 2006 Nov 1;41(9):1413-24. • Ghosh S, Kewalramani G, Yuen G, Pulinilkunnil T, An D, Innis SM, Allard MF, Wambolt RB, Qi D, Abrahani A, Rodrigues B.• Division of Pharmacology and Toxicology, Faculty of Pharmaceutical Sciences, The University of British Columbia, Vancouver, British Columbia, Canada V6T 1Z3. PubMed 17023268.

662   Omega-3 fatty acids and cardiovascular disease: a case for omega-3 index as a new risk factor.• Pharmacol Res. 2007 Mar;55(3):217-23. Epub 2007 • Jan 25 Harris WS. • Nutrition and Metabolic Disease Research Institute, Sanford Research/USD, Sanford School of Medicine of the University of South Dakota, 1400 West 22nd Street, Sioux Falls, SD 57105, USA. PubMed 17324586.

663   Prevention of Cardiac Arrhythmia by Dietary (n-3) Polyunsaturated Fatty Acids and Their Mechanism of Action • The Jnl. of Nutrition Vol. 127 No. 3 March 1997, pp. 383-393 • Sudheera S. D. Nair, James W. Leitch, John Falconer, and Manohar L. Garg Discipline of Nutrition and Dietetics, • University of Newcastle, Callaghan, NSW, Dept. of Cardiology and Discipline of Reproductive Medicine, John Hunter Hospital, NSW Australia.

664   Dietary omega-3 polyunsaturated fatty acid supplementation and airway hyperresponsiveness in asthma.• J Asthma. 2005 Jun;42(5):305-14 • Mickleborough TD.• Dept. of Kinesiology, Indiana University, Bloomington, Indiana 47401. PubMed 16036405.

665   Protective effect of fish oil supplementation on exercise-induced ronchoconstriction in asthma. • Chest. 2006 Jan;129(1):39-49 • Mickleborough TD, Lindley MR, Ionescu AA, Fly AD. • Human Performance and Exercise Biochemistry Laboratory, Dept. of Kinesiology, Indiana University, 1025 E Seventh St, Bloomington, USA. PubMed 16424411.

666   Role of breast milk in a mouse model of maternal transmission of asthma susceptibility.• J Immunol. 2006 Jan 15;176(2):762-9 • Leme AS, Hubeau C, Xiang Y, Goldman A, Hamada K, Suzaki Y, Kobzik L.• Dept. of Environmental Health, Harvard School of Public Health. PubMed 16393959.

667   Diet and obstructive lung diseases.• Epidemiol Rev. 2001;23(2):268-87 Romieu I, Trenga C.• Pan American Health Organization and National Institute of Public Health, Center for Population Studies, Cuernavaca, Morelos, Mexico. PubMed 12192737.

668   Breast milk fatty acids may link innate and adaptive immune regulation: analysis of soluble CD14, prostaglandin E2, and fatty acids • Pediatr Res. 2006 May;59(5):723-7. • Laitinen K, Hoppu U, Hämäläinen M, Linderborg K, Moilanen E, Isolauri E. • Dept. of Paediatrics, Turku University Central Hospital, Finland. PubMed 16627889.

669   N-3 polyunsaturated fatty acids and atopy in Korean preschoolers. • Lipids. 2007 Apr;42(4):345-9• Hwang I, Cha A, Lee H, Yoon H, Yoon T, Cho B, Lee S, Park Y. Dept. of Preventive and Occupational Medicine, College of Medicine, Pusan National University, Pusan, South Korea. PubMed 17406929.

670   Oxidative stress in autism. - Pathophysiology. 2006 Aug;13(3):171–81. - Chauhan A, Chauhan V. - NYS
      Institute for Basic Research in Developmental Disabilities, NY USA. PubMed 16766163.

671   Omega-3 fatty acids supplementation in children with autism: See 671 above.

672   Essential fatty acids and phospholipase A2 in autistic spectrum disorders. - Prostaglandins Leukot Essent
      Fatty Acids. 2004 Oct;71(4):201–4. Bell JG, MacKinlay EE, Dick JR, MacDonald DJ, Boyle RM, Glen AC.
      - Lipid Nutrition Group, Institute of Aquaculture, University of Stirling, Stirling, Scotland, FK9 4LA, UK.
      PubMed 15301788.

673   Healthy intakes of n–3 and n–6 fatty acids: See 1 Above.

674   Dietary n–3 PUFA deprivation alters expression of enzymes of the arachidonic and docosahexaenoic
      acid cascades in rat frontal cortex - Mol Psychiatry. 2007 Feb;12(2):151–7. - Rao JS, Ertley RN, DeMar JC,
      Rapoport SI, Bazinet RP, Lee HJ.Brain - Physiology and Metabolism Section, National Institute on Aging,
      National Institutes of Health, Bethesda, MD 20892, USA. PubMed 16983392.

675   Ratio of n–6 to n–3 fatty acids and bone mineral density in older adults: the Rancho Bernardo Study
      American - Jnl. of Clinical Nutrition, Vol. 81, No. 4, 934–938, April 2005 - Lauren A Weiss, Elizabeth Barrett-
      Connor and Denise von Mühlen - Dept. of Family and Preventive Medicine, University of California.

676   Polyunsaturated fatty acids in the central nervous system: evolution of concepts and nutritional implications
      throughout life. - Reprod Nutr Dev. 2004 Nov–Dec;44(6):509–Alessandri JM, Guesnet P, Vancassel S,
      Astorg P, Denis I, Langelier B, Aïd S, Poumès-Ballihaut C, Champeil-Potokar G, Lavialle M. - Neurobiologie
      des Lipides, Laboratoire de Nutrition et Sécurité Alimentaire, INRA, France. PubMed 15762297.

377   Controversial Nutrients That Potentially Affect Preterm Neurodevelopment - Essential Fatty Acids and Iron
      Pediatric Research. Issue. 57(5 Part 2):99R–103R, May 2005. - Georgieff, Michael K.; Innis, Shelia M.

678   Astrocytes in culture require docosahexaenoic acid to restore the n–3/n–6 polyunsaturated fatty acid
      balance in their membrane phospholipids. - J Neurosci Res. 2004 Jan 1;75(1):96–106 - Champeil-Potokar G,
      Denis I, Goustard-Langelier B, Alessandri JM, Guesnet P, Lavialle M. - Laboratoire de Nutrition et Sécurité
      Alimentaire, Institut National de la Recherche Agronomique, Jouy-en-Josas, France. PubMed 14689452.

679   Roles of unsaturated fatty acids in the brain at various ages and during ageing. See 336.

680   Cognitive aging, childhood intelligence, and the use of food supplements: possible involvement of n–3
      fatty acids - American Jnl. of Clinical Nutrition, Vol. 80, No. 6, 1650–1657, December 2004 - Lawrence J
      Whalley, Helen C Fox, Klaus W Wahle, John M Starr and Ian J Deary - University of Aberdeen Dept.
      of Mental Health Royal Cornhill Hospital, the Robert Gordon University Dept. of Life Sciences, the
      University of Edinburgh, Dept. of Geriatric Medicine, Royal Victoria Hospital, the University of Edinburgh,
      Dept. of Psychology.

681   Nutrigenomic explanation for the beneficial effects of fish oil on cognitive function - American Jnl. of
      Clinical Nutrition, Vol. 81, No. 6, 1453–1454, June 2005 - Celia M Ross.

682   Membrane phospholipid composition and membrane fluidity of human brain tumour: a spin label study. -
      Neurol Res. 1987 Mar;9(1):38–43 - Hattori T, Andoh T, Sakai N, Yamada H, Kameyama Y, Ohki K, Nozawa
      Y. PubMed 2883605.

683   Phospholipids and fatty acids in human brain tumors. - Acta Physiol Hung. 1992;79(4):381–7 - Ledwozyw
      A, Lutnicki K. - Dept. of Pathophysiology, Veterinary Faculty of Agricultural Academy, Lublin, Poland.
      PubMed 1343190.

684   The fatty acid composition of human gliomas differs from that found in nonmalignant brain tissue. -
      Lipids. 1996 Dec;31(12):1283–8. - Martin DD, Robbins ME, Spector AA, Wen BC, Hussey DH. - Dept. of
      Radiology, University of Iowa Hospitals and Clinics, Iowa City 52242, USA.

685   Long-chain n–3-to-n–6 polyunsaturated fatty acid ratios in breast adipose tissue from women with
      and without breast cancer. - Nutr Cancer. 2002;42(2):180–5. - Bagga D, Anders KH, Wang HJ, Glaspy JA.
      - Division of Hematology-Oncology, Dept. of Medicine, University of California, Los Angeles School of
      Medicine, Los Angeles, CA 90095, USA. PubMed 12416257.

686   n–3 PUFAs reduce VEGF expression in human colon cancer cells modulating the COX–2/PGE2 induced
      ERK-1 and -2 and HIF-1alpha induction pathway. - Carcinogenesis. 2004 Dec;25(12):2303–10 - Calviello G,
      Di Nicuolo F, Gragnoli S, Piccioni E, Serini S, Maggiano N, Tringali G, Navarra P, Ranelletti FO, Palozza P.
      - Institute of General Pathology, Catholic University, L.go F. Vito, 1, 00168 Rome, Italy PubMed 15358633.

687   N–3 fatty acids and lipid peroxidation in breast cancer inhibition - Br J Nutr. 2002 Mar;87(3):193–8 - Stoll
      BA. - Oncology Dept., St Thomas' Hospital, London, UK. PubMed 12064327.

688   Study of COX-2, Ki67, and p53 expression to predict effectiveness of 5-flurouracil, epirubicin and
      cyclophosphamide with celecoxib treatment in breast cancer patients. - Biomed Pharmacother. 2005
      Oct;59 Suppl 2:S298–301 - L.W.C. Chow W.T.Y. Loo, C.C.Y. Wai, E.L.H. Lui, L. Zhu and M. Toi - Hung
      Chao Hong Integrated Center for Breast Diseases, Dept. of Surgery, The University of Hong Kong
      Medical Center, Queen Mary Hospital, Pokfulam, China. PubMed 16507397.

689   Dietary omega-3 fatty acids and ionizing irradiation on human breast cancer xenograft growth and angiogenesis · Cancer Cell Int. 2005; 5: 12 · W Elaine Hardman, LuZhe Sun, Nicholas Short, and Ivan L Cameron · Pennington Biomedical Research Center, Louisiana State University System, Louisiana University of Texas Health Science Center at San Antonio, Dept. of Cellular and Structural Biology, San Antonio, Texas USA. PubMed 1097743.

690   Reduced prostaglandin synthesis by renal and aortic tissues from adult rats fed essential fatty acid-deficient diet after food deprivation. · Prostaglandins Leukot Med. 1985 May;18(2):183-92 · Sakr HM, Dunham EW. PubMed 3892546.

691   Essential fatty acid deficiency delays the onset of puberty in the female rat. See 211 above.

692   Eicosapentaenoic acid inhibits UV-induced MMP-1 expression in human dermal fibroblasts · Jnl. of Lipid Research, Vol. 46, 1712-1720, August 2005 · Hyeon Ho Kim, Chung Min Shin, Chi-Hyun Park, Kyu Han Kim, Kwang Hyun Cho, Hee Chul Eun and Jin Ho Chung · Dept. of Dermatology, Seoul National University College of Medicine, Laboratory of Cutaneous Aging Research, Clinical Research Institutes, Seoul National University Hospital, Institute of Dermatological Science, Seoul National University, Seoul, Korea.

693   Adipose tissue omega-3 and omega-6 fatty acid content and breast cancer in the EURAMIC study. · European Community Multicenter Study on Antioxidants, Myocardial Infarction, and Breast Cancer. · Am J Epidemiol. 1998 Feb 15;147(4):342-52 · Simonsen N, van't Veer P, Strain JJ, Martin-Moreno JM, Huttunen JK, Navajas JF, Martin BC, Thamm M, Kardinaal AF, Kok FJ, Kohlmeier L. · University of North Carolina, Chapel Hill 27599, USA. PubMed 9508101.

694   Differential Effects of Delivery of Omega-3 Fatty Acids to Human Cancer Cells by Low-Density Lipoproteins versus Albumin · Clin Cancer Res. 2004 Dec 15;10(24):8275-83 · Iris J. Edwards, Isabelle M. Berquin, Haiguo Sun, Joseph T. O'Flaherty, Larry W. Daniel, Michael J. Thomas, Lawrence L. Rudel, Robert L. Wykle and Yong Q. Chen · Dept. of Pathology, Wake Forest University, School of Medicine North Carolina USA. PubMed 15623603.

695   Mechanisms of action of dietary fatty acids in regulating the activation of vascular endothelial cells during atherogenesis · Nutrition Reviews, Aug 2003 · Christon, Raymond A.

696   Docosahexaenoic acid induces ciap1 mRNA and protects human endothelial cells from stress-induced apoptosis. · Am J Physiol Heart Circ Physiol. 2006 Jun;290(6):H2178-86. · Pfrommer CA, Erl W, Weber PC. PubMed 16473961.

697   Overweight, obesity and elevated blood pressure in children and adolescents. · Eur J Med Res. 2006 Mar 27;11(3):97-101. · Schiel R, Beltschikow W, Kramer G, Stein G.Inselklinik Heringsdorf GmbH, · Dept. of Diabetes and Metabolic Diseases, Setheweg 11, D-17424 Seeheilbad Heringsdorf, Germany. PubMed 16751109.

698   Cardiovascular risk factors in overweight German children and adolescents: relation to gender, age and degree of overweight. · Nutr Metab Cardiovasc Dis. 2005 Jun;15(3):181-7 Reinehr T, Andler W, Denzer C, Siegried W, Mayer H, Wabitsch M. · Dept. of Pediatrics, University of Witten-Herdecke, Dr. F. Steiner Str. 5, 45711 Datteln, Germany. PubMed 15955466.

699   Type 1 diabetes compromises plasma arachidonic and docosahexaenoic acids in newborn babies · Lipids. 2004 Apr;39(4):335-42 Ghebremeskel K, Thomas B, Lowy C, Min Y, Crawford MA. · Institute of Brain Chemistry and Human Nutrition, London Metropolitan University, London, N7 8DB, United Kingdom. PubMed 15357021.

700   Dietary macronutrient intake and five-year incident cataract: the blue mountains eye study. · Am J Ophthalmol. 2007 Apr 23; : 17459316 · Townend BS, Townend ME, Flood V, Burlutsky G, Rochtchina E, Wang JJ, Mitchell · P. Centre for Vision Research, Dept. of Ophthalmology and the Westmead Millennium Institute, Westmead, Australia.

701   Serum n3 polyunsaturated fatty acids are depleted in Crohn's disease. · Dig Dis Sci. 1997 Jun;42(6):1137-41. · Kuroki F, Iida M, Matsumoto T, Aoyagi K, Kanamoto K, Fujishima M.Second · Dept. of Internal Medicine, Faculty of Medicine, Kyushu University, Fukuoka, Japan. PubMed 9201073.

702   Usefulness of omega-3 fatty acid supplementation in addition to mesalazine in maintaining remission in pediatric Crohn's disease: a double-blind, randomized, placebo-controlled study. World J Gastroenterol. 2005 Dec 7;11(45):7118-21. · Romano C, Cucchiara S, Barabino A, Annese V, Sferlazzas C. · Pediatric Dept., University of Messina. PubMed 16437657.

703   Increased intake of n-3 polyunsaturated fatty acids elevates the level of apoptosis in the normal sigmoid colon of patients polypectomized for adenomas/tumors. · Cancer Lett. 2003 Apr 10;193(1):17-24. · Cheng J, Ogawa K, Kuriki K, Yokoyama Y, Kamiya T, Seno K, Okuyama H, Wang J, Luo C, Fujii I, Ichikawa H, Shirai T, Tokudome S. · Dept. of Health Promotion and Preventive Medicine, Nagoya City University Graduate School of Medical Sciences, Mizuho-ku, Nagoya, Japan. PubMed 12691819.

704 n–6 and n–3 polyunsaturated fatty acids differentially modulate oncogenic Ras activation in colonocytes. ⁃ Am J Physiol Cell Physiol. 2001 May;280(5):C1066–75 ⁃ Collett ED, Davidson LA, Fan YY, Lupton JR, Chapkin RS. ⁃ Molecular and Cell Biology Group, Faculty of Nutrition, and Center for Environmental and Rural Health, Texas A&M University. PubMed 11287318.

705 Fish oil increases mitochondrial phospholipid unsaturation, upregulating reactive oxygen species and apoptosis in rat colonocytes ⁃ Carcinogenesis, Vol. 23, No. 11, 1919–1926, November 2002 ⁃ Mee Young Hong, Robert S. Chapkin, Rola Barhoumi Robert C. Burghardt Nancy D. Turner, Cara E. Henderson, Lisa M. Sanders, Yang-Yi Fan, Laurie A. Davidson, Mary E. Murphy, Christine M. Spinka, Raymond J. Carroll and Joanne R. Lupton.

706 Effects of Omega–3 Polyunsaturated Fatty Acids on Inflammatory Markers in COPD ⁃ Chest. 2005;128:3817–3827. ⁃ Wataru Matsuyama, MD, PhD; Hideo Mitsuyama, MD; Masaki Watanabe, MD, PhD; Ken-ichi Oonakahara, MD; Ikkou Higashimoto, MD, PhD; Mitsuhiro Osame, MD, PhD and Kimiyoshi Arimura, MD, PhD ⁃ Division of Respiratory Medicine, Respiratory and Stress Care Center, Kagoshima University Hospital, Kagoshima, Japan.

707 In chronic fatigue syndrome, the decreased levels of omega–3 poly-unsaturated fatty acids are related to lowered serum zinc and defects in T cell activation. ⁃ Neuro Endocrinol Lett. 2005 Dec;26(6):745–51 ⁃ Maes M, Mihaylova I, Leunis JC. ⁃ Care4U Outpatient Clinics, and the Clinical Research Center for Mental Health, Antwerp, Belgium. PubMed 16380690.

708 Effect of an 8-month treatment with omega–3 fatty acids (eicosapentaenoic and docosahexaenoic) in patients with cystic fibrosis. ⁃ JPEN J Parenter Enteral Nutr. 2003 Jan–Feb;27(1):52–7 ⁃ De Vizia B, Raia V, Spano C, Pavlidis C, Coruzzo A, Alessio M. ⁃ Dept. of Pediatrics, University Federico II, Napoli, Italy. PubMed 12549599.

709 Potential role of dietary n–3 fatty acids in the prevention of dementia and macular degeneration. ⁃ Am J Clin Nutr. 2006 Jun;83(6 Suppl):1494S–1498S ⁃ Johnson EJ, Schaefer EJ. ⁃ Carotenoid & Health and Lipid Metabolism Laboratories, Jean Mayer U.S. Dept. of Agriculture Human Nutrition Research Center on Aging at Tufts University, Boston, MA 02111, USA. PubMed 16841859.

710 Depression and adipose and serum cholesteryl ester polyunsaturated fatty acids in the survivors of the seven countries study population of Crete European ⁃ Jnl. of Clinical Nutrition (2006) 60, 1016–1023. ⁃ Mamalakis G, Jansen E, Cremers H, Kiriakakis M, Tsibinos G, Kafatos A. ⁃ Dept. of Social Medicine Preventive Medicine and Nutrition, School of Medicine, University of Crete, Iraklion, Crete, Greece

711 Omega–3 fatty acids and neuropsychiatric disorders. ⁃ Reprod Nutr Dev. 2005 Jan–Feb;45(1):1–28 ⁃ Young G, Conquer J. Human Biology and Nutritional Sciences, University of Guelph, Guelph, Ontario, Canada. PubMed 15865053.

712 Effects of fish oil on the central nervous system: a new potential antidepressant? ⁃ Nutr Neurosci. 2004 Apr;7(2):91–9. Naliwaiko K, Araújo RL, da Fonseca RV, Castilho JC, Andreatini R, Bellissimo MI, Oliveira BH, Martins EF, Curi R, Fernandes LC, Ferraz AC. ⁃ Laboratorio de Fisiologia e Farmacologia do Sistema Nervoso Central, Departamento de Fisiologia e Farmacologia, Universidade Federal do Paraná, Curitiba, Brazil. PubMed 15279495.

713 Selective Deficits in the Omega–3 Fatty Acid Docosahexaenoic Acid in the Postmortem Orbitofrontal Cortex of Patients with Major Depressive Disorder. ⁃ Biol Psychiatry. 2007 Jul 1;62(1):17–24. Epub 2006 Dec 22 ⁃ McNamara RK, Hahn CG, Jandacek R, Rider T, Tso P, Stanford KE, Richtand NM. ⁃ Dept. of Psychiatry, University of Cincinnati College of Medicine. PubMed 17188654.

714 Omega 3 fatty acids and the brain: review of studies in depression ⁃ Asia Pac J Clin Nutr. 2007;16 Suppl 1:391–7. ⁃ Sinclair AJ, Begg D, Mathai M, Weisinger RS. ⁃ School of Exercise and Nutrition Sciences, Deakin University, Victoria 3125, Australia. PubMed 17392137.

715 Omega–3 Treatment of Childhood Depression: A Controlled, Double-Blind Pilot Study ⁃ Am J Psychiatry 163:1098–1100, June 2006 ⁃ Hanah Nemets, M.D., Boris Nemets, M.D., Alan Apter, M.D., Ziva Bracha, M.D. and R.H. Belmaker, M.D.

716 Fatty acid composition in major depression: decreased omega 3 fractions in cholesteryl esters and increased C20: 4 omega 6/C20:5 omega 3 ratio in cholesteryl esters and phospholipids. ⁃ J Affect Disord. 1996 Apr 26;38(1):35–46 ⁃ Maes M, Smith R, Christophe A, Cosyns P, Desnyder R, Meltzer H. Clinical Research Center, University Dept. of Psychiatry, Antwerp, Belgium. PubMed 8735157.

717 Lipids, depression and suicide ⁃ Encephale. 2003 Jan–Feb;29(1):49–58 ⁃ Colin A, Reggers J, Castronovo V, Ansseau M. Université de Liège, CUP La Clairière, Bertrix. ⁃ PubMed 12640327.

718   Hibbeln, Joseph R. - Fish consumption and major depression. - The Lancet, Vol. 351, April 18, 1998, pp. 1213
        719 Selective deficits in the omega–3 fatty acid docosahexaenoic acid in the postmortem orbitofrontal
        cortex of patients with major depressive disorder. - Biol Psychiatry. 2007 Jul 1;62(1):17–24. - McNamara
        RK, Hahn CG, Jandacek R, Rider T, Tso P, Stanford KE, Richtand NM. - Dept. of Psychiatry, University of
        Cincinnati College of Medicine. PubMed 17188654.

719   Hibbeln, Joseph R. Fish consumption and major depression. The Lancet, Vol. 351, April 18, 1998, pp. 1213
        (correspondence)

720   Clinical review Type I diabetes: recent developments - BMJ 2004;328:750–754 (27 March), doi:10.1136 /
        bmj.328 .7442.750 - Devasenan Devendra, Edwin Liu, George S Eisenbarth, Barbara Davis - Center for
        Childhood Diabetes, University of Colorado Health Sciences Center, Denver, 80262 CO, USA.

721   Use of cod liver oil during the first year of life is associated with lower risk of childhood-onset type I
        diabetes: a large, population-based, case-control study American - Jnl. of Clinical Nutrition, Vol. 78, No.
        6, 1128–1134, December 2003 - Lars C Stene, Geir Joner - and The Norwegian Childhood Diabetes Study
        Group Diabetes Research Centre, Aker and Ullevål University Hospitals Ullevål University Hospital, and
        Division of Epidemiology, Norwegian Institute of Public Health, Oslo.

722   Elevated C-Reactive Protein Levels in the Development of Type I Diabetes Diabetes - 53:2569–2573,
        2004 H. - Peter Chase, Sonia Cooper, Iris Osberg, Lars C. Stene, Katherine Barriga, Jill Norris, George S.
        Eisenbarth, and Marian Rewers Dept. of Pediatrics, - The Barbara Davis Center for Childhood Diabetes
        and General Clinical Research Center Laboratory, University of Colorado Health Sciences Center, Denver
        and Dept. of Preventive Medicine and Biometrics, University of Colorado Health Sciences Center,
        Denver, Colorado.

723   Hepatic delta9, delta6, and delta5 desaturations in non-insulin-dependent diabetes mellitus eSS rats.
        - Lipids. 2003 Aug;38(8):827–32. - Montanaro MA, Rimoldi OJ, Igal RA, Montenegro S, Tarres MC,
        Martinez SM, Brenner RR. - Instituto de Investigaciones Bioquímicas de La Plata, Universidad Nacional
        de La Plata-Consejo Nacional de Investigaciones Científicas y Técnicas, Facultad de Ciencias Médicas,
        UNLP, La Plata, Argentina. PubMed 14577661.

724   Expression and Regulation of D5-Desaturase, D6-Desaturase...See 195 above,

725   Prevention of diabetes in the BB rat by essential fatty acid deficiency. Relationship between physiological
        and biochemical changes. - Journal of Experimental Medicine, Vol 171, 729-743J -Lefkowith, G Schreiner,
        J Cormier, ES Handler, HK Driscoll, D Greiner, JP Mordes and AA Rossini - Department of Medicine,
        Washington University School of Medicine, St. Louis, Missouri 63110. .

726   Dietary (n–3) and (n–6) Polyunsaturated Fatty Acids Rapidly Modify Fatty Acid Composition and Insulin
        Effects in Rat Adipocytes - The Jnl. of Nutrition Vol. 128 No. 3 March 1998, pp. 512–519 - Maria Fickova, Pierre
        Hubert, Gérard Crémel, and Claude Leray - Institute of Experimental Endocrinology, Slovak Academy
        of Sciences, 83306 Bratislava, Slovakia; INSERM U. 338, F-67084 and INSERM U. 311, F-67065 Strasbourg,
        France.

727   N–3 long chain polyunsaturated fatty acids: a nutritional tool to prevent insulin resistance associated
        to type 2 diabetes and obesity? - Reprod Nutr Dev. 2004 May–Jun;44(3):289–99. - Delarue J, LeFoll C,
        Corporeau C, Lucas - D.EA-948 Oxylipides, Faculté de Médecine, 29200 Brest, France. PubMed 15460168.

728   Brief episode of STZ-induced hyperglycemia produces cardiac abnormalities in rats fed a diet rich in n–6
        PUFA - Am J Physiol Heart Circ Physiol 287: H2518–H2527, 2004 - Sanjoy Ghosh, Dake Qi, Ding An,
        Thomas Pulinilkunnil, Ashraf Abrahani, Kuo-Hsing Kuo, Richard B. Wambolt, Michael Allard, Sheila
        M. Innis, and Brian Rodrigues - Division of Pharmacology and Toxicology, Faculty of Pharmaceutical
        Sciences, and Dept.s of Anatomy, Pathology and Laboratory Medicine, and Pediatrics, University of
        British Columbia, Vancouver, British Columbia, Canada.

729   Fatty Acids in Dyslexia, Dyspraxia and ADHD Can Nutrition Help? - Alexandra J. Richardson - Mansfield
        College and University Lab. of Physiology, Oxford.

730   Relation between dietary n–3 and n–6 fatty acids and clinically diagnosed dry eye syndrome in women
        - American Jnl. of Clinical Nutrition, Vol. 82, No. 4, 887–893, October - Biljana Miljanovi , Komal A
        Trivedi, M Reza Dana, Jeffery P Gilbard, Julie E Buring and Debra A Schaumberg - Division of Preventive
        Medicine, Brigham and Women's Hospital, Boston, MA the Schepens Eye Research Institute, and the
        Dept. of Ophthalmology, Massachusetts Eye and Ear Infirmary and the Dept. of Ambulatory Care and
        Prevention Harvard Medical School, and the Dept. of Epidemiology, Harvard School of Public Health,
        Boston, 2005.

731   The role of omega–3 long-chain polyunsaturated fatty acids in health and disease of the retina. - Prog
        Retin Eye Res. 2005 Jan;24(1):87–138. - SanGiovanni JP, Chew EY. - Division of Epidemiology and Clinical
        Research, National Eye Insitute, NIH 31 Center Drive, Building 31, Bethesda, MD USA. PubMed 15555528.

732 Anti-inflammatory Effect of Docosahexaenoic Acid on Cytokine-Induced Adhesion Molecule Expression in Human Retinal Vascular Endothelial Cells · Investigative Ophthalmology and Visual Science. 2005;46:4342–4347. · Weiqin Chen, Walter J. Esselman, Donald B. Jump, and Julia V. · Busik Dept.s of Microbiology and Molecular Genetics and Physiology, Michigan State University.

733 Effects of altering dietary fatty acid composition on prostaglandin synthesis and fertility. · Prostaglandins Leukot Essent Fatty Acids. 1999 Nov;61(5):275–87 · Abayasekara DR, Wathes DC. · Reproduction and Development Group, Dept. of Veterinary Basic Sciences, Royal Veterinary College, London, UK. PubMed 10670689.

734 Unique lipids of primate spermatozoa: desmosterol and docosahexaenoic acid. · J Lipid Res. 1993 Mar;34(3):491–9 · Lin DS, Connor WE, Wolf DP, Neuringer M, Hachey DL.Division of Endocrinology, Metabolism, and Clinical Nutrition, · Oregon Health Sciences University, Portland. PubMed 8468532.

735 Effects of supplemented DHA on phospholipid DHA levels in infertile male seminal plasma and sperm. · G.V.Skuladottir, S Thorsteinsdottir, A L Petursdottir, A Gisladottir A Hauksson and H Bjorgvinsson. · University of Iceland, Landspitali University Hospital, Reykjavik Health Care Centre Iceland.

736 Uneven distribution of desmosterol and docosahexaenoic acid in the heads and tails of monkey sperm. · J Lipid Res. 1998 Jul;39(7):1404–11. · Connor WE, Lin DS, Wolf DP, Alexander M · Dept. of Medicine, Oregon Health Sciences University, Portland 97201, USA. PubMed 9684743.

737 Primary open-angle glaucoma patients have reduced levels of blood docosahexaenoic and eicosapentaenoic acids. · Prostaglandins Leukot Essent Fatty Acids. 2006 Mar;74(3):157–63. · Ren H, Magulike N, Ghebremeskel K, Crawford M. · Institute of Brain Chemistry and Human Nutrition, London Metropolitan University, North Campus, London, UK, and Dept. of Ophthalmology, University of Nigeria Teaching Hospital, Enugu, Nigeria. PubMed 16410047.

738 Fatty acid use in glaucomatous optic neuropathy treatment · Acta Ophthalmol Scand Suppl. 1998;(227):41–2. · Cellini M, Caramazza N, Mangiafico P, Possati GL, Caramazza R. · Oculistics Clinic, University of Bologna. PubMed 9972342.

739 Omega-3 Fatty Acid Effect on Alveolar Bone Loss in Rats · J Dent Res 85(7):648–652, 2006 L. · Kesavalu, B. Vasudevan, B. Raghu, E. Browning, D. Dawson, J. M. Novak, M.C. Correll, M.J. Steffen, A. Bhattacharya, G. Fernandes, and J.L. Ebersole · Center for Oral Health Research, College of Dentistry, 159 HSRB, University of Kentucky, Lexington, KY, USA; and Dept. of Medicine, University of Texas Health Science Center at San Antonio,

740 Relationship between upper body obesity and periodontitis. · J Dent Res. 2001 Jul;80(7):1631–6. Saito T, Shimazaki Y, Koga T, Tsuzuki M, Ohshima A. · Dept. of Preventive Dentistry, Kyushu University Faculty of Dental Science, Fukuoka, Japan. PubMed 11597023.

741 Content and composition of fatty acids in normal and inflamed gingival tissues. · Prostaglandins Leukot Essent Fatty Acids. 2005 Mar;72(3):147–51. · Ciçek Y, Ozmen I, Canakçi V, Dilsiz A, Sahin F. · Dept. of Periodontology, Ataturk University, Faculty of Dentistry, Erzurum, Turkey. PubMed 15664298.

742 Effect of the nature and amount of dietary energy on lipid composition of rat gingival tissue. · Br J Nutr. 1983 Mar;49(2):187–92 · Das SK, Elliott ML, King HC PubMed 6830747.

743 Arachidonic acid, prostaglandin E2 and leukotriene C4 levels in gingiva and submandibular salivary glands of rats fed diets containing n–3 fatty acids. · Lipids. 1991 Nov;26(11):895–900 · Alam SQ, Bergens BM, Alam BS. · Dept. of Biochemistry and Molecular Biology, LSU Medical Center, New Orleans 70119 PubMed 1805093.

744 Therapeutic versus prophylactic plus therapeutic administration of omega–3 fatty acid on endotoxin-induced periodontitis in rats. · Jnl. of Periodontology December 2004, Vol. 75, No. 12, Pages 1640–1646 · Dr. Saynur Vardar Eralp Buduneli Oya Türkoglu School of Dentistry, Dept. of Periodontology, Afig Hüseyinov Berdeli Haluk Baylas Ege University, Dept. of Pediatrics, Molecular Medicine Laboratory Haluk Baylas School of Dentistry, Dept. of Periodontology Aykut Ba kesen SSK Tepecik Hospital, Clinical Biochemistry Laboratory Gül Atilla, Ege University, School of Dentistry, Dept. of Periodontology, zmir, Turkey.

745 Tissue n–3 and n–6 fatty acids and risk for coronary heart disease events. Atherosclerosis. · 2007 Jul;193(1):1–10. Epub 2007 May 15 · Harris WS, Poston WC, Haddock CK. · Sanford School of Medicine, University of South Dakota, Sioux Falls, USA PubMed 17507020.

746 Effects of fish-oil supplementation on myocardial fatty acids in humans · Am J Clin Nutr. 2007 May;85(5):1222–8 · Metcalf RG, James MJ, Gibson RA, Edwards JR, Stubberfield J, Stuklis R, Roberts-Thomson K, Young GD, Cleland LG. · Rheumatology Unit and the School of Medicine, University of Adelaide, Adelaide, Australia. PubMed 17490956.

747 Role of prescription omega–3 fatty acids in the treatment of hypertriglyceridemia. · Pharmacotherapy. 2007 May;27(5):715–28. · McKenney JM, Sica D. · School of Pharmacy, Virginia Commonwealth University, Richmond, Virginia, USA. 17461707.

748   A review of omega–3 ethyl esters for cardiovascular prevention and treatment of increased blood triglyceride levels. · Vasc Health Risk Manag. 2006;2(3):251–62. · von Schacky C. · Medizinische Klinik and Poliklinik Innenstadt, University of Munich. PubMed 17326331.

749   n–3 Fatty acids and 5–y risks of death and cardiovascular disease events in patients with coronary artery disease American · Jnl. of Clinical Nutrition, Vol. 78, No. 1, 65–71, July 2003 · Arja T Erkkilä, Seppo Lehto, Kalevi Pyörälä and Matti IJ Uusitupa · Dept. of Clinical Nutrition, University of Kuopio and Kuopio University Hospital, Kuopio, and the Dept. of Medicine, University of Kuopio, Kuopio, Finland.

750   Omega–3 fatty acids and cardiovascular disease: A case for omega–3 index as a new risk factor · Pharmacol Res. 2007 Mar;55(3):217–23. Epub 2007 Jan 25 · Harris WS. · Nutrition and Metabolic Disease Research Institute, Sanford Research/USD, Sanford School of Medicine of the University of South Dakota, 1400 West 22nd Street, Sioux Falls, SD 57105, United States. PubMed 17324586.

751   Eicosanoids and renal vascular function in diseases. · Clin Sci (Lond). 2006 Jul;111(1):21–34 Imig JD. · Vascular Biology Center, Dept. of Physiology, Medical College of Georgia, Augusta, GA 30912, USA. PubMed 16764555.

752   Development of alcoholic fatty liver and fibrosis in rhesus monkeys fed a low n–3 fatty acid diet · Alcohol Clin Exp Res. 2004 Oct;28(10):1569–76 · Pawlosky RJ, Salem N. · Laboratory of Membrane Biochemistry and Biophysics, National Institute on Alcohol Abuse and Alcoholism, Division of Intramural Clinical and Biological Research, National Institutes of Health. PubMed 15597091.

753   The effects of low dietary levels of polyunsaturates on alcohol-induced liver disease in rhesus monkeys. · Hepatology. 1997 Dec;26(6):1386–92 · Pawlosky RJ, Flynn BM, Salem N. · National Institute on Alcoholism and Alcohol Abuse, Division of Intramural Clinical and Biological Research, Rockville, MD 20852, USA.

754   Decreased n–6/n–3 fatty acid ratio reduces the invasive potential of human lung cancer cells by downregulation of cell adhesion/invasion-related genes · Carcinogenesis 2005 26(4):779–784; · Shu-Hua Xia, Jingdong Wang and Jing X. Kang · Dept.s of Medicine, Massachusetts General Hospital and Harvard Medical School.

755   Nutritional intervention with omega–3 Fatty acids in a case of malignant fibrous histiocytoma of the lungs · Nutr Cancer. 2005;52(2):121–9. · Pardini RS, Wilson D, Schiff S, Bajo SA, Pierce R. · Dept. of Biochemistry, College of Agriculture, Biotechnology and Natural Resources, University of Navada, Reno, NV 89557, USA. PubMed 16201843.

756   Inhibitory Effects of Oleic and Docosa-hexaenoic Acids on Lung Metastatic Colony Formation and Matrix Metalloproteinase (MMP) Activity · National Cancer Center Research Institute Japan.

757   Effects of an eicosapentaenoic and docosahexaenoic acid concentrate on a human lung carcinoma grown in nude mice. · Lipids. 1991 Nov;26(11):866–70 de Bravo MG, de Antueno RJ, Toledo J, De Tomás ME, Mercuri OF, Quintans C. · Instituto de Investigaciones Bioquimicas de La Plata, Facultad de Medicina, UNLP, Argentina. PubMed 1839563.

758   Macular Degeneration By Marilyn Haddrill; reviewed by Dr. Charles Slonim.

759   The role of omega–3 long-chain polyunsaturated fatty acids in health and disease of the retina · Prog Retin Eye Res. 2005 Jan;24(1):87–138 · SanGiovanni JP, Chew EY. · Division of Epidemiology and Clinical Research, National Eye Insitute, NIH, Bethesda, MD. PubMed 15555528.

760   Reduced G protein-coupled signaling efficiency in retinal rod outer segments in response to n–3 fatty acid deficiency. · J Biol Chem. 2004 Jul 23;279(30):31098–104 · Niu SL, Mitchell DC, Lim SY, Wen ZM, Kim HY, Salem N Jr, Litman BJ. · Laboratory of Membrane Biochemistry and Biophysics, National Institute on Alcohol Abuse and Alcoholism, Rockville, Maryland 20852, USA. PubMed 15145938.

761   The DHA Story Robert Abel Jnr MD.

762   Association of Adipose and Red Blood Cell Lipids With Severity of Dominant Stargardt Macular Dystrophy (STGD3) Secondary to an ELOVL4 Mutation Arch · Ophthalmol. 2006;124:257–263. · Amy F. Hubbard, MS; E. Wayne Askew, PhD; Nanda Singh, PhD; Mark Leppert, PhD; Paul S. Bernstein, MD, PhD.

763   Cell cycle arrest and apoptosis of melanoma cells by docosahexaenoic acid: association with decreased pRb phosphorylation. · Cancer Res. 2000 Aug 1;60(15):4139–45 · Albino AP, Juan G, Traganos F, Reinhart L, Connolly J, Rose DP, Darzynkiewicz Z. · The American Health Foundation, Valhalla, New York 10595, USA PubMed 10945621.

764   Role of omega–3 polyunsaturated fatty acids on cyclooxygenase–2 metabolism in brain-metastatic melanoma · J Lipid Res. 2005 Jun;46(6):1278–84. Epub 2005 Mar 16. · Denkins Y, Kempf D, Ferniz M, Nileshwar S, Marchetti D. · Dept. of Comparative Biomedical Sciences, School of Veterinary Medicine, Louisiana State University, Baton Rouge, LA 70803, USA PubMed 15772428.

765   Omega–3 fatty acids in inflammation and autoimmune diseases. See above 344.

766 Red blood cell and adipose tissue fatty acids in mild inactive multiple sclerosis. Acta Neurol Scand. 1990 Jul;82(1):43–50. - Nightingale S, Woo E, Smith AD, French JM, Gale MM, Sinclair HM, Bates D, Shaw DA. - Dept. of Neurology, Royal Victoria Infirmary, Newcastle upon Tyne. PubMed 2239137.

767 Cancer Reseach UK http://www.cancerhelp.org.uk/help/default.asp?page=2656.

768 Prostate tumor growth and recurrence can be modulated by the omega–6:omega–3 ratio in diet: athymic mouse xenograft model simulating radical prostatectomy - Neoplasia. 2006 Feb;8(2):112–24 - Kelavkar UP, Hutzley J, Dhir R, Kim P, Allen KG, McHugh K. - Dept. of Urology and Cancer Institute, University of Pittsburgh. PubMed 16611404.

769 Prostate cancer risk and consumption of fish oils: a dietary biomarker-based case-control study. - Br J Cancer. 1999 Dec;81(7):1238–42. - Norrish AE, Skeaff CM, Arribas GL, Sharpe SJ, Jackson RT. - Dept. of Community Health, University of Auckland, New Zealand. PubMed 10584888.

770 The yin and yang of 15-lipoxygenase-1 and delta-desaturases: Dietary omega–6 linoleic acid metabolic pathway in prostate - J Carcinog. 2006; 5: 9. - Uddhav Kelavkar, Yan Lin, Doug Landsittel, Uma Chandran, and Rajiv Dhir - Dept. of Urology and University of Pittsburgh Cancer Institute, Pittsburgh, PA, USA Dept. of Biostatistics, Graduate School of Public Health, University of Pittsburgh, Dept. of Mathematics and Computer Science, Duquesne University, Dept. of Pathology and University of Pittsburgh Cancer Institute, USA. PubMed 16566819.

771 Arachidonic acid, an omega–6 fatty acid, induces cytoplasmic phospholipase A2 in prostate carcinoma cells Cancer - Carcinogenesis 2005 26(9):1520–1526 - Millie Hughes-Fulford, Raymond R. Tjandrawinata, Chai-Fei Li and Sina Sayyah - Laboratory of Cell Growth, Dept. of Medicine, Northern California Institute for Research and Education and Veterans Affairs Medical Center, University of California-San Francisco, USA.

772 Arachidonic Acid Activates Phosphatidylinositol 3-Kinase Signaling and Induces Gene Expression in Prostate Cancer Research - 66, 1427–1433, February 1, 2006 - Millie Hughes-Fulford, Chai-Fei Li, Jim Boonyaratanakornkit and Sina Sayyah - Dept. of Veterans Affairs Medical Center; Northern California Institute for Research and Education; and University of California, San Francisco, California.

773 Omega–3 fatty acids and inflammation. - Curr Atheroscler Rep. 2004 Nov;6(6):461–7. - Mori TA, Beilin LJ. - School of Medicine and Pharmacology–Royal Perth Hospital Unit, The University of Western Australia, Medical Research Foundation Building, Perth. PubMed 15485592.

774 Omega–3 fatty acids in inflammation and autoimmune diseases. See 344 above.

775 Omega–3 fatty acid-based lipid infusion in patients with chronic plaque psoriasis: results of a double-blind, randomized, placebo-controlled, multicenter trial. - J Am Acad Dermatol. 1998 Apr;38(4):539–47 - Mayser P, Mrowietz U, Arenberger P, Bartak P, Buchvald J, Christophers E, Jablonska S, Salmhofer W, Schill WB, Krämer HJ, Schlotzer E, Mayer K, Seeger W, Grimminger F. - Dept. of Dermatology and Andrology, Justus Liebig University Giessen, Germany. PubMed 9555791.

776 n–3 fatty acids in psoriasis. - Br J Nutr. 2002 Jan;87 Suppl 1:S77–82 - Mayser P, Grimm H, Grimminger F. - Dept. of Dermatology and Andrology, Justus Liebig University, Giessen, Germany. PubMed 11895157

777 Parenteral Nutrition with Fish Oil Modulates Cytokine Response in Patients with Sepsis - American Jnl. of Respiratory and Critical Care Medicine Vol 167. pp. 1321–1328, (2003) - Konstantin Mayer, Stephanie Gokorsch, Christine Fegbeutel, Katja Hattar, Simone Rosseau, Dieter Walmrath, Werner Seeger and Friedrich Grimminger. - Medizinische Klinik II, Justus Liebig University, Giessen; and Medizinische Klinik mit Schwerpunkt Infektiologie, Charité, Humboldt University, Berlin, Germany.

778 Docosahexaenoic acid administered in the acute phase protects the nutritional status of septic neonates. Nutrition. -2006 Jul–Aug;22(7–8):731–7. Epub 2006 Jun 5 - Lopez-Alarcon M, Bernabe-Garcia M, Del Prado M, Rivera D, Ruiz G, Maldonado J, Villegas R. - Medical Nutrition Research Unit, Pediatric Hospital, Centro Medico Nacional "Siglo XXI," Mexican Institute of Social Security, Mexico City, Mexico. PubMed 16750345.

779 Lipoproteins in inflammation and sepsis. Clinical aspects - Wendel, Martina; Paul, Rüdiger; Heller, Axel Source - Intensive Care Medicine, Vol 33, No 1, Jan 2007, pp. 25–35(11).

780 Effect of dietary fish oil on plasma thromboxane B2 and 6-keto-prostaglandin F1 alpha levels in septic rats. - Arch Surg. 1991 Feb;126(2):179–82. - Muakkassa FF, Koruda MJ, Ramadan FM, Kawakami M, Meyer AA. - Dept. of Surgery, University of North Carolina, Chapel Hill. PubMed 1992995.

781 Preoperative oral supplementation with long-chain Omega–3 fatty acids beneficially alters phospholipid fatty acid patterns in liver, gut mucosa, and tumor tissue. - JPEN J Parenter Enteral Nutr. 2005 Jul–Aug;29(4):236–40 - Senkal M, Haaker R, Linseisen J, Wolfram G, Homann HH, Stehle P. - Dept. of Surgery, St. Josef Hospital, Ruhr University, Bochum, Germany. PubMed 15961678.

782 Supplementation of omega–3 fatty acids in parenteral nutrition beneficially alters phospholipid fatty acid pattern · JPEN J Parenter Enteral Nutr. 2007 Jan–Feb;31(1):12–7 · Senkal M, Geier B, Hannemann M, Deska T, Linseisen J, Wolfram G, Adolph M. · Dept. of Surgery, Ruhr-University Bochum, St. Josef Hospital, Germany. PubMed 17202435.

783 Steady-state haemoglobin level in sickle cell anaemia increases with an increase in erythrocyte membrane n–3 fatty acids. · Prostaglandins Leukot Essent Fatty Acids. 2005 Jun;72(6):415–21 · Ren H, Obike I, Okpala I, Ghebremeskel K, Ugochukwu C, Crawford M. · Institute of Brain Chemistry and Human Nutrition, London Metropolitan University, London. PubMed 15876528.

784 The fatty acid composition of the serum phospholipids of children with sickle cell disease in Nigeria. · Prostaglandins Leukot Essent Fatty Acids. 2002 Oct;67(4):217–22. · Glew RH, Casados JK, Huang YS, Chuang LT, VanderJagt DJ.Dept. of Biochemistry and Molecular Biology, University of New Mexico School of Medicine, Albuquerque, USA. PubMed 12401435.

785 Decreased antioxidant enzymes and membrane essential polyunsaturated fatty acids in schizophrenic and bipolar mood disorder patients. · Psychiatry Res. 2003 Dec 1;121(2):109–22 · Ranjekar PK, Hinge A, Hegde MV, Ghate M, Kale A, Sitasawad S, Wagh UV, Debsikdar VB, Mahadik SP. · National Chemical Laboratory, Homi Bhabha Road, Pune 411008, India. PubMed 14656446.

786 Potential role of dietary omega–3 essential fatty acids on some oxidant/antioxidant parameters in rats' corpus striatum. · Prostaglandins Leukot Essent Fatty Acids. 2003 Oct;69(4):253–9 · Sarsilmaz M, Songur A, Ozyurt H, Ku I, Ozen OA, Ozyurt B, Sö üt S, Akyol O. · Dept. of Anatomy, Faculty of Medicine, Firat University, Elazi, Turkey. PubMed 12907135.

787 Abnormalities in the fatty acid composition of the postmortem orbitofrontal cortex of schizophrenic patients: gender differences and partial normalization with antipsychotic medications · Schizophr Res. 2007 Mar;91(1–3):37–50. · McNamara RK, Jandacek R, Rider T, Tso P, Hahn CG, Richtand NM, Stanford KE.· Dept. of Psychiatry, University of Cincinnati College of Medicine, Cincinnati USA. PubMed 17236749.

788 Respiratory and allergic diseases: from upper respiratory tract infections to asthma. · Jaber R. · Division of Wellness and Chronic Illness, Dept. of Family Medicine, University Hospital and Medical Center, Health Sciences Center, State University of New York at Stony Brook, Stony Brook, NY 11794–8461, USA. PubMed 12391710.

789 Nutritional supplements as adjunctive therapy for children with chronic/recurrent sinusitis: pilot research. · Int J Pediatr Otorhinolaryngol. 2004 Jun;68(6):785–93 · Linday LA, Dolitsky JN, Shindledecker RD. Dept. of Otolaryngology, The New York Eye and Ear Infirmary, NY. PubMed 15126020.

790 The relationship between dietary n–3 and n–6 fatty acids and clinically diagnosed dry eye syndrome in women · Biljana Miljanovi, Am J Clin Nutr. 2005 October; 82(4): 887–893 · Komal A. Trivedi, M. Reza Dana, Jeffery P. Gilbard, Julie E. Buring, and Debra A. Schaumberg. PubMed 1360504.

791 Essential fatty acid status in cell membranes and plasma of patients with primary Sjogren's syndrome. Correlations to clinical and immunologic variables using a new model for classification and assessment of disease manifestations. · Prostaglandins Leukot Essent Fatty Acids. 1998 Oct;59(4):239–45. · Oxholm P, Asmussen K, Wiik A, Horrobin DF. · Copenhagen Sjögren's Syndrome Research Centre, Dept. of Rheumatology U, Copenhagen County Hospital in Gentofte, Hellerup, Denmark. PubMed 9849649.

792 Eicosapentaenoic acid inhibits UV-induced MMP-1 expression (see 701).

793 Omega–3 polyunsaturated essential fatty acid status as a predictor of future suicide risk · Am J Psychiatry. 2006 Jun;163(6):1100–2 · Sublette ME, Hibbeln JR, Galfalvy H, Oquendo MA, Mann JJ. · Dept. of Neuroscience, NY State Psychiatric Institute, Columbia University, New York, USA. Pubmed 16741213.

794 In humans, the seasonal variation in poly-unsaturated fatty acids is related to the seasonal variation in violent suicide and serotonergic markers of violent suicide. · Prostaglandins Leukot Essent Fatty Acids. 2004 Jul;71(1):13–8 · De Vriese SR, Christophe AB, Maes M. · Division of Nutrition, Ghent University Hospital, Belgium. PubMed 15172679.

795 Suicide attempt and n–3 fatty acid levels in red blood cells: a case control study in China. See 381.

796 Causes of Peroxisomal Disorders. · Manuela Martinez Foundation.

797 A Ray of Hope: DHA Therapy and Nutrition. · Manuela Martinez Foundation.

ABOUT THE AUTHOR

Who am I. Good question. I have been trying to work that out myself! I was once described as Eeyore, the Winnie the Pooh character.

I have an enquiring and analytical mind, a need for answers, time, and on occasion nerdish qualities of application. I have had a long term on and off interest in diet and nutrition.

Like most of us I plod on as a carbon consuming unit, asking what it is all about. I do believe life is truly wondrous, we are part of something bigger, humans have a greater potential, but the choices are ours.

I have no glittering career in the field of science. I qualified as a Chartered Accountant after more than one attempt. I learned with help a little carpentry, plumbing, and general "Do It Yourself'. I have installed a kitchen or two.

I cycle locally in preference to driving when circumstances permit. I enjoy skiing when I can.

I am currently in litigation as part of quest to find out if I am the illegitimate child of Princess Margaret. In my naivety I believed that once I had summoned up the courage to ask, I would get either a sharp no, or a yes, sorry that was just the way it had to be. I should have known better.

At the time of writing, I am trying to have the wills of Princess Margaret and Her Majesty The Queen Mother opened, as a step in my investigation, which is turning into a saga. I debated if I should tell of my pursuit of possible Royal identity for fear of detracting from the book, but the issue was bound to arise, and without these events this book would not have happened.

One way of dealing with the spare time, uncertainties, isolation, and avoiding the negative emotional consequences of my quest, was to keep my mind occupied, between court hearings and judgements. I had found a captivating subject. As I became fascinated, the idea of a book formed. The project, was positive in spirit, largely in my control, made me feel I was involved in something worthwhile, and kept my mind busy. Three years and much nerding later, here is my offering.

Very many thanks to you for reading this book. I hope it helps you see the life altering importance of Omega 3 and 6. Understanding has helped my fitness, radically improved my digestion and sleep, and kept my equilibrium intact,

Robert Andrew Brown.

Printed in the United Kingdom by
Lightning Source UK Ltd., Milton Keynes
136664UK00001B/27-28/P